Fundamentals of Applied Animal Nutrition

Fundamentals of Applied Animal Nutrition

Gordon McL. Dryden

Adjunct Associate Professor, School of Agriculture and Food Sciences,
The University of Queensland, Australia
Dryden Animal Science

CABI

CABI is a trading name of CAB International

CABI
Nosworthy Way
Wallingford
Oxfordshire OX10 8DE
UK

Tel: +44 (0)1491 832111
Fax: +44 (0)1491 833508
E-mail: info@cabi.org
Website: www.cabi.org

CABI
WeWork
One Lincoln St
24th Floor
Boston, MA 02111
USA

Tel: +1 (617)682-9015
E-mail: cabi-nao@cabi.org

A catalogue record for this book is available from the British Library, London, UK.

References to Internet websites (URLs) were accurate at the time of writing.

ISBN-13: 9781786394453 (paperback)
9781786394460 (ePDF)
9781786394477 (ePub)

DOI: 10.1079/9781786394453.0000

Commissioning Editor: Alexandra Lainsbury
Editorial Assistant: Lauren Davies
Production Editor: Marta Patiño

Typeset by SPi, Pondicherry, India

Contents

Preface

Fundamentals of Applied Animal Nutrition is written for undergraduates taking courses in animal nutrition. In addition, farmers and advisors who want to broaden their understanding of animal feeding and management, and scientists who would like to see how their research interests mesh into practical animal feeding, will also find this text useful.

This is a book about the application of nutrition science. Even if we understand the basic concepts of animal nutrition – its biochemistry and physiology (which are described in *Animal Nutrition Science*, also published by CAB International) – it is difficult to use that information in animal feeding. The basic concepts, and their practical application, are really quite different areas of knowledge. *Fundamentals* is intended to bridge this gap.

Animal nutrition is a remarkably diverse discipline, as it deals with animal nutrient requirements, feed nutritive value, the effects of feeding methods and feeds on animal health, feed processing, and the practical management of animal feeding. We have to consider animal welfare and behaviour, and how to optimize the quality of a wide range of products, and to do that while minimizing the impact of animals on the environment. Each domestic animal species, and each production system, has its own characteristics and must be managed in different ways, and it is impossible to adequately deal with all aspects of the practical feeding of sheep, goats, horses, dairy and beef cattle, pigs, and poultry in one volume. But there are general principles. These are described in this book, with discussions about how these concepts are modified for different animal types. As well, to help in their application, in each chapter there are pointers which indicate how we can apply these concepts.

Fundamentals of Applied Animal Nutrition is organized into 10 parts. In these we discuss:

- Why animals need nutrients including water, and how different feeds provide these.
- How animals digest feeds, and how ruminant and monogastric digestive systems affect the release and nature of nutrients.
- Where we can find data on feed nutrient contents, and the characteristics of different types of feeds.
- Factors which regulate feed intake, how we can estimate likely feed consumptions, and how to identify nutritionally efficient animals.
- Feed additives such as enzymes, supplements, acidity regulators and probiotics.
- Feed-related factors which affect animal health, such as secondary substances and feed-borne disease organisms, and how some feeds and feeding methods can adversely affect health.
- How animal nutrient requirements are described and quantified, and how we can combine information on nutrient requirements and feed nutritive values to devise feed mixtures which supply the animals' requirements.
- Grazing animal nutrition including diet selection, factors which influence the nutritive value of pasture, grazing systems, assessing the nutritional status of grazing animals, and providing nutrient supplements.
- Methods of processing feeds to improve their digestibility, nutrient content and handling characteristics; and equipment and methods for storing, handling and feeding animal feeds.
- The influence of the environment on animal nutrient requirements, and how animal nutrition can affect the environment.

Textbooks are not usually read from start to finish; instead, readers search for the topic that they are interested in at that time. While this can be time-efficient, there is a risk that concepts or terminology may be misunderstood unless the reader has the necessary prior knowledge. To help with this, there is a degree of repetition in this text so that readers can find supporting information that they may need *in situ*, rather than having to refer to other chapters. There are cross-references to other chapters where the topic or concept is discussed in detail, and there is a glossary of the terms commonly used in animal nutrition. There are also pointers to additional information in *Animal Nutrition Science*, and in a range of research papers included in the bibliographies in each chapter.

Enjoy!

Gordon McL. Dryden
The University of Queensland, Australia
Dryden Animal Science
10 March 2021

Acknowledgements

Parts of this book were reviewed by Xiuhua Li, Karen Harper, Rafat Al Jassim and Dennis Poppi (University of Queensland), Lex Turner (Queensland Department of Agriculture and Fisheries) and Geoff Niethe. I am grateful for their very helpful comments. Of course, any errors of omission or interpretation are mine.

To the very helpful CABI editorial staff, and to my wife and family who have given me continued support – my sincere thanks.

1 Nutrients and important feed constituents and their functions

Introduction

Almost the first thing that we think about when we have animals to care for or manage is 'How should I feed them?' And the answer to that question starts with answering two other questions: 'Why do animals need feed?' and 'What actually is feed?' These topics are discussed in this chapter.

Terms used to describe animal feed:

- 'Food' is a term which is often reserved for human foodstuffs, while animal feed is usually called 'feed'. This usage is arbitrary and either word can be used to refer to animal feed.
- 'Ingredient' is a term used to describe individual feeds and is often used to refer to the components of rations. 'Feedstuff' has a similar meaning.
- 'Diet' and 'ration' often have the same meaning in animal nutrition. The term 'ration' is usually reserved for a mixture of feed ingredients which has been formulated to provide specific amounts of nutrients. 'Diet' usually means the same as 'ration', or even 'feed', but it can also imply a particular type and/or amount of feed or mixture of ingredients.
- 'Concentrates' are feeds which have little fibre and usually a fairly high level of starch and/or protein (Chapter 6). They are plant seeds and fruits, and by-products made from these, and feeds made from animal tissues and products.
- 'Roughages' are feeds which contain relatively high levels of fibre (Chapter 6). They are often forages, i.e. the vegetative parts of pasture plants. 'Roughage' is used in human nutrition to mean indigestible fibre, but this is an incorrect usage in animal nutrition.

Why do animals need feed?

There are five reasons why animals need feed:

- If an animal is growing or otherwise producing, it needs external sources of the components of body tissue (for growth), and of its products (such as eggs, milk, etc.).
- Body cell components and metabolites are continually synthesized and broken down. Many of these constituents are synthesized from recycled precursors, but there is some inevitable wastage. This has to be made up by materials obtained from feed.
- Animals need energy to fuel the biochemical reactions and physiological processes which keep them alive, healthy and productive.
- Animal cells use a wide variety of chemical substances in their metabolism. Most of these are made by the animal itself but there is a range of compounds which animals cannot make. These include minerals, most vitamins, and some amino acids and fatty acids. These must be supplied from external sources, i.e. the animal's feed.
- Some feed constituents promote wellbeing, e.g. fibre supports digestive tract function and health, tannins help to control intestinal parasites, some minerals have pharmacological effects, and ruminally degradable protein (RDP) is essential for rumen micro-organisms.

The chemical composition of feeds

Feed analysis begins with measuring the feed's water and dry matter (DM) contents. Within the DM we have the organic matter (OM) and minerals; and the OM can be further divided into fibre, non-fibrous (non-structural) carbohydrates, protein, fat, vitamins and non-nutrient substances.

The analytical methods used to determine these fractions are briefly described in Table 1.1. The basic method used is the proximate analysis (developed in the latter part of the 19th century) which identifies DM, crude protein, crude fibre, crude fat (ether extract) and crude minerals (ash). The proximate analysis is now supported by newer methods, including detergent extraction for measuring fibre, atomic absorption spectroscopy for the individual minerals and chromatography for measuring fatty acids, amino acids and vitamins. These

DOI: 10.1079/9781786394453.0001

Table 1.1. Methods of measuring the nutritionally important constituents of feeds.

Food constituent	Analytical method
Dry matter (DM)	Measured by heating the feed, usually at 100°C for several hours; fresh forages may be dried at 50–60°C to avoid heat damage to proteins and loss of carbohydrates and other constituents
Organic matter (OM)	Determined as the loss of mass after ashing (see below)
Fibre (acid detergent fibre, ADF; neutral detergent fibre, NDF; and crude fibre, CF)	ADF and NDF are the residues which are resistant to the actions of either acid detergent (cetyltrimethylammonium bromide in sulphuric acid) or neutral detergent (sodium dodecyl sulphate in a pH 7 solution). Early methods of fibre analysis used a sequential extraction with acid and alkali to give a residue called CF. This analysis is now not often used and has been replaced with the more reliable detergent methods
Protein (crude) (CP or Prot.)	Determined by measuring the total N content (using the Kjeldahl or Dumas methods) and multiplying this by 6.25. This method assumes that all the feed N is from protein, and that all proteins contain 16% N. Neither of these assumptions is completely correct, so CP values often overestimate the actual protein content. The individual amino acids which make up proteins are measured by chromatography
Non-structural carbohydrates (NSC) or water-soluble carbohydrate (WSC)	These are carbohydrates which are not part of the plant cell wall. NSC includes starch and WSC. WSC is simple sugars (see text), β-glucans and fructans. These compounds are measured by polarimetry, ethanol extraction, and enzymatic methods
Fat (crude) (EE, for 'ether extract')	Diethyl ether, petroleum ether, or hexane are used to extract fats and other substances such as phospholipids, waxes, fat-soluble vitamins, and pigments. This constituent is also called 'ether extract'. Individual fatty acids are measured by chromatography
Minerals (ash)	Ash is measured by burning a sample at 500°C or more for several hours. The ash contains most of the minerals – although some are lost by volatilization; this analysis is now more used for determining the organic matter content (see text). Data on individual minerals, rather than the total ash, is needed to properly describe a feed. Individual minerals are measured by photometry and atomic absorption spectroscopy
Vitamins	Measured by chromatography, microbial bioassays, and other methods

methods are fully described in Nielsen (2017) and AOAC (2019).

Water in feeds occurs in several different forms:

- water from rain, irrigation, dew, water added in processing, etc., which either adheres to the feed particles or is adsorbed onto them;
- water in the xylem and phloem vessels of forages, cytoplasmic water (water in the cell contents), and water in the pores of cell walls; or
- water of crystallization (associated with minerals).

Feeds of plant origin can have between 5% and 90% water (see below). Feeds made from animal tissue (e.g. meat meals) are used as air-dry meals, and their water content is about 10%.

Dry matter is the non-water part of feed; it contains all the constituents listed in Table 1.1 and Fig. 1.1. The DM content of air-dry feeds (feeds which feel dry to the touch and are stable in storage) is usually between 85% and 95%. Published values (NRC, 1982) vary between 85% and 97% for hays and straws, and 87% and 92% for cereal grains. The DM contents of fresh forages (i.e. pasture plants, freshly cut plant material and silages) are much lower than those of air-dry feeds. Fresh immature forages can have as little as 10–15% DM, although values are usually about 25% in more mature pasture, and up to 45% in ripened, dried-off pasture.

The concept of dry matter is sometimes confused with feed type. DM is a feed component; it is not a nutrient, or roughage, or straw, hay, or mature (over-ripe or dried-off) pasture (which are examples of roughages), or air-dry feed.

The main uses for feed DM data are to:

- Provide a stable basis for expressing the contents of nutrients and other constituents of feeds. The water content of feeds varies with factors such as air humidity and rain, and feed processing

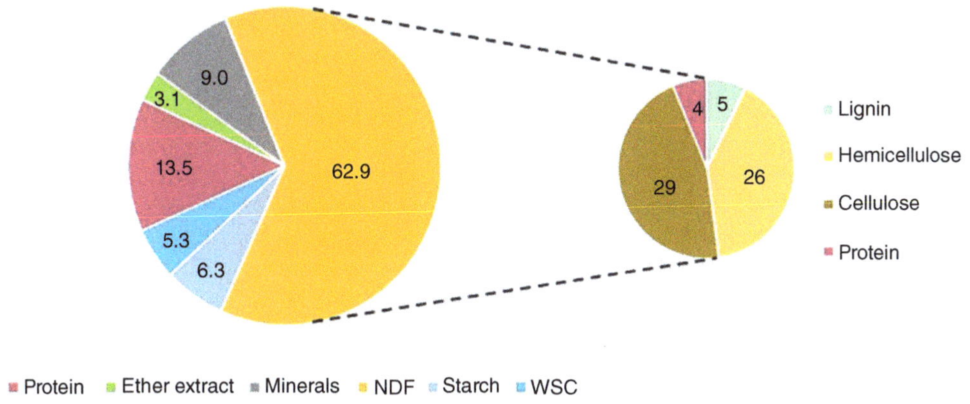

Fig. 1.1. The composition (% dry matter basis) of cocksfoot grass (orchard grass; *Dactylis glomerata*) showing the composition of neutral detergent fibre. (Copyright: Gordon McL. Dryden.)

and storage methods, so describing a feed's composition by using the total feed (DM plus water) as the basis can give very variable values.

- Give a general measure of how much feed an animal is probably able to eat or should be offered. Animals do not have a 'requirement' for DM, even though an owner might ask that question. The question should be: 'How much DM is my pig/cow/bird/horse… likely to be able to eat?' This is a sensible question because animals do have upper limits to their DM intake.

Organic matter is the organic (non-mineral) part of the feed (i.e. the carbohydrates, fats, proteins, vitamins, etc.). Like DM, there is no specific animal requirement for OM, although its constituents are required by animals in different amounts. The main uses for OM data are to:

- Indicate the likely energy content of a feed if we are not able to measure the energy content directly. For feeds with low fat and ash contents, the OM content is a good predictor of the total energy content.
- Avoid bias in measurements of feed intake and digestibility when the samples can be contaminated by extraneous minerals, e.g. soil ingested when grazing animals eat pasture.

Non-structural carbohydrates (NSC) include the water-soluble carbohydrates (WSC) and polysaccharides such as starch. WSC in plant material consists of simple sugars (monosaccharides; single sugar molecules like glucose, galactose and fructose), disaccharides (two joined sugar molecules, like lactose, sucrose and maltose) and fructans (chains of fructose molecules). Starch is also part of the NSC (but is not included in the WSC). It consists of two polysaccharides – amylopectin (about 75% of starch) and amylose (about 25%). Starch polysaccharides are large, complex carbohydrate molecules which are made from joining many glucose molecules in either linear (straight) or branched chains. Starches provide carbon and energy reserves for the developing plant embryo. Pectins (Chapter 4) are constituents of plant cell walls and are water soluble but are not classed within the WSC fraction.

Fibre is the plant cell wall (Chapter 4) of plant-origin feeds, and consists of the carbohydrates cellulose, hemicelluloses and pectins, a non-carbohydrate polymer lignin, and a small amount of protein (see Fig. 1.1). The external walls of plant tissues are covered with a cuticle which is made of various waxes. Apart from pectins, these constituents are all resistant to solubilization by the neutral detergent reagent.

In those feeds which are based on animal tissue, such as meat and bone meals, feather meal or insect meals, the detergent-resistant constituents include bone chips, pieces of feather or hair, connective tissue and chitin. These are also reported as part of the feed fibre.

Neutral detergent fibre (NDF) and acid detergent fibre (ADF) are measures of the fibrosity of feeds. Extraction of the feed with acid detergent gives values for ADF (actually cellulose + lignin) which are somewhat similar to the older crude fibre (CF) analysis, but ADF is a much better-defined chemical entity. NDF (mainly cellulose + hemicellulose + lignin, with some protein and some mineral) is the residue after extraction with neutral detergent and is most of the cell wall material in plant feeds. NDF is also chemically well defined. CF is essentially lignin and cellulose, although the reagents used actually extract some of both of these constituents. The chemical composition of CF varies between different feeds.

Proteins are assemblages of hundreds or thousands of amino acids formed into chains. These chains are often coiled into spirals or globules, or sometimes organized into sheets. Some proteins contain sugar molecules; these are called glycoproteins. Proteins are constituents of cell membranes, of hair, skin and muscle cells, enzymes, and some hormones.

Fats are molecules which combine three fatty acids (FA) attached to a glycerol backbone. There are variants of this, especially in plants, where a sugar molecule replaces one of the FA; these are called glycolipids. Animal cell membranes contain phospholipids, where a phosphate radical replaces one of the FA. FA are considered as 'long chain' if they have 14 or more C atoms joined together. 'Volatile' fatty acids (VFA) include acetic, propionic and butyric acids and typically have less than six C atoms. An unsaturated fatty acid has double bonds between some of its C atoms, due to the absence of H atoms which would otherwise take up (saturate) the vacant bonding positions on the C atoms (Fig. 1.2). *Cis* and *trans* fatty acids are unsaturated fatty acids where the C atoms on either side of the double bond are either both on the same side of the bond or are on different sides.

N-free extract (NFE) is the remainder after the feed's protein, CF and ether extract contents have been subtracted from the OM. It was part of the original proximate analysis and was always estimated by calculation rather than by chemical analysis. NFE is an undefined fraction which has been superseded by more modern analyses and it should not be used to describe feeds. Instead, we should determine the contents of the individual carbohydrates (which in NFE includes some of the cellulose and hemicellulose), vitamins, secondary substances and other constituents which contribute to the NFE.

Minerals comprise the non-organic part of the feed DM. There is a wide range of minerals in animal feed, examples in plant-origin feeds are P which is a component of nucleic acids and cell membranes (in both plant and animal tissue), Mg, which is a component of chlorophyll, and Cu, which is an enzyme cofactor. In feeds made from animal sources Ca, P, Na, Cu, Fe, I, Mg and S are found in association with proteins (e.g. enzymes, thyroid hormones), porphyrins (e.g. haem), enzymes including those required for keratin (hair protein) synthesis and for oxidative phosphorylation, and in bone minerals (e.g. Ca and P in hydroxyapatite).

Vitamins are a group of chemically unrelated substances. They are present either as the active vitamin, such as the B group vitamins (including thiamine, riboflavin, niacin, etc.) or as precursors, such as β-carotene which is a precursor of vitamin A.

Other substances: This is a collection of substances like plant pigments, alkaloids (e.g. gossypol in cottonseed), tannins, waxes, trypsin inhibitor, phytin, goitrogens, oxalate, etc. These can limit the utility of the feed, especially for monogastric animals (secondary substances are further discussed in Chapter 12).

Animal feed as a source of nutrients

Nutrients are the substances in feed which the animal obtains and uses to carry out its metabolic functions (see Table 1.2).

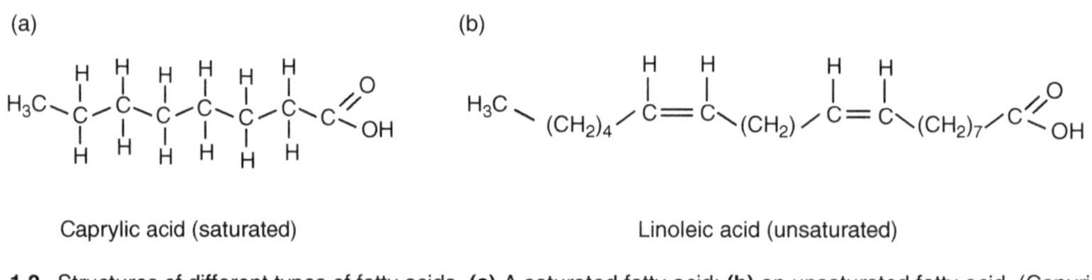

Fig. 1.2. Structures of different types of fatty acids. **(a)** A saturated fatty acid; **(b)** an unsaturated fatty acid. (Copyright: Gordon McL. Dryden.)

Table 1.2. Nutrient groups and their functions.

Nutrient group	Usual form in feeds	Function	Example functions
Amino acids	Proteins	Structural	Synthesis of the structural proteins of cells, e.g. proteins in cell membranes, actin and myosin in muscle cells, and in connective tissue, bone, etc.
		Energy	When surplus amino acids are deaminated and their carbon skeletons are oxidized, yielding ATP (an energy-rich compound)
		Regulatory	When used to synthesize enzymes or peptide hormones
Fatty acids	Fats	Structural	Synthesis of cell membranes
		Energy	When oxidized through the β-oxidation reactions
		Regulatory	When used to synthesize steroid hormones and prostaglandins
Carbohydrates	Plant fibre, starches, monosaccharides and disaccharides	Structural	Constituents of glycoproteins, glycolipids and cartilage constituents
		Energy	When oxidized through reactions such as the glycolytic and pentose phosphate pathways, yielding ATP
Minerals	In complexes with other minerals (e.g. bone); as components of enzymes, haemoglobin, thyroxine, chlorophyll	Structural	Mineralization of bone tissue; in haemoglobin and thyroxine
		Regulatory	When used as enzyme cofactors and as constituents of hormones
Vitamins	As active vitamins, or as provitamins	Regulatory	When used as enzyme cofactors or in gene expression (e.g. the action of vitamin D in promoting the synthesis of Ca-binding proteins)
Water	Free water (cellular and adhering water), water of crystallization	Structural	As a major constituent of lean tissue, blood, lymph and milk
		Regulatory	As the medium in which the chemical reactions of the body take place, in the control of body temperature by sweating and panting, and used in excreting waste

Nutrients generally occur in feed as components of larger, more chemically complex substances (i.e. as components of proteins, fats, complex carbohydrates and mineral complexes). They are released from these complex substances by the process of digestion (Chapter 3).

Nutrients are used:

- as materials for building cells, cell organelles and cell products;
- to provide the energy needed to drive the animal's metabolism; and
- to regulate and facilitate the body's metabolism.

The six types of nutrient required to build animal tissue and products, and as sources of energy, are listed in Table 1.2. Energy is not listed in Table 1.2 because, strictly speaking, energy is not a nutrient – it is obtained by the animal as it oxidizes amino acids, fatty acids or carbohydrates. However, it has become a convenient convention in animal nutrition to talk about 'energy' as though it is a nutrient (see below).

How animals use nutrients

Water comprises about 70% of an animal's lean tissue mass. Water provides a medium for biochemical reactions, carries nutrients and waste products in blood and lymph, and transports enzymes in digestive tract secretions. It is also used to control body temperature, assist in waste removal (e.g. in urine), and is a component of the body's cells, and of milk and other animal products. Requirements for water are described in Chapter 2.

Energy: When carbohydrates, amino acids and fatty acids are oxidized in the body's cells, some of the energy in these molecules is released and is captured as adenosine triphosphate (ATP). This energy-rich ATP is used to support the synthesis of tissues and products, and physiological processes such as muscle contraction, nerve impulse transmission, etc.

It is extremely difficult to estimate the ATP-generation potential of feed constituents (although modern Dutch and Danish feeding standards attempt to do this), so we usually take another approach. This is to measure the total chemical energy in a feed by burning it, thus changing the chemical energy of the feed's carbohydrates, fats, proteins and other organic constituents into heat which is easily measured.

This heat energy is an (approximate) estimate of the amount of ATP energy which the feed can potentially supply and is called the feed's gross (or total) energy.

Amino acids are the building blocks of peptides and proteins and are involved in the synthesis of nucleic acids and a wide variety of other substances.

Animal bodies contain about 16% protein. Examples of proteins in animal tissue are:

- the proteins in muscle fibres (e.g. actin, myosin and the troponins);
- transport proteins in cell membranes;
- enzymes involved in digestion (e.g. the pepsins, trypsin and lactase) and intermediary metabolism (e.g. glyceraldehyde-3-phosphate dehydrogenase and RNA polymerase);
- peptide hormones (e.g. insulin, glucagon and parathyroid hormone);
- haemoglobin; and
- protein constituents of milk and eggs and in wool and hair fibres.

These proteins are made in the animal's cells from amino acids. All of the amino acids which are used to make proteins come from the feed, either directly in the case of the essential amino acids (see below for a discussion of 'essential nutrients'), or indirectly in the case of the non-essential ones which are made in the animal's cells from nitrogenous precursors supplied by the feed.

An animal's proteins are made from 21 different amino acid residues. Of these, about 12 are essential (see below). The list of essential amino acids varies according to animal species and age. Table 1.3 lists the essential and non-essential amino acids for pigs; this list also applies (in the specific amino acids but not in the amounts needed) to most other animals. Young animals need larger amounts of essential amino acid than adults, as is shown in Table 1.3 and NRC (1994).

Poultry and cats are two species which have different requirements to other domestic animals: taurine is essential for cats (to make the bile acid taurocholic acid, and it has other important physiological functions), and serine and glycine can be limiting for poultry. Poultry need glycine to form uric acid (their main way of excreting waste N), and serine to make nucleic acids, and both to make many other important substances. They may need a feed source of these amino acids if they do not eat enough cystine or threonine (glycine is made in the bird's tissues from these amino acids).

Ruminants have similar needs as pigs, horses and poultry for essential amino acids. They usually do not need these supplied in the feed because they are obtained from the digestion of microbial protein produced in the rumen. However, while rumen microbial metabolism delivers a wide range of amino acids, both essential and non-essential, the host animal's requirements for some essential amino acids (e.g. methionine, lysine, arginine and histidine) may not be fully met from rumen bacterial protein. In practice, methionine, lysine and histidine can be limiting amino acids for high-producing lactating dairy cows, and cyst(e)ine and methionine for wool-producing sheep.

Table 1.3. The amino acids needed by pigs. (From Dryden, 2008; reprinted with permission.)

Essential amino acids		Non-essential amino acids	
Arginine[a]	Methionine[c,d]	Alanine	Glutamine
Cyst(e)ine[b,c,d]	Phenylalanine[c]	Asparagine	Hydroxyproline
Histidine	Threonine	Aspartic acid	Proline
Isoleucine	Tryptophan	Glycine[e]	Taurine[e]
Leucine	Tyrosine[c]	Glutamic acid	
Lysine	Valine	Serine[e]	

[a]Synthesized in the urea cycle at rates sufficient for maintenance in the pig.
[b]Includes cystine and cysteine.
[c]Cystine can provide 50–80% of the requirement for sulphur amino acids, and tyrosine can provide 50% of the tyrosine + phenylalanine requirement of pigs.
[d]Cystine, cysteine and methionine are S-containing amino acids; cystine consists of two cysteine molecules.
[e]Taurine, glycine and serine are not essential for the pig, but can be limiting for felines and poultry (see the text).

Microbial protein is synthesized in the horse and pig large intestines but it is not digested there by the animal's intrinsic digestive enzymes and so does not provide any absorbable amino acids.

For information on the actual amino acid requirements of any specific animal type, check the relevant feeding standards (see Chapter 8).

Amino acids that are present in excess of the amount that the animal needs for the synthesis of proteins, nucleic acids, peptide hormones and other substances can be deaminated (i.e. the amino, -NH_2, group is removed), their carbon skeletons oxidized, and the energy which this process yields trapped in ATP. The carbon skeleton of some amino acids can be used as the starting point of glucose synthesis. This is especially important for ruminants because most feed glucose, or sources of glucose, is fermented by rumen micro-organisms and glucose is thus lost to the host animal.

Fatty acids are used to make cell membranes, prostaglandins, steroid hormones and other metabolically active molecules. Fatty acids are also used as an energy source.

All animals need certain long-chain, unsaturated fatty acids in their diet. Non-ruminant animals (e.g. pigs, horses and poultry) and new-born ruminants (especially lambs) need these nutrients in their feed, while adult ruminants are less demanding (Palmquist, 2010).

The most important of these are arachidonic acid (an unsaturated 20 C molecule, i.e. a fatty acid with 20 carbon atoms), linoleic acid and α-linolenic acid (LA and ALA; both unsaturated 18 C molecules). These fatty acids are found in high concentrations in vegetable oils and grass lipids. LA, ALA and arachidonic acids are most likely to be deficient in grain-rich diets because of the low fat content of cereal grains.

LA and ALA can be used to make three other important long-chain, unsaturated fatty acids: arachidonic acid from LA, and eicosapentaenoic acid (EPA) and docosapentaenoic acid (DHA) from ALA. If there is a high demand for arachidonic acid, DHA or EPA, or if there is not enough LA or ALA in the diet, then arachidonic acid, DHA and EPA will have to be supplied in the feed. These fatty acids are needed for the synthesis of biologically active substances such as prostaglandins and hormones.

The requirements of individual animal types for long-chain, unsaturated fatty acids vary. Check the relevant feeding standards (see Chapter 8).

Carbohydrates in feeds are either structural (fibrous) or non-structural (see Table 1.1). Fibrous carbohydrates are digested by microbes in the rumen and large intestine by a process that yields VFA (Chapter 3) which are used by the host animal as energy sources. Non-structural carbohydrates are monosaccharides or disaccharides, or the complex polysaccharide starch. When these are digested the simple sugars which they are made of are released and absorbed from the digestive tract. As well as using them as energy sources, animals use carbohydrates as structural components, e.g. in lactose (glucose and galactose), nucleic acids (ribose) and glycoproteins. Glycoproteins are widely distributed in animal tissue and are components of cartilage and mucus, cell membranes, and biologically active substances such as hormones and immunoglobulins.

Minerals are classed as either 'major' (or 'macro-)' or 'trace' (or 'micro-') depending on whether the daily requirement for them is large (g/day) or small (mg/day). Some authorities use the term 'ultra-trace' for those few minerals which are required in very small amounts. All of these minerals are essential nutrients. There are seven major and ten trace minerals which are known to be required for good health and production, and another ten which appear to have beneficial effects on animal metabolism. Minerals are constituents of biologically important macromolecules such as haemoglobin, thyroxine, various coenzymes, nucleic acids, phospholipids, bone minerals, etc. Some minerals are used to regulate body fluid osmolarity and pH, and to carry nerve impulses. These functions are described in Dryden (2008).

Vitamins are a group of unrelated chemicals which have essential functions in the animal's biochemistry. They are classed as either fat-soluble or water-soluble (Table 1.4). Most vitamins are used as enzyme cofactors, i.e. they assist the function of enzymes, often by helping to bind substrates to the enzyme. Other vitamins have a hormonal role. Vitamin A occurs as its precursor β-carotene in many feeds.

Essential and non-essential nutrients

In animal nutrition, essential means 'essential in the diet', i.e. the nutrient must be supplied in the animal's feed. Some authorities refer to 'essential' nutrients as 'indispensable' nutrients. These terms mean the same thing.

Table 1.4. A list of water-soluble and fat-soluble vitamins. (Adapted from Dryden, 2008; reprinted with permission.)

Common name	Other names	Common name	Other names
Water-soluble vitamins			
Vitamin C	Ascorbic acid		
B group vitamins			
B12	Cobalamin	Pantothenic acid	B5
Biotin	B7, vitamin H	Pyridoxine	B6
Choline		Riboflavin	B2
Folic acid	Folacin, folate, B9 or B11	Thiamine	B1
Niacin	Nicotinic acid, B3		
Fat-soluble vitamins			
Vitamin A	Retinol, retinoic acid, retinoids β-Carotene (the precursor)	Vitamin E	Tocopherol (α, β, γ and δ)
Vitamin D	D2, ergocalciferol D3, cholecalciferol	Vitamin K	Menaquinone, phylloquinone

A nutrient is essential when either:

- It cannot be made at all within the animal's cells, e.g. the essential amino acids listed in Table 1.3, α-linolenic and linoleic fatty acids, all the minerals needed by animals and almost all vitamins (there are some individual species differences); or
- It can be made but not rapidly enough to meet the animal's current need for it, e.g. in some circumstances, the amino acid arginine.

A list of essential nutrients is given in Table 1.5.

Nutrients which can be synthesized within animal body cells are called non-essential nutrients. This does not mean that they are not needed in the animal's metabolism, just that they do not have to be provided in the animal's feed. However, the feed must supply those substances which the animal needs as starting points to synthesize non-essential nutrients.

Examples of non-essential nutrients are:

- The amino acid asparagine, which is made by transferring an amino group from a glutamic acid molecule that the animal does not immediately need to aspartic acid (another amino). About ten (see Table 1.3) amino acids can be made in this way and are therefore non-essential.
- A wide range of fatty acids and fatty acid derivatives, including phospholipids, can be synthesized in animal cells.
- Glucose is needed for many synthetic processes, e.g. synthesis of lactose; and it is also needed as an energy source for the brain. It can be made from propionic acid, and from several amino acids.

Deficient and limiting nutrients

A nutrient is deficient when it is present in the diet at a concentration which is less than that needed for optimum animal health and production.

In practice, essential nutrients are sometimes present in the animal's feed at less than the concentrations needed to support life, health and/or production. Generally, there is one nutrient which is the 'most deficient' in comparison to the animal's requirement for it, and which consequently has the greatest effect on the animal's metabolism and its ability to thrive and produce. This nutrient is called the 'limiting nutrient'.

Note that a limiting nutrient is:

- an essential nutrient, which is
- deficient in the diet, and
- a supplement of that nutrient gives a positive animal response.

Table 1.5. Essential and potentially limiting nutrients in conventional animal feeds. (Adapted from Dryden, 2008; reproduced with permission).

Nutrient group	Individual nutrients	Look for potential limiting nutrients in these situations
Amino acids	See Table 1.3 for a list of essential amino acids	Insufficient available lysine in pig or poultry diets which are based on cereal grains, and insufficient lysine in horse diets. Deficiencies of methionine for lactating dairy cows, or cystine for sheep or goats (see text for more possible deficiencies)
Fatty acids	Possibly limiting: linoleic acid The other essential FA are the long-chain, ω3 and ω6 unsaturated FA, including α-linolenic, arachidonic, eicosapentaenoic (EPA), and docosahexaenoic (DHA) acids	Pig and poultry diets which are based on cereal grains and which contain little vegetable oil. Embryonic development in cattle may respond to Ca salts of ω6 FA
Minerals[a]	Possibly limiting: Ca, Co, Cu, I, Fe, Mg, P, Se, Na Other essential minerals are Cr, Mn, Mo, K, Si, S and Zn As, B, Br, F, Li, Ni, Rb, Sn and V may be essential but are not limiting	Pig and poultry diets usually contain large quantities of cereal grains and their by-products; these have low concentrations of available Ca and P. Pasture may have little P or trace minerals depending on their stage of maturity and the soils they grow on
Vitamins	Possibly limiting: vitamin A (retinol), thiamine (vitamin B1), cobalamin (vitamin B12), biotin, vitamin D Other vitamins include niacin, riboflavin (vitamin B2), pantothenic acid, pyridoxine (vitamin B6), folic acid, vitamin E and vitamin K	Vitamin A deficiency may restrict the performance of animals fed unsupplemented grain-based diets, or graze over-mature pastures for a lengthy period. Vitamin E and vitamin K are not likely to be limiting in practical diets. Vitamin C (ascorbic acid) may be needed by animals of some species and/or ages, e.g. the young pig. Additional dietary choline may be useful in the diets of newborn lambs and dairy calves and lactating dairy cattle may respond to additional ruminally protected choline
Water	Sometimes limiting	In droughts, or if the animals' water supply fails, or if the water is very cold, hot or saline; sometimes animals (e.g. horses) are reluctant to drink 'foreign-tasting' water

[a]Calcium (Ca), cobalt (Co), copper (Cu), iodine (I), iron (Fe), magnesium (Mg), phosphorus (P), selenium (Se), sodium (Na); chromium (Cr), manganese (Mn), molybdenum (Mo), potassium (K), silicon (Si), sulphur (S), zinc (Zn); arsenic (As), boron (B), bromine (Br), fluorine (F), lithium (Li), nickel (Ni), rubidium (Rb), tin (Sn), vanadium (V).

Animals will respond to a supplement of a limiting nutrient but may not respond to supplements of other deficient nutrients if the limiting nutrient deficiency is not corrected.

The 'leaky bucket' analogy is often used to illustrate this situation (Fig. 1.3). The production level attainable (demonstrated by the higher water level in the bucket) when the limiting nutrient deficiency is corrected is determined by the effect of the next-limiting deficiency.

If we only correct a non-limiting deficiency, then the animal's performance will still be limited by the limiting nutrient deficiency.

Nutrient toxicities

Nutrients are essential to an animal's health and productivity, but some can have adverse effects if they are eaten in excessive amounts.

Energy in excess will increase fat deposition and this can lead to lower carcase quality, although the actual outcome depends on the animal's genotype and its environment.

Similarly, excess RDP, or urea given as a feed supplement, lead to excessive amounts of ammonia (NH_3) which is absorbed from the rumen. High concentrations in the blood can overcome the blood–brain barrier and cause a range of symptoms including incoordination and weakness, and often death.

In practice, mineral and vitamin excesses cause the most commonly experienced nutrient toxicities. A short list of problematic nutrients is given in Table 1.6.

Functional and pharmacological roles of feed constituents

There are several feed constituents which have important functional and/or pharmacological roles in addition to any nutrients that they may supply.

Plant fibre is fermented in the rumen and large intestine by microbes with the production of VFA as end-products. These VFA are absorbed and used as energy sources by the host animal; they are important energy sources for ruminants and herbivorous birds, and horses and pigs can also get up to a third of their energy requirement from the VFA produced by intestinal bacteria.

Fibre has an important role in maintaining digestive tract health (Chapter 13). Pigs and horses need fibre to prevent ulcers developing in the oesophagus and upper part of the stomach and to maintain

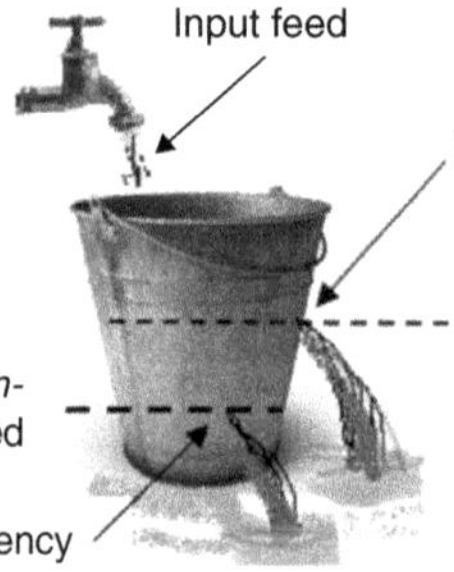

Fig. 1.3. The *leaky bucket* analogy illustrates the effect of supplementing a limiting nutrient. (Copyright: Gordon McL. Dryden.)

Table. 1.6. Some nutrients which are toxic when eaten in excess.

Nutrient	Situation
Ruminally available N	'Urea poisoning' occurs when ruminant animals (sheep, goats, cattle and deer, among others) degrade protein or urea and release excess amounts of NH_3 in the rumen. Most commonly a result of feeding excess urea; see Chapter 13
Amino acids	Appetite depression in pigs and poultry fed diets which contain an excess of a particular amino acid, especially methionine and cysteine
Unsaturated fatty acids	Muscular myopathy can result from feeding excess unsaturated fatty acids, especially if antioxidants such as vitamin E are deficient
Ca	Excess Ca reduces the ability of the animal to absorb other nutrients. Pigs may suffer from parakeratosis (a Zn deficiency disorder) if the diet Ca concentration is above 1.2%
Cu	Excess Cu causes jaundice, haemolysis of red blood cells, and often death. There is considerable species variation in susceptibility to Cu poisoning. Sheep are the most susceptible of the common domestic animals and their upper level of tolerance is about 25 ppm in the diet. Cattle (100 ppm) and pigs (250 ppm) are more tolerant, and horses (800 ppm) are very tolerant of high Cu levels
Se	A potentially very poisonous mineral. Symptoms include hair loss, lameness, difficulty breathing, then death. Toxicity may occur at 2 ppm of the diet for sheep, horses and beef cattle, and at 5 ppm for pigs
S	Excess can be poisonous to ruminants if it is converted to H_2S in the rumen. The recommended upper limit in the diet is 0.4%
Vitamin A	Pigs suffer from foetal abnormalities, and fragile and overgrown bones
Vitamin D	Excess vitamin D causes calcification of soft tissues (e.g. heart and blood vessels), extensive kidney damage, and brittle and deformed bones

a flow of digesta through the tract. The saliva produced when fibrous feed is chewed helps to keep the rumen pH near 6.5 and thus avoid rumen acidosis, and the abrasive effect of fibrous particles rubbing on the rumen wall helps to prevent rumenitis. Physically effective fibre (peNDF) is a measure used to predict how effectively feed fibre will promote chewing and saliva production, and abrasion in the rumen. A feed's peNDF is the amount of plant cell wall (NDF) which is contained in feed particles which are not likely to pass from the rumen without being chewed by rumination (this particle size is 1.18 mm) (Mertens, 1997). Cattle need feeds which contain 28–30% peNDF (Cooke *et al.*, 2020). Finely milled roughages (small particles) have less 'fibre effect' than longer pieces as they need less chewing to form into a bolus, and this promotes less saliva production.

Effective fibre (eNDF) is the amount of NDF which will maintain milk fat contents in dairy cattle. Dairy cows must have a minimum digestible plant fibre content in their feed as they use acetate (a VFA produced in the rumen when fibre is fermented) as the starting point for milk fat synthesis. If the eNDF level is too low rumen pH will fall, with reductions in DM intake, passage of undigested feed from the rumen and microbial protein yield. The concepts of eNDF and peNDF are described in more detail in NRC (2001).

Condensed tannins: These bind to protein and increase the feed's bypass protein content. They also reduce the likelihood of rumen bloat, can have an anthelmintic effect on intestinal worms (helminths), and may reduce CH_4 emissions. Tannins are further discussed in Chapter 6.

Trace minerals: In some cases, trace minerals can have both a nutritional and a pharmacological role. Cu can be used to control intestinal parasites in pigs. This practice stopped when it was realized that the large amount of Cu which these animals excreted was an environmental hazard. Minerals like F which hardens teeth but is toxic in large amounts, V which has anti-tumour effects and Li which has a neuroprotective function, appear to have a pharmacological role but not a straightforward nutritional one. These aspects of mineral nutrition are described in Dryden (2008).

Plant pigments: A variety of different substances which reflect different wavelengths of visual light, and which serve a variety of functions in plant biochemistry, including photosynthesis. Some have effects on animal products, e.g. carotene and xanthophyll improve the colour of egg yolks (if we like richly coloured, yellow/orange yolks) and may colour the fat of grazing cattle, and others have anti-microbial or anti-inflammatory properties.

Ruminally degradable protein: To adequately feed ruminants we have to correctly nourish the rumen microbiota – the bacteria, archaea, protozoa and fungi. NH_3 is an essential nutrient for bacteria, especially those which digest plant fibre, and is obtained from that part of the feed protein which is able to be degraded by microbial action in the rumen.

Secondary substances

These are substances which are found in feeds and which can adversely affect animal health and product quality (see Chapters 6 and 12). Examples are gossypol in cottonseeds, trypsin inhibitor in soybeans and other grain legumes, and erucic acid in rapeseed. Plants produce these substances to protect themselves against browsing by animals, and from pathogenic micro-organisms. While they help the plant, they have adverse effects on the animals which eat them.

Important examples are:

- Phytin is a phosphorus-rich substance which is widely distributed in plants and particularly in seeds where it is about 75% of the total phosphorus. Phytate-P is essentially unavailable to pigs.
- Oxalate is found in the tissues of some grasses (e.g. kikuyu, etc.). It binds to feed Ca, making it unavailable to animals.
- Aromatic substances (indole and skatole) and short-chain alkenes (allyl sulphides) that are produced by rumen micro-organisms or are present in some feeds (e.g. onion and garlic, peppergrass, silage, etc.) will taint milk.
- Gossypol is a polyphenolic substance in cottonseed which impairs reproduction in male animals.
- Inhibitors of proteases (enzymes which digest proteins), such as pepsin and trypsin inhibitors in legume seeds.

References

AOAC (2019). *Official Methods of Analysis*, 21st edn. Rockville, Maryland, USA: AOAC.

Cooke, R.F., Daigle, C.L., Moriel, P., Smith, S.B., Tedeschi, L.O. and Vendramini, J.M.B. (2020). Cattle adapted to tropical and subtropical environments: social, nutritional, and carcass quality considerations. *Journal of Animal Science* 98(2): skaa014. DOI: https://doi.org/10.1093/jas/skaa014.

Dryden, G.McL. (2008). *Animal Nutrition Science*. Wallingford, UK: CAB International.

Mertens, D.R. (1997). Creating a system for meeting the fiber requirements of dairy cows. *Journal of Dairy Science* 80: 1463–1481.

National Research Council (NRC) (1982). *United States–Canadian Tables of Feed Composition*, 3rd rev. Washington, DC: National Academies Press. Available at: www.nap.edu/catalog/1713/united-states-canadian-tables-of-feed-composition-nutritional-data-for (accessed 23 December 2020).

National Research Council (NRC) (1994). *Nutrient Requirements of Poultry*, 8th rev. edn. Washington, DC: National Academies Press. Available at: www.nap.edu/catalog/19397/nutrient-requirements-of-poultry-eighth-revised-edition-1984 (accessed 23 December 2020).

National Research Council (NRC) (2001). *Nutrient Requirements of Dairy Cattle*, 7th rev. edn. Washington, DC: National Academies Press. Available at: www.nap.edu/catalog/9825/nutrient-requirements-of-dairy-cattle-seventh-revised-edition-2001 (accessed 23 December 2020).

Nielsen, S.S. (ed.) (2017). *Food Analysis*, 5th edn. Cham, Switzerland: Springer International.

Palmquist, D.L. (2010). Essential fatty acids in ruminant diets. *Proceedings of the 21st Annual Ruminant Nutrition Symposium*, Gainesville, FL, pp. 127–141. Institute of Food and Agricultural Sciences, University of Florida, Gainesville. Available at: www.researchgate.net/publication/228397452_Essential_fatty_acids_in_ruminant_diets (accessed 23 December 2020).

2 Water

Water is a sometimes under-appreciated nutrient. Animals usually have access to plenty of water and we do not concern ourselves much about providing it. But when we put animals into intensive housing, or natural water sources fail during droughts or for any other reason, then the importance of water, and the consequences of water deficiency, immediately become obvious.

Functions and sources of water

Animals use water for a wide variety of functions. We can group these as follows:

- Transport: water helps to carry undigested feed (digesta) through the digestive tract, keeps faeces moist so that they can be easily excreted, and is the main constituent of urine, and so is essential in the excretion of waste products. Water is responsible for the transport of absorbed nutrients in blood and lymph. Water also carries body secretions, e.g. saliva and enzymes secreted into the digestive tract in pancreatic juice.
- A component of body tissues (70% or more of body cells), and animal products (e.g. about 88% of cows' milk, and about 75% of eggs).
- Physiological functions and chemical reactions: water dissolves oxygen in the lungs, lubricates (e.g. tears) and cushions joints against shocks (e.g. synovial fluid in joints). It is an intermediate or product of chemical reactions, e.g. the reactions which are carried out within cells when energy sources are oxidized, or when molecules such as fatty acids are synthesized.
- Body temperature control: animals get rid of surplus heat from their bodies by sweating and/or panting. The heat is removed from the body when the water in sweat and exhaled breath is vaporized.
- A component of body tissues and animal products: water is a constituent of body cells (it can be 70% or more of body cells), milk (about 88% of cows' milk) and other products.

Sources of water – metabolic water, feed water and drinking water: There are three ways that animals get the water they need.

- Metabolic water is made in the animal's body cells as they oxidize sugars, amino acids and fatty acids to release the chemical energy that these substances can provide. Metabolic water is not a large water source.
- Water in the feed: plant-derived feeds contain water, depending on whether they are fresh (the leafy parts of pasture grasses and legumes can have 60–90% water) or air-dry (cereal grains and protein meals will contain 5–15% water). Water in feed can be part of the plant cells (Chapter 1), or it may be rain or irrigation water which adheres to plant material when it is eaten, or water may be mixed with the air-dry feed to form a gruel (e.g. in some pig feeding systems; Chapter 17). A dairy cow eating 20 kg of dry matter/day from temperate grass pasture will ingest about 80 kg/day of plant cell water. A growing pig eating 2.25 kg/day of a typical air-dry commercial feed will consume some 220 g/day of feed water.
- Drinking water supplies the difference between the animal's water requirement and the amount of water it gets from metabolic and feed sources.

Animals get most of their water from external sources, either in their feed or from drinking water. The amount of drinking water that an animal needs depends on:

- Its physiological state: whether it is pregnant or lactating, or not; its age and thus the type of body components (bone, lean tissue or fat) that are being laid down as it grows, and how fast it is growing.
- The environment: the ambient temperature, wind speed, and humidity; the presence of shade.
- The type of water it has to drink: if the drinking water is saline this will increase the amount that the

 Fundamentals of Applied Animal Nutrition (G.McL. Dryden)
DOI: 10.1079/9781786394453.0002

animal must drink to meet its water requirement; the water temperature also affects consumption – animals may drink less warm or cold water.

These factors are summarized in Fig. 2.1.

Because of the many factors which influence the amount of drinking water an animal needs, it is not easy to give exact recommendations on water requirements. But if we assume that the drinking water that we have available has a suitable salinity (i.e. the level of dissolved solids is less than the animal's tolerance level), and if there are no extremes of ambient temperature, or other environmental factors which would increase the water requirement, then we can make the recommendations given in Table 2.1. The beef cattle recommendations are for *Bos taurus* animals; *Bos indicus* cattle drink a little less, except when temperatures rise to 30°C or more.

Toxic levels of some water contaminants: Depending on the soil type, groundwater can carry variable loads of dissolved minerals. ANZECC (2000) recommends upper limits for Cu in drinking water of 0.5 mg/L for sheep, 1 mg/L for cattle and 5 mg/L for pigs and poultry. Fluoride levels should not exceed 2 mg/L, and Ca should be less than 1000 mg/L provided that Mg and Na levels are not excessive and that the diet provides adequate P. Sulphate concentrations up to 1000 mg/L are not likely to cause problems, but levels up to 2000 mg/L may adversely affect young or lactating animals. Levels of dissolved Se and Zn should not exceed 0.02 and 20 mg/L, respectively.

Nitrates and nitrites can occur in drinking water. ANZECC (2000) recommends maximum nitrate levels of 400 mg/L in drinking water and no more than 30 mg/L of nitrite.

Saline water can affect animal health and performance

Water can contain dissolved salts – principally Ca, Na and Mg carbonates, bicarbonates, chlorides, phosphates and sulphates – and other substances such as nitrates. The total of mineral salts is called the total dissolved solids (TDS). When the concentration of TDS exceeds the animal's ability to excrete these then it begins to suffer from the effects of water salinity ('saline water' is a general term for water which contains amounts of dissolved solids, irrespective of what these solids are).

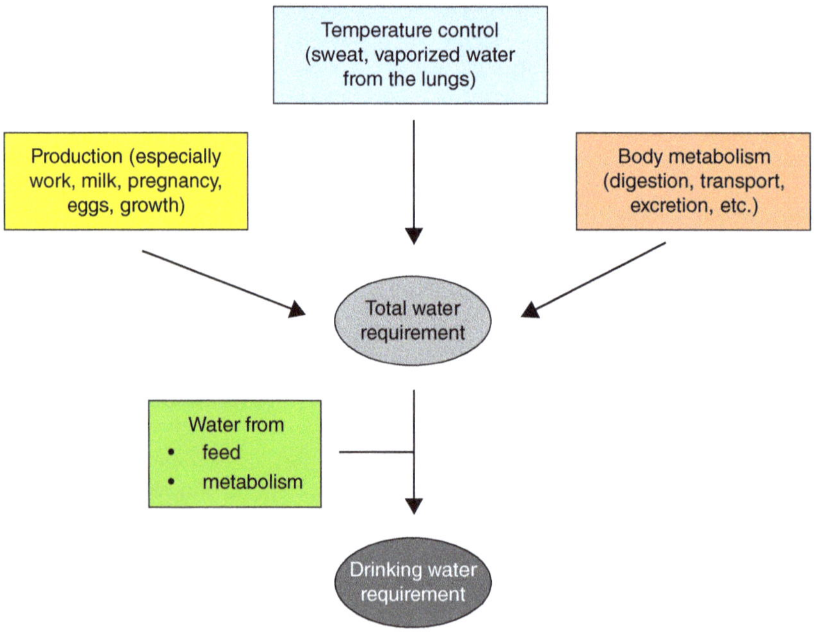

Fig. 2.1. Factors which influence the drinking water requirements of animals. (From Dryden, 2008; reproduced with permission.)

Table 2.1. Water requirements and salinity tolerances of domestic animals. (From ANZECC, 2000; Poultry CRC, 2021, and references in Dryden, 2008.)

Animal	Water requirement (L/day)	Maximum salinity (mg TDS/L)
Beef cattle:		
Lactating cow	43–60	4500–6000
Growing heifer, steer	15–57	5000–10 000
Mature dry cow	22–78	5000–10 000
Dairy cattle:		
Lactating cow	70–105	2500–7000
Dry adult cow	45–60	
Calf (1 to 4 weeks)	1–4.5	2500–7000
Calf (weaned)	22–30	
Deer:		
Red deer hinds	4.5	9200
Rusa deer stags	7	8500
Goats:		
Dry adults	1.5–4	15 000–20 000
Lactating does	6–15	10 000–14 000
Horses:		
Working	55–70	1000–5000
Resting	20–45	5000–7000
Foals (6 to 10 weeks)	4–5.5	1000–5000
Pigs:		
Dry and breeding sows	20–40	4000–8000
Growers and finishers	3.5–14	4000–8000
Weaners	0.5–9	4000–8000
Sheep:		
Lactating ewe	9–14	4500–6000
Dry ewe, wether	5–7	10 000–13 000
Lamb	1.5–2.5	3500–4000
Poultry:[a]		
Chicks (1 week)	0.07–0.11	2000–3500
Broilers (8 weeks)	0.37–0.56	2000–3500
Laying hens	0.22–0.33	2000–3500

[a]Data are from Poultry CRC (2021); they are not warranted to be accurate, complete or up to date.

The TDS concentration can be easily and quickly measured by determining the water's electrical conductivity (EC) and converting this reading to TDS:

$$\text{TDS (mg/L)} = \text{EC } (\mu\text{S/cm}) \times 0.67$$

Why water salinity causes problems: Saline water can have serious adverse effects on health and productivity. When TDS levels exceed the animal's salinity tolerance feed intake falls, its ability to cope with heat stress is compromised, production decreases and the animal may die.

When an animal drinks saline water we have the sequence of events that is illustrated in Fig. 2.2. As the TDS content of drinking water increases, the animal needs more water to excrete wastes in the urine. As these wastes include excess dissolved substances in the drinking water, we get into the vicious cycle shown in the box in Fig. 2.2.

As more drinking water is used to excrete excess salts, there is progressively less water for the animal's metabolism, production and temperature control. When the amount of water needed to maintain general metabolism, production and temperature control (A in Fig. 2.2) is more than the amount of water available for these purposes (B in Fig. 2.2) the animal can no longer function.

Tolerance of saline water: In most cases animals are adversely affected by high levels of dissolved salts. However, the effect can be modified by slowly adapting animals to water with high TDS levels.

Approximate limits to salinity tolerance of different species are given in Table 2.1. Where a range is given, the lower level is what the animal or bird is expected to tolerate without any adverse effects, and the mid-range should be tolerated after initial reluctance to drink but animals should adapt to these levels (ANZECC, 2000).

The factors which influence the response to saline water can be grouped into 'animal' and 'environmental' factors.

The animal factors are:

- Species and breed: Table 2.1 shows clearly the different tolerances of different animal species.
- Physiological state: whether the animal is growing, lactating, pregnant, actively working, etc. Those with higher water requirements are less tolerant of water salinity.
- Animal age: older animals are more tolerant of saline water than young ones.
- The animal's ability to concentrate its urine, i.e. to reduce the amount of water which it uses to excrete soluble wastes. Species like sheep which can produce more concentrated urine (e.g. compared to cattle) are more tolerant of saline water.
- Adaptation to salinity: sheep and pigs have been shown to adapt to increased salinity if they are gradually exposed to increasing TDS levels. However, this behaviour does not protect them

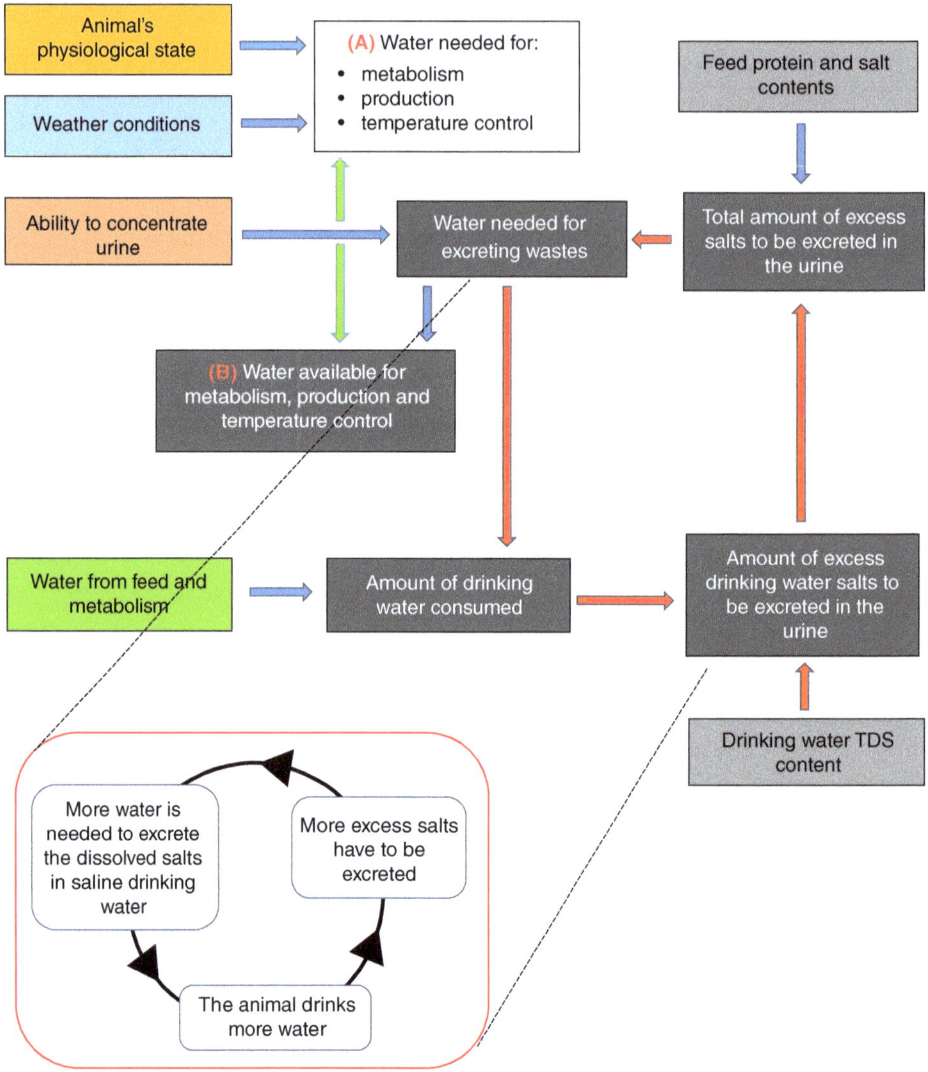

Fig. 2.2. How water salinity affects animals (the sequence shown by the red arrows and in the red box is the 'vicious cycle' mentioned in the text). (Copyright: Gordon McL. Dryden.)

from very high TDS levels (at or above the upper ends of the ranges shown in Table 2.1) and we should not rely on this.

The environmental factors include:

- Climatic conditions: air temperature, wind speed, humidity, and access to shade influence the animal's need for water.
- The type of feed being eaten, especially the protein and salts contents which influence the amounts of wastes needed to be excreted in the urine.
- The type of dissolved ions: Na salts are tolerated better than Mg salts, and sulphates and chlorides are tolerated better than carbonates.

How animals respond to high levels of salinity: One of the animal's first responses to saline water is to drink more water. This behaviour persists until the salt load becomes too great. When given water with TDS levels near the salinity tolerance limit, water and feed intakes can become erratic – changing markedly from day to day. Take this as an important warning that TDS levels are becoming too high. When TDS is too high and exceeds the animal's salinity tolerance, water and feed intakes fall to very low levels. Animals will show occasional diarrhoea and general weakness.

Avoiding salinity problems: Always check the TDS content of drinking water. It is important that we get the water supply checked not only for TDS content (as is shown by its electrical conductivity) but also for the concentrations of carbonates and Mg salts.

Water from rivers or dams will often have low TDS contents. But do not assume that this is true in every case – rivers collect water which has flowed through soil and picked up salts as it did so.

The TDS content of any given water supply can change between seasons. This is especially so if we move from surface water (rivers, streams, dams) to underground water from wells or bores in periods of low rainfall.

Practical considerations about giving water to animals

Water can be provided from several types of source. Each of these has its own advantages and potential problems.

Dams, ponds and streams: These have the advantage of very low cost (unless they are fenced and water is pumped from them into troughs), and the water quality is usually acceptable. The main difficulties with these are the possible collapse of banks, and dams beginning to dry up which then makes animals walk through mud to reach the water and possibly become bogged. This can cause serious issues when the animal is being rescued – it is best to get help from a veterinarian or other professional to avoid injuring hooves and legs. If possible, isolate the dam behind a fence and pump the water into a trough.

Evaporation of water from dams is a real issue in hot climates. Evaporation can be reduced but not eliminated, by covering the dam. There are several ways of doing this, including sheltering the dam from wind and sun, using shade cloth, or covering the water surface with plastic balls.

Algal growth occurs in still water, e.g. in troughs or dams in warm conditions, and especially if the water is exposed to sunlight. In many cases the growth is unsightly but does not deter animals from drinking (but see 'blue-green algae' below). Non-poisonous algae can be controlled by using a copper sulphate block; the block is simply placed in the trough and Cu slowly leaches from the block and poisons the algae. However, be very careful when using these blocks as the treated water contains added Cu, and sheep in particular are very susceptible to excess Cu. ANZECC (2000) recommends that water for grazing animals contains no more than 0.5 mg/L Cu for sheep and 1 mg/L Cu for cattle.

'Blue-green algae' (cyanobacteria) sometimes grow in open water storages and in slow-flowing streams. If algae are present in or on the water, check the type – it is important to identify if they are cyanobacteria. If a blue-green algal bloom has occurred before, be especially vigilant. All cyanobacteria can produce toxins which will kill animals. If blue-green algae are present, animals should be prevented from using the water. The risks posed by blue-green algae, and how to deal with them, are well described by CSIRO (2019), but in brief (ANZECC 2000; Water Quality Australia, undated):

- Cyanobacteria produce poisons which damage liver and nerve cells, the kidneys, digestive tract and blood vessels.
- Poisons can be ingested when animals drink infested water or eat dried mats of cyanobacteria.
- If algae are present, assume that they are poisonous until they have been tested.

Troughs are used in many situations, e.g. for grazing animals where paddocks do not have adequate surface water, and for intensively housed animals other than poultry.

Troughs are made from plastic, these are light and easily moved when empty, but they can be broken by cattle; or concrete, and are solid but heavy and difficult to move; or galvanized steel, usually sound but prone to rust when the galvanizing begins to fail. In all troughs the water flow is controlled by a float valve.

Water troughs allow flexible water point placement, and they can be sited within a fence so that they can serve two areas.

Nipple and cup drinkers: These are used in intensive housing; they dispense water from a valve controlled by a spring-loaded nipple, plate or button, and the valve is often situated over a bowl which catches excess water. This allows animals to drink from the bowl and also prevents water from soiling the bedding.

Monitoring water supplies: Check water supplies regularly; this should be done every day in hot, dry weather when water intakes are at their highest. Animals succumb to water deprivation more quickly than to lack of feed. If needed to oversee remote locations, install cameras which can be monitored via the internet.

When managing water supplies, look for these things:

- Faulty float valve action, including overflow caused by snakes, toads or other wildlife sitting on the float.
- Electrical hazard from electric fence wires which have become in contact with steel troughs or pipes, or with the water. Animals receive a shock which deters them from drinking.
- Build-up of scale in pipes servicing troughs: some types of water will deposit scale and eventually block the pipe, especially if the water system is also used to provide urea or phosphate nutritional supplements.
- Water freezing in pipes in winter: several methods of preventing this are described by NSAIS (2010).
- Changes in water salinity between seasons.
- Monitor trough and dam water salinity in hot weather; there are reports of cattle suffering from salinity poisoning as the dissolved solids content of the water increases with evaporation. This problem is usually restricted to grazing animals, but housed animals can also be affected if the water comes from an on-farm supply.
- Wearing away of soil around troughs leading to young or small animals being unable to reach over the lip of the trough.
- Wet soil around dams which may bog animals.
- Algal growth.
- Gates or other access to water shut or blocked – blocked access to water can be an unexpected problem if spear gates are used to direct animals towards water over a walk-over weighing device, and these gates fail for some reason.
- Make sure that there are enough water points for the number of animals or birds, and that these are all operational.
- Horses taken to events away from home may not drink if the water tastes differently to what they are accustomed to.

Water point placement for grazing animals: Animals will graze for limited distances from water, and this can influence the amount of grazing land which they use. This is discussed in greater detail in Chapter 15.

References

Australian and New Zealand Environment and Conservation Council (ANZECC) /Agriculture and Resource Management Council of Australia and New Zealand (2000). *Australian and New Zealand Guidelines for Fresh and Marine Water Quality*. Volumes 1 and 3. Available at: www.waterquality.gov.au/anz-guidelines/resources/previous-guidelines/anzecc-armcanz-2000 (accessed 23 December 2020).

Commonwealth Scientific and Industrial Research Organisation (CSIRO) (2019). *What are blue-green algae*? Available at: www.csiro.au/en/Research/Environment/Water/Blue-green-algae/What-are-blue-green-algae (accessed 3 March 2021).

Dryden, G.McL. (2008). *Animal Nutrition Science*. Wallingford, UK: CAB International.

National Sustainable Agriculture Information Service (NSAIS) (2010). *Freeze Protection for Livestock Watering Systems*. Available at: https://attra.ncat.org/product/freeze-protection-for-livestock-watering-systems/ (accessed 18 March 2021).

Poultry CRC (2021). *Water consumption rates for chickens*. Poultry Hub. Available at: https://www.poultryhub.org/all-about-poultry/nutrition (accessed 14 March 2021).

Water Quality Australia (undated). *Cyanobacteria (Blue-Green Algae) and Water Quality*. Available at: www.waterquality.gov.au/issues/blue-green-algae (accessed 23 December 2020).

3 Digestion of feeds

Feeding behaviour and digestive physiology

We can separate animals and birds into several different types, depending on what type of feed they typically use and how their digestive tract functions. Almost all our domestic animals are herbivores. The pig, and some birds, are omnivores and are the only common farm animals which are not herbivores.

- Herbivores typically eat forages (roughages, fibre-rich plant feeds), although they will also eat concentrate feeds such as grains, molasses and plant protein meals. We often give these animals cereal grain milling and brewing by-products (e.g. dried distiller's solubles, millrun, bran, maize gluten meal). Milk processing by-products (e.g. skim milk powder, buttermilk powder, casein, whey powder) are used in milk replacers fed to unweaned young. These are not natural feeds for herbivores, but they are accepted by these animals and can form useful parts of their feed.
- Omnivores naturally eat both plant- and animal-origin feeds. While they use a wide range of feeds when they live naturally (in the wild), these animals are typically given plant-origin feeds when they are managed under farm conditions. As well, pigs and poultry are fed meat meals or fish meals as sources of essential amino acids.

If we know whether our animal is naturally a herbivore or an omnivore this will help us to identify the feedstuffs that it is most likely to accept and be able to eat without suffering from digestive disorders.

There are several ways of classifying animals according to their nutritional characteristics. Because these overlap, it is best to discuss each of the main animal types separately.

- Horses and donkeys are grazing animals which have evolved to eat plant material, especially forages (roughages, pasture, vegetative plant material), as their main feed type. However, they will eat, and often eat avidly, concentrate feeds such as grains, protein meals, molasses and fats. The plant fibre (plant cell wall material) in their feeds is digested (or 'fermented') by micro-organisms which inhabit their colon and caecum (the lower parts of the digestive tract). Accordingly, equines are referred to as 'hind-gut fermenters'.
- Cows, goats, sheep, buffalo, and deer and other ruminants have evolved to eat the same types of feed as equines, i.e. forages, and they also eat concentrates when they have access to these. Ruminants graze quickly and later regurgitate large feed particles from their reticulo-rumen and re-chew these in a process called rumination. Like equines, they rely on micro-organisms to digest the fibre in their feed. They have microbial populations in their fore-stomach – the reticulum, rumen, and omasum – and also in their hind gut – the caecum and colon. Because of the presence of microbes in the reticulo-rumen and omasum these animals are referred to as 'fore-gut fermenters'. This terminology reflects the importance of the microbial population in the reticulo-rumen, even though these animals also have a second microbial population in their large intestine.
- Llamas, alpacas and camels are members of the camelid family, and have a three-compartment stomach (compared to the four compartments of ruminants). They are fore-gut fermenters and, like ruminants, they have microbial populations in both their stomach and their large intestine. Like ruminants, they ruminate and eruct (belch) gases produced by microbial fermentation. Camelids are sometimes called pseudo-ruminants because they have stomach compartments which function similarly to the reticulo-rumen but are not exact replicates of these ruminant animal organs.
- Pigs are monogastrics, i.e. they have a simple, glandular stomach which empties into their small intestine. Pigs have a population of micro-organisms

 Fundamentals of Applied Animal Nutrition (G.McL. Dryden)
DOI: 10.1079/9781786394453.0003

in their caecum and colon, and this can contribute to the energy sources (mainly volatile fatty acids, VFA) which are made available to the animal by digestion. When they are intensively managed, pigs are fed a low-fibre (usually less than 5% plant fibre), concentrate-rich feed. Under these conditions the micro-organisms of the large intestine make only a small contribution to feed digestion. However, grazing pigs eat a much more fibrous diet and the contribution of the hind-gut microbes is much greater.

- Birds vary in their types of natural feed. Some birds are obligate carnivores; others rely almost entirely on plant-origin feed. Most, including domestic poultry, are omnivores. Herbivorous birds have a population of microbes in their caeca which digests plant fibre.
- Kangaroos and wallabies are not domestic animals but are included here for completeness. These animals are pseudo-ruminants (a term which is also applied to camelids). They have a stomach compartment which has a population of micro-organisms between their oesophagus and their glandular stomach. These animals do not ruminate; instead, they chew their feed very finely as they eat it. They also have a smaller population of micro-organisms in their caecum and colon.

Digestive tract function – intrinsic and microbial digestion

All animals have their own, intrinsic, digestive enzymes which attack the carbohydrates, proteins and fats in feed and release their constituent molecules to be absorbed. These enzymes are secreted from salivary, gastric and duodenal glands, and from the pancreas. The small intestinal epithelium also has enzymes which are not secreted into the lumen of the tract but which are located in the membranes of the epithelial cells of the villi lining the tract.

As described above, there are several places in the digestive tract that host populations of microbes – protozoa, archaea, bacteria, fungi, yeasts – which are also involved in digestion: the reticulo-rumen (in ruminants), C1 and C2 stomach compartments (of camelids), caecum and colon (some birds, ruminants, horses, pigs, camelids), and the *saccus caecus* part of the simple stomach (horses and pigs; although the micro-organisms here have little effect on digestion). The microbes which inhabit the digestive tract exist in symbiosis with their host animal or bird. The host supplies the microbes' feed and a secure place for them to live (controlled pH and temperature, continuous supply of feed and continuous removal of the end-products of their metabolism); while the end-products of microbial metabolism (e.g. VFA, vitamins and amino acids) supply nutrients to the host which they might not otherwise be able to get.

● The sequence of microbial and intestinal digestion is very important because it determines the types of nutrients which are absorbed from the digestive tract.

For best use of the results of microbial cell growth, this should occur before the digesta flows to a region where the animal's own enzymes operate as this digestive sequence allows the microbial cells to be digested. Thus ruminants and camelids make better use of bacterial metabolism than horses and other hind-gut fermenters.

On the other hand, to get the best use of the non-fibre constituents in foods, intestinal digestion should precede microbial digestion. Bacteria destroy some feed amino acids, alter the chemistry of fatty acids and sometimes destroy vitamins. Horses and pigs make better use than ruminants of starch, soluble sugars, proteins which have large concentrations of essential amino acids, and unsaturated fatty acids.

Anatomy of the digestive tract

The digestive tract (or gastrointestinal tract) is a tube running from a food-gathering and pre-processing organ – the mouth or beak – to an orifice through which waste is voided – the anus in animals and the cloaca in birds.

The digestive tract is not simply a conduit, but is also a place where digesta is held, exposed to various physical and chemical processes (chewing, mixing, separation of particles, chemical buffering, and enzymatic hydrolysis), and where the end-products of digestion are absorbed.

● Digestive tracts have several parts. In order, from the mouth to the anus, we have:

1. Mouth: buccal cavity, lips, teeth, tongue, salivary glands (in mammals); beak, tongue and salivary glands (in birds).
2. Oesophagus; plus the crop (a feed storage organ) in birds.

3. In ruminants and camelids, places where digestive micro-organisms are located: the C1 and C2 compartments (camelids) and reticulum, rumen and omasum (ruminants).
4. Glandular stomach: this is also called the gastric stomach and is called the abomasum in ruminants and the proventriculus in birds.
5. Gizzard (in most birds, but not in mammals); also called the ventriculus.
6. Small intestine: consisting of the duodenum, jejunum and ileum.
7. Large intestine: consisting of the caecum (two caeca in birds), colon and rectum; habitat for digestive micro-organisms.
8. Anus (animals) or cloaca (birds).

The digestive tracts of representative animals and domestic poultry are shown diagrammatically in Fig. 3.1.

The parts of the digestive tract have several functions

Prehension: The lips, teeth and tongue in mammals, and the beak and tongue in birds, are used to prehend feed, i.e. to collect feed and take it into the mouth. Birds are able to select and pick-up small pieces of feed with their beaks. Cattle use their tongues, horses, sheep and goats their lips, and pigs their muzzle, to find and prehend selected pieces of feed. All domestic mammals have incisor teeth which are used in prehension – horses and pigs have upper and lower incisors (i.e. in both jaws) while ruminants have lower incisors and a dental pad in the upper jaw; all mammals have premolars and molars in both jaws which are used for chewing. When feed has to be broken away from the bulk of material presented to the animal, such as grass plants or tufts of hay in a bale, the feed is trapped between the incisors, or the incisors and the dental pad, and breaks as it is pulled away from the mass.

Particle size reduction: The premolar and molar teeth in mammals, and the gizzard in birds, are used to reduce the particle size of the prehended feed. Herbivores chew their feed with a sideways motion which grinds feed pieces between the top and lower molars. Some mammals, including horses and sheep, chew their feed quite finely as they prehend it, while others, such as cows, deer and alpaca, only chew as much as is needed to form a bolus. All ruminants (cows, sheep, goats, deer, etc.) and camelids (camels, alpaca, llama, etc.) are able to return large pieces of roughage feed from the rumen to the mouth and re-chew these particles. This process is called rumination. Because of the way that the ruminant and camelid fore-stomachs are able to retain large feed particles, and the effect of rumination, the average size of undigested feed particles voided in faeces is smaller for fore-gut fermenters than for hind-gut fermenters such as the horse (Clauss *et al.*, 2015).

Birds do not chew their feed; instead, domestic poultry reduce the size of large particles in the gizzard (Fig. 3.1c; some bird species do not have a gizzard). Pieces of feed such as whole grains are crushed as the muscular walls of the gizzard contract against each other. This physical breakage of feed particles is helped by the presence of small stones which are swallowed by the bird and lodge in the gizzard.

Storage: The bird's crop is an enlargement at the end of the oesophagus. It stores feed and releases it slowly into the proventriculus. The reticulo-rumen and gastric stomach serve a similar purpose, as well as being places where digestion begins.

Digestion: This is the breaking up of large macromolecules into their individual molecules – glucose and other monosaccharides in the case of polysaccharides, amino acids in the case of proteins, and fatty acids, acyl glycerols and glycerol in the case of fats. Digestion is discussed in greater detail in the next section of this chapter.

Absorption: This is the movement of digestion products through the epithelial cells which line the intestinal tract and into the blood. Absorption occurs by three different mechanisms: (i) active transport which is an energy-demanding process (see below); (ii) facilitated diffusion; and (iii) simple diffusion which is driven by a concentration gradient (movement from regions of higher to lower concentration).

Excretion: The rectum stores undigested feed wastes before they are eliminated through the anus. In the bird's cloaca, undigested feed and uric acid from the kidneys are mixed and then eliminated.

Nutrient recycling: Ammonia-N is absorbed through the rumen wall and detoxified by converting it to urea in the liver (Lapierre and Lobley, 2011). About half of this urea is returned to the reticulo-rumen through the saliva and by passage through the

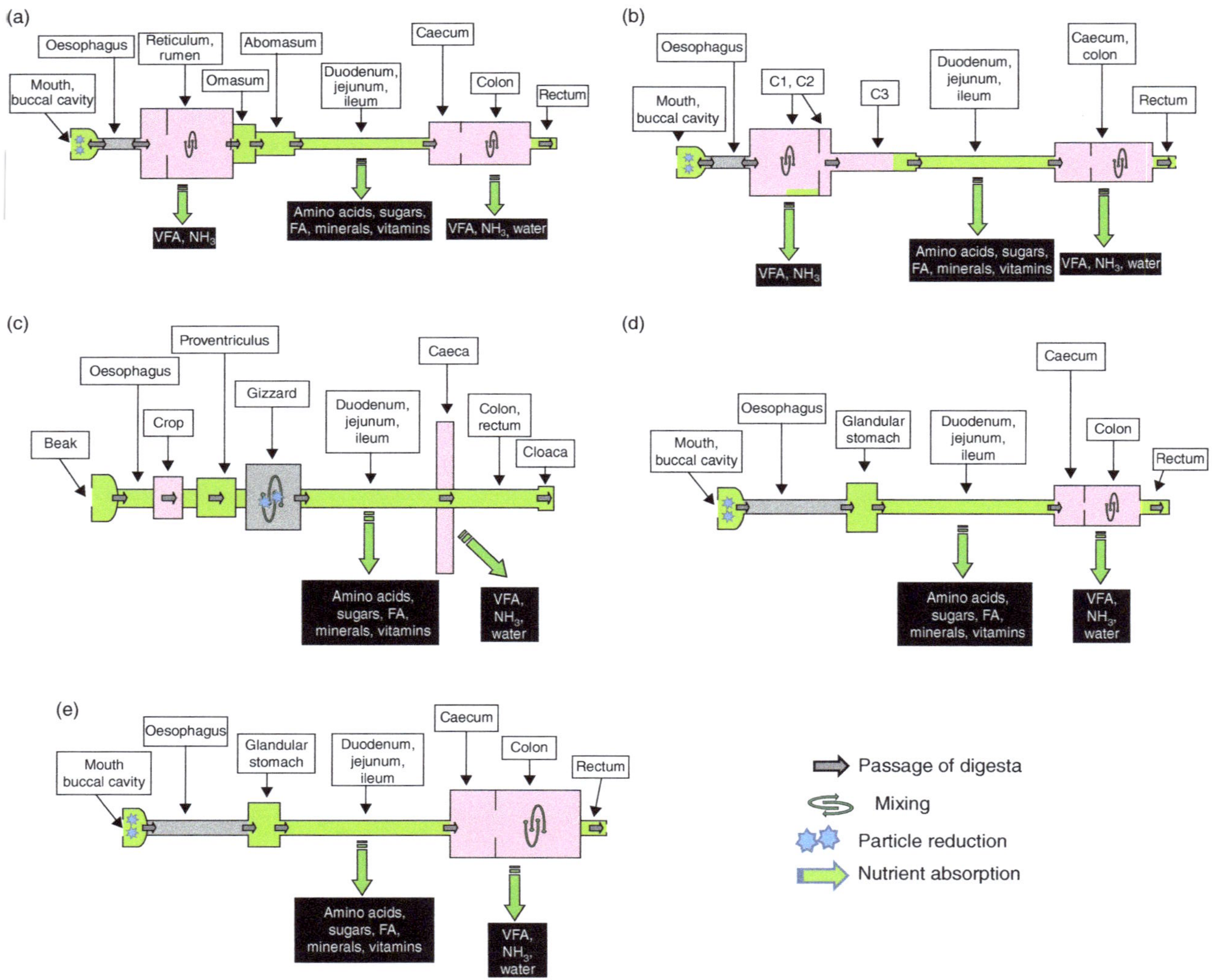

Fig. 3.1. The digestive tracts of **(a)** ruminants, **(b)** camelids, **(c)** poultry, **(d)** pig and **(e)** horse. (Adapted from Dryden, 2008; reproduced with permission.)

rumen wall; this recycled urea helps to maintain the level of ruminally available N, especially when the animal is eating a low-protein feed. Phosphorus is also returned to the rumen via saliva and this may provide half of the P required by rumen micro-organisms.

Bile salts synthesized in the liver are secreted into the proximal duodenum in the bile, then reabsorbed in the terminal ileum and recycled to the liver.

Signalling to the brain about hunger: Ghrelin is a peptide hormone which is secreted from epithelial cells in the stomach and is carried in the blood to the hypothalamus (a region of the brain). Ghrelin signals that the animal is hungry and this initiates meal eating. As well as signalling hunger, ghrelin regulates bone growth and prevents muscle atrophy.

Ancillary organs are important in digestion: Several ancillary organs are involved in digesting feed and absorbing the released nutrients. Salivary glands in the mouth secrete water and mucus which lubricate the bolus and allow it to be easily swallowed. These glands also secrete enzymes which begin starch digestion (α-amylase in pigs, horses and sheep; but not in cattle or goats) and fat digestion (e.g. in pre-ruminant calves and in pigs). While the fat-digesting enzyme in saliva may have a digestive role, it is very unlikely that the relatively small and varying levels of α-amylase in saliva make much contribution to overall starch digestion.

Saliva also contains phosphates and bicarbonates; these constitute a chemical buffering system. In non-ruminants this buffer maintains the pH of the buccal cavity at 6 to 8. Ruminants secrete large amounts of saliva (50 to 150 L per day) during chewing, and the buffers in the swallowed saliva help to maintain the pH of the reticulo-rumen at about 6.5.

The pancreas is situated at the start of the duodenum (the proximal duodenum); it synthesizes and secretes enzymes into the duodenum which are responsible for most of the preliminary digestion of proteins and starches, and for the digestion of fats.

The liver secretes bile salts and bile pigments. These help in the digestion and absorption of fats and fatty acids. In some animals and birds (e.g. pigs, cattle, sheep, goats and poultry, but not horses, camels or red deer) bile is stored in a gall bladder and is secreted into the proximal duodenum when digesta is present there.

Why does feed have to be digested?

Animals obtain nutrients from feeds through two sequential processes:

1. Digestion: the breaking up of large molecules so that the smaller products of digestion are of a size that can be absorbed.
2. Absorption: the passage of these small molecules through the epithelial cells and into the blood or lymph.

To appreciate why these processes are important we should understand something about the structure of the small intestine and its epithelium. There are three sections: the duodenum, which begins at the pyloric sphincter in the gastric stomach or abomasum, the jejunum, and then the ileum which ends at the ileo-caecal junction. The intestine is suspended in a mesentery that carries arteries which supply oxygen and nutrients; and veins, particularly the hepatic portal vein which carries absorbed nutrients from the intestines to the liver. The internal surface of the small intestine is raised into small finger-like projections called 'villi', and the cells of the intestinal epithelium (i.e. the cells which line the lumen or inside space of the intestine) are, in turn, lined with microvilli (Fig. 3.2).

The epithelial cells have two functions: (i) they are involved in digestion of feed and absorption of nutrients; and (ii) they protect the animal by controlling the way that substances pass from the lumen of the digestive tract to the blood. This last function is just as important as the digestion/absorption function because feeds often contain materials that we would not want to have absorbed into the body (see Chapter 12).

The micro-anatomy of this epithelium is well described by Goff (2018). These cells have:

- Tight junctions between them which prevent large molecules from slipping between the cells and entering the extracellular fluid or blood. These tight junctions can be relaxed and admit water, mineral ions such as Na and Mg, and small amino acids.
- Transport proteins in the membranes of the luminal surfaces of the epithelial cells which actively bind to and absorb their target substances. There are different transport proteins for different digestion products. This active transport has two important characteristics: the transport proteins bind to only their specific target substance, and the process requires

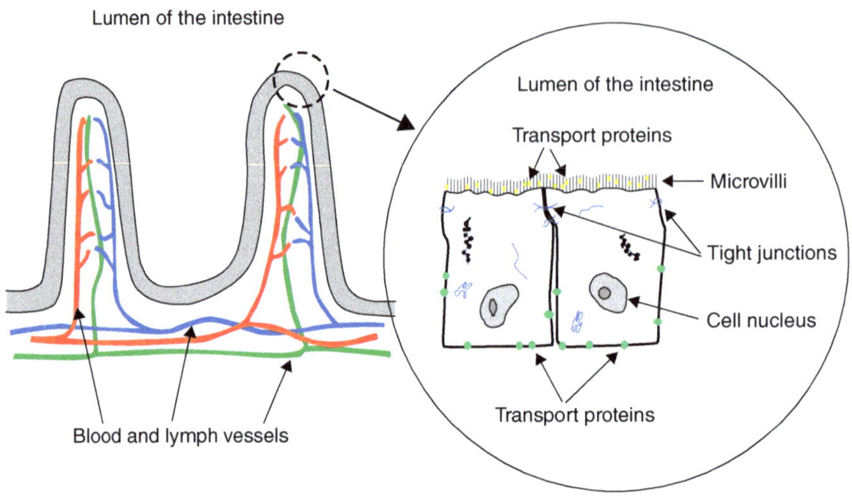

Fig. 3.2. Diagram of the small intestinal villi showing the fine structure of the epithelium: microvilli and active transport proteins, tight junctions between the epithelial cells, and passive transport proteins in the lateral and basal cell surfaces. (Copyright: Gordon McL. Dryden.)

the loaded transport protein to change its shape and thus bring the substance being transported through the cell membrane. This is an energy-demanding process.

- Transport proteins in the lateral and basal surfaces of the epithelial cells which actively bind to their substrate molecule but in this case, the transport of the substance through the cell membrane is driven by the concentration gradient – higher concentration inside the cell and lower concentration outside.

Why does feed have to be digested? The proteins, and most of the carbohydrates and fats, in feeds are very large molecules, or 'macromolecules'. Macromolecules are amalgamations of smaller molecules. Proteins are good examples: they are composed of amino acids (small, simple molecules) bonded together to form a chain (a macromolecule). These chains are coiled or folded into a ball or sheet, and often several of these balls are grouped into an even larger formation.

Molecules which have a mass of more than about 1 kDa cannot pass through the membranes of the intestinal epithelial cells, or through the tight junctions between these cells. A Dalton (Da) is the unit used to denote molecular weight; for macromolecules the molecular weight is given in kDa (1 kDa = 1000 Da).

The large macromolecules in feeds (Fig. 3.3) have molecular weights of several hundred or thousand kDa and so are much too big to be able to be absorbed. They have to be reduced to their constituent, simple molecule, parts.

The very abundant plant protein rubisco (possibly the most widely distributed of all proteins) has a molecular weight of 560 kDa. Tristearin, which is a macromolecule made from three 18-carbon stearic acid molecules joined to a glycerol backbone, has a molecular weight of 0.891 kDa. Starch constituents, and especially amylopectin, vary considerably depending on the type of starch and how it has been processed, but amylopectin can have molecular weights between 74 000 and 270 000 kDa. The simple molecules which make up these macromolecules are very much smaller. For example, amino acids range from 0.075 kDa (glycine) to 0.204 kDa (tryptophan); most fatty acids have molecular weights less than 0.35 kDa (e.g. stearic acid at 0.285 kDa, and arachidonic acid at 0.304 kDa); the molecular weight of glucose is 0.18 kDa; glycerol is 0.092 kDa; and vitamin A has a molecular weight of 0.287 kDa.

Large macromolecules are broken into their constituent parts during digestion. This chemical process is carried out by the action of digestive enzymes.

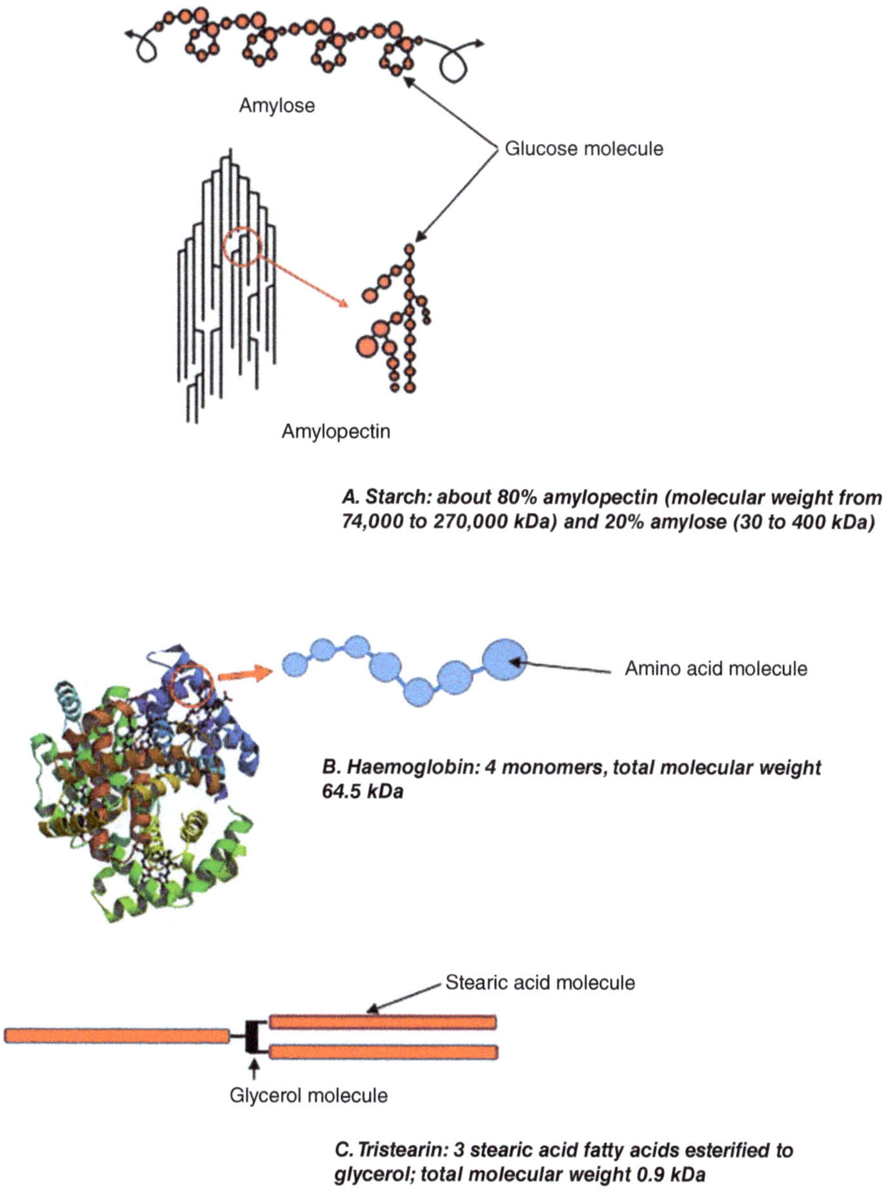

Fig. 3.3. Diagrammatic representations of important feed constituents; the different macromolecules are not drawn to scale. (Haemoglobin molecule from Richard, *et al.*, 1993, from the RSCB Protein Data Bank; others copyright: Gordon McL. Dryden.)

Feed digestion by animal (intrinsic) enzymes

Protein digestion: Protein-digesting enzymes attack either the central parts of the protein macromolecule (these are called 'endo-peptidase' enzymes), or they release individual amino acids from the ends of the amino acid chains (the 'exo-peptidases').

Feed passing through the animal and bird digestive tracts is first exposed to pepsins, which are protein-digesting enzymes secreted in the glandular stomach, abomasum and proventriculus. Pepsins are endo-peptidases so the product of pepsin digestion is a number of protein molecules which are smaller than the original macromolecules but which are still too large to be absorbed.

The next steps in the protein digestion sequence are carried out by several pancreatic enzymes – trypsin, the chymotrypsins, and elastase (all endo-peptidases), and the carboxypeptidases (which are exo-peptidases). Finally, there are several peptidases which are located in the small intestinal epithelial cell membranes which break dipeptides and tripeptides into their constituent amino acids. The overall process is illustrated in Fig. 3.4.

Amino acids are absorbed from the small intestine as described above.

Digestion of feed carbohydrates: There are several different types of carbohydrates in animal feeds. We find polysaccharides made from monosaccharides linked with β1-4 glycosidic bonds in plant cell walls (these are cellulose and the hemicelluloses; Chapter 4), α1-4- and α1-6-linked polysaccharides used as plant energy stores (starch in the endosperm of seeds and in the young leaves of grasses), and smaller disaccharides and monosaccharides in plant leaves and by-products such as molasses and bakery waste.

Starches and pectins are the only plant polysaccharides which can be digested by the animal's intrinsic digestive enzymes, because these are the only ones which contain large amounts of α1-4 bonds, the type of chemical linkage that the main animal carbohydrate-digesting enzyme, α-amylase, can attack.

Starch digestion proceeds in a series of steps. The first step is digestion by salivary amylase, but this continues for only a short while until the HCl secreted in the glandular stomach penetrates into the centre of the swallowed bolus and the pH falls below the optimum for salivary amylase activity.

The second and subsequent steps occur in the small intestine. First, α-amylase is secreted from the pancreas and attacks starch as it enters the duodenum. There are three products of α-amylase digestion of starch: maltose (which is a glucose–glucose disaccharide), maltotriose (glucose–glucose–glucose) and a 'limit dextrin'. The limit dextrin is a small macromolecule formed as amylopectin is digested. It is made of α1-4-linked glucose molecules which are surrounded by glucose molecules linked by α1-6 bonds. These bonds are the branch points in the amylopectin macromolecules (see Fig. 3.3) and they remain intact because α-amylase cannot break α1-6 bonds.

When the products of α-amylase digestion contact the intestinal epithelial cells, they are further digested by enzymes which, like the peptidases, are located in the epithelial cell membranes. The sequence of starch digestion is shown in Fig. 3.5.

Some feeds contain disaccharides; these are molecules which consist of two simple sugars. Examples are sucrose (glucose–fructose) in molasses and the leaves of temperate grasses, and lactose (glucose–galactose) in milk. These disaccharides are too large to pass through the epithelial cell membrane and are

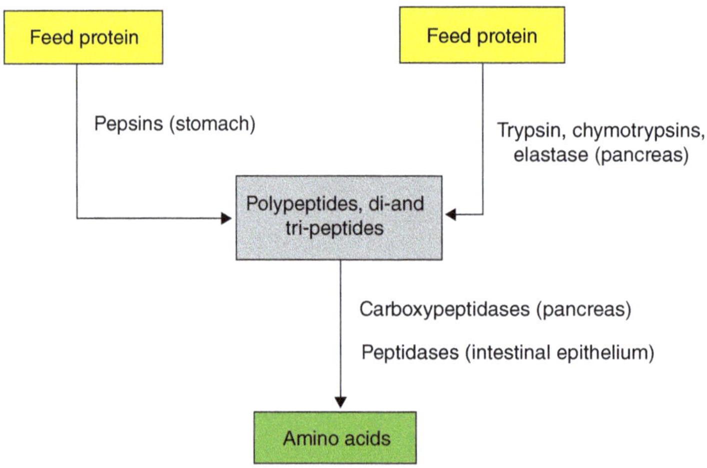

Fig. 3.4. The sequence of protein digestion in the glandular stomach and small intestine. (Copyright: Gordon McL. Dryden.)

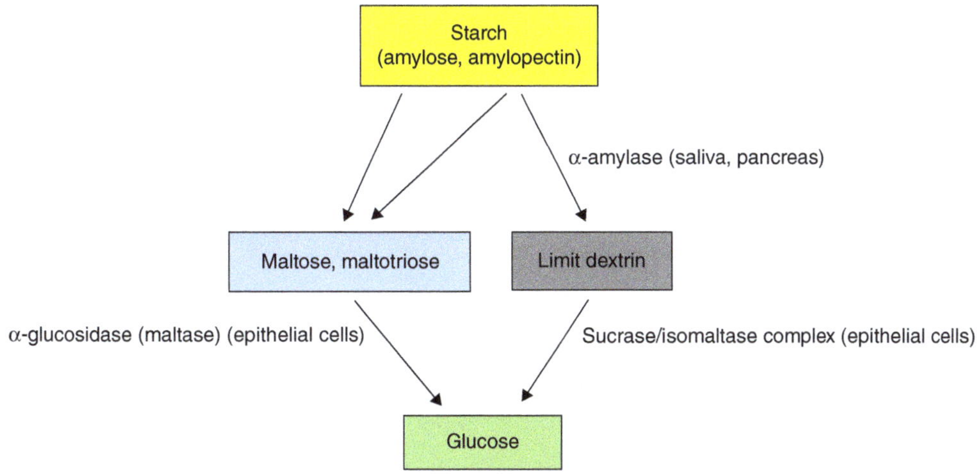

Fig. 3.5. The sequence of starch digestion in animals. (Copyright: Gordon McL. Dryden.)

digested by disaccharidases – sucrose by the sucrase/isomaltase complex and lactose by β-galactosidase (lactase) – located in the epithelial cell membranes.

Monosaccharides are absorbed through the intestinal epithelial cells as discussed previously.

Fat digestion: Feed lipids are usually neutral fats (glycerol molecules which carry three fatty acid molecules – these macromolecules are called triacyl glycerols or triglycerides) or phospholipids (a diacyl glycerol which has a phosphate group attached to the glycerol molecule instead of a third fatty acid – these are an important part of animal cell membranes) or galactolipids (diacyl glycerols which have a galactose sugar molecule attached to the glycerol molecule – these are a major type of plant lipid and are important in the plant's chloroplasts).

When fats leave the glandular stomach, they have been partially digested by salivary and gastric lipases (fat-digesting enzymes). The partially digested and undigested lipid passes into the duodenum where it is mixed with bile and pancreatic lipase. Bile contains bile salts (Na and K salts of taurocholic and glycocholic acids), cholesterol and lecithin. These substances emulsify the feed fat and divide it into smaller droplets which are more easily attacked by lipase, assisted by colipase which is also produced in the pancreas.

Lipase gradually removes the fatty acids from their attachments to glycerol (Fig. 3.6). This gives first, a diacyl glycerol, then a monoacyl glycerol, and eventually some fat is digested to free fatty acids and glycerol.

There are specific enzymes which digest phospholipids (phospholipases) and galactolipids (pancreatic lipase related protein 2; PLRP2). Phospholipase is present in all animals and birds, PLRP2 occurs in non-ruminant herbivores but not in pigs.

Fatty acid absorption: The action of lipase on feed fat is not complete, about 70% of the fatty acids are absorbed as 2-monoacyl glycerols, about 6% as 3-monoacylglycerols and 20% as free fatty acids.

The products of lipase action are absorbed into the cells of the small intestinal epithelium in a package called a micelle. Micelles have a fatty acid core (mostly monoacyl glycerol; i.e. glycerol with a single fatty acid attached) which is covered with an envelope of bile salts, lecithin and cholesterol. The envelope protects the core from the watery environments of the epithelial cell cytoplasm, lymph and blood.

When the micelle has been absorbed into the epithelial cell most of the fatty acids are re-esterified (joined to glycerol again) into triacyl glycerol molecules. These are then formed into chylomicrons which protect the triacyl glycerol molecules so that they can be transported in blood and lymph to the body cells.

Microbial digestion and metabolism

Microbial digestion and metabolism take place in the fore and hind parts of the digestive tract, depending on the type of digestive system that we are dealing with. This discussion of how microbes digest and metabolize feeds, and the types of end-products that

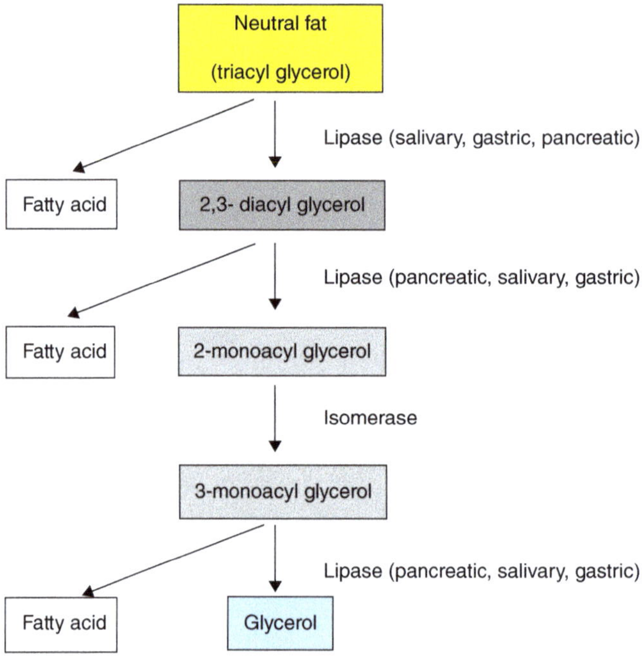

Fig. 3.6. Action of lipase on neutral feed fats. (Copyright: Gordon McL. Dryden.)

are produced will focus on events in the reticulo-rumen.

Types of organisms in the reticulo-rumen: There are six main types of micro-organisms:

- Bacteria: about 10^{10} bacteria/mL (described in Vasta *et al.*, 2019).
- Archaea: make up 3–4% of the rumen microbial mass; most are methanogens (organisms that produce CH_4).
- Protozoa: about 10^5 protozoa/mL, making up about 50% of the total microbial mass.
- Fungi: may make up 8 to 20% of the rumen microbial mass.
- Viruses and yeasts are also present in smaller numbers.

At any time, 30–40% of the bacteria (mainly those species which digest starch and protein) are free in the rumen liquor, 60–70% (mainly fibre digesters) are attached to feed particles, and about 1% are located on the rumen wall. Methanogenic archaea may live in close association with protozoa so that they can harvest the H which is excreted from the protozoal cells. Protozoa and fungi compete for feed: normally, fungi colonize highly lignified fibrous material, although how much this contributes to the digestion of plant fibre is not established. When the rumen is defaunated (the protozoa are removed), the fungi proliferate and rapidly occupy the niche which had been occupied by the protozoa.

The rumen is well adapted to hosting symbiotic micro-organisms:

- The microbes have a continual supply of substrate: fibrous feed is digested slowly (e.g. 1–5%/h) so there is almost always substrate available for microbial metabolism. The regular contractions of the muscles in the walls of the reticulum and rumen make sure that the rumen liquor and the undigested feed is continually being mixed, so that undigested feed particles are always being made available to the microbes.
- The host animal maintains the rumen pH at between 5.5 and 7.5 in roughage-fed animals, although if we over-feed starch-rich ingredients the pH can fall below 5.5. The rumen pH is kept within its usual range because of the phosphate and carbonic acid/carbonate buffers secreted in saliva, and through the continuous absorption of VFA and NH_3.

- The rumen is effectively oxygen free; rumen bacteria are mostly obligate anaerobes (bacteria which cannot live in the presence of oxygen).
- The temperature is kept at approximately 39°C, except when the animal drinks cold water, but this effect lasts for only several minutes.
- The osmotic pressure is normally close to isotonic.
- The host animal removes microbial wastes (these are the end-products of nutrient metabolism by the bacteria, protozoa and fungi). Waste removal occurs by passage to the lower digestive tract, absorption through the rumen wall, and by eructation of gases formed during bacterial fermentation, especially CH_4.

Each species of bacteria has specific types of feed that they can digest and metabolize. We can group bacteria into four types:

- Starch digesters: such as *Streptococcus bovis*, *Ruminobacter amylophilus*, *Prevotella ruminicola* and *Prevotella amylophilus*. These bacteria digest starch and produce formic, acetic, propionate, succinic and butyric acids; *S. bovis* also produces lactic acid which can contribute to rumen acidosis in ruminants fed starch-rich rations.
- Fibre digesters: *Fibrobacter succinogenes*, *Ruminococcus flavefaciens*, *Ruminococcus albus* and *Butyrivibrio fibrisolvens* are typical examples of these. These bacteria have enzymes which are able to digest the β1-4 bonds of cellulose and hemicelluloses and are the key types of bacteria which allow herbivores to get nutrients from forages. These bacteria produce formic and acetic acids as major metabolic end-products, and also succinic and butyric acids.
- Protein digesters: *Ruminobacter amylophilus*, *Prevotella ruminicola*, *Butyrivibrio fibrisolvens* and *Streptococcus bovis*, and other bacteria.
- Bacteria which use the end-products of other bacteria: *Megasphaera elsdenii* and *Selenomonas ruminantium* subsp. *lactilytica* both utilize lactic acid as an energy source; succinic acid produced by *Fibrobacter* is an energy substrate for *Selenomonas*, which produces some of the CO_2 used by *Fibrobacter*; *Prevotella ruminicola* digests protein to dipeptides which are used by other bacteria; non-cellulolytic bacteria synthesize vitamin B12 (cobalamin) which is needed by protozoa and the cellulolytic (fibre-digesting) bacteria; and protein-metabolizing bacteria produce NH_3 which is an essential nutrient for fibre-digesting bacteria.

Methanogens are archaea which use formic acid or CO_2 and H_2 to drive the synthesis of adenosine triphosphate (Deppenmeier *et al.*, 1996; ATP is an energy storage molecule). This process results in CH_4 as a by-product. Protozoa and bacteria produce large amounts of H when they oxidize nutrients as energy sources. Some methanogens live on the cell membrane of protozoa – this is a good ecological niche for methanogens because they can harvest the H excreted by the protozoa.

Some of the inter-relationships between rumen bacteria, protozoa and archaea are illustrated in Fig. 3.7.

Rumen microbial metabolism provides nutrients for the host animal but affects animal products and the environment

There are several things that rumen and other digestive tract microbes do which affects animal performance – sometimes beneficially, in other cases to our disadvantage. We can make use of, or deal with the effects of, or prevent, some of these but others have inescapable outcomes.

Microbial digestion and metabolism: Bacteria, protozoa and fungi have enzymes which can digest the cellulose and hemicelluloses in plant fibre (the process is described by Dryden, 2008). They secrete the enzymes onto feed particles and absorb the digestion products into their cells.

Metabolism of these absorbed nutrients occurs in two stages; in the first stage the monosaccharides are oxidized via the glycolytic and pentose phosphate pathways (which usually means the removal of H rather than the addition of O). This process breaks the monosaccharide molecule up and is associated with the synthesis of ATP and the production of H, a microbial waste product. Pyruvic acid is the end-product of this primary metabolism.

Secondary metabolism uses pyruvic acid as a starting point for VFA synthesis. Acetate, propionate and butyrate are the main VFA end-products of microbial fermentation. The metabolic pathways which generate ATP for the microbes, and yield CH_4 and VFA as end-products, are illustrated in Fig. 3.8.

Rumen microbial metabolism provides nutrients for the host animal: Cattle and sheep eating roughages have 65–75% acetate, 15–20% propionate and 10–15% butyrate in the mix of VFA produced in the rumen (Blaxter, 1962). Similar microbial digestion

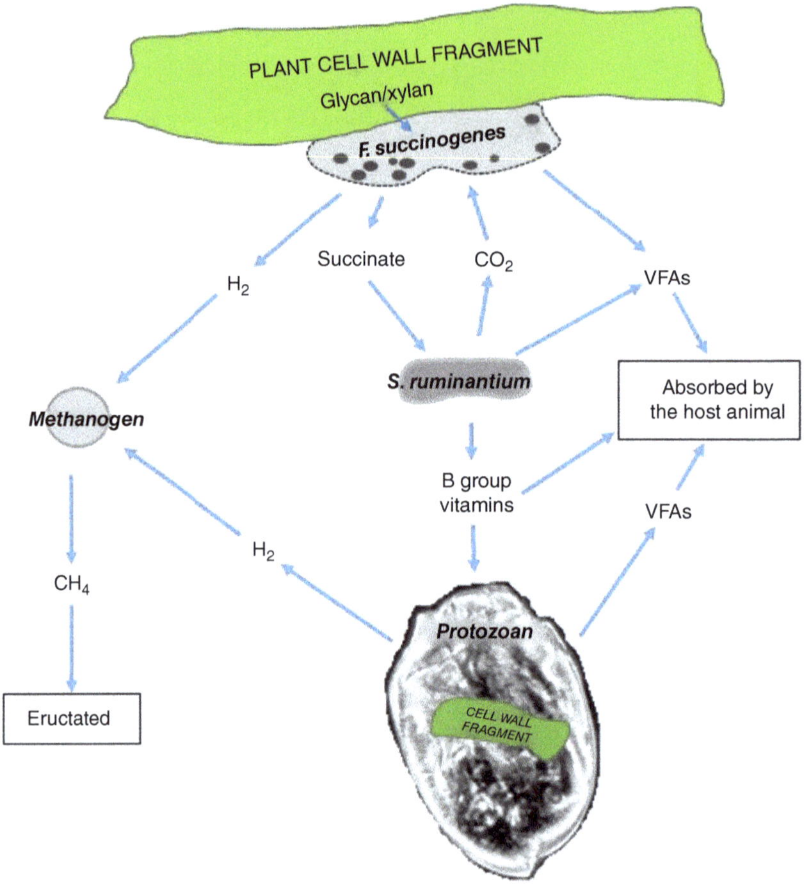

Fig. 3.7. Microbial ecology in the rumen: examples of interactions between different bacteria, archaea (methanogens) and protozoa. (Copyright: Gordon McL. Dryden.)

occurs in the large intestine. These VFA are absorbed and used as energy sources by the host animal.

Animals like horses, cattle, sheep, grazing pigs and herbivorous poultry are thus able to use forages as an energy source even though none of them have any intrinsic digestive enzymes which can break β-glycosidic bonds between the glucoses, xyloses and other monosaccharides which make up the constituents of plant cell walls (see Chapter 4). If these animals did not have a symbiotic relationship with digestive tract micro-organisms they would have to subsist on the starches, monosaccharides and disaccharides, fats and proteins in seeds, grains and immature vegetation. In doing this, they would compete for feed with other organisms, including omnivores such as humans.

Bacterial synthesis of B group vitamins makes the host animal largely independent of a dietary supply of these essential nutrients.

Microbial metabolism produces large amounts of hydrogen: The microbial metabolism of plant cell wall constituents is accompanied by the production of large amounts of H. Dietary unsaturated fatty acids, VFA synthesis, and CH_4 synthesis are used as 'H sinks'. This gives two adverse outcomes:

- H is used by archaea to synthesize CH_4, which is a potent global warming agent (see Chapter 19).
- The saturation of dietary fatty acids has the consequences that are described below.

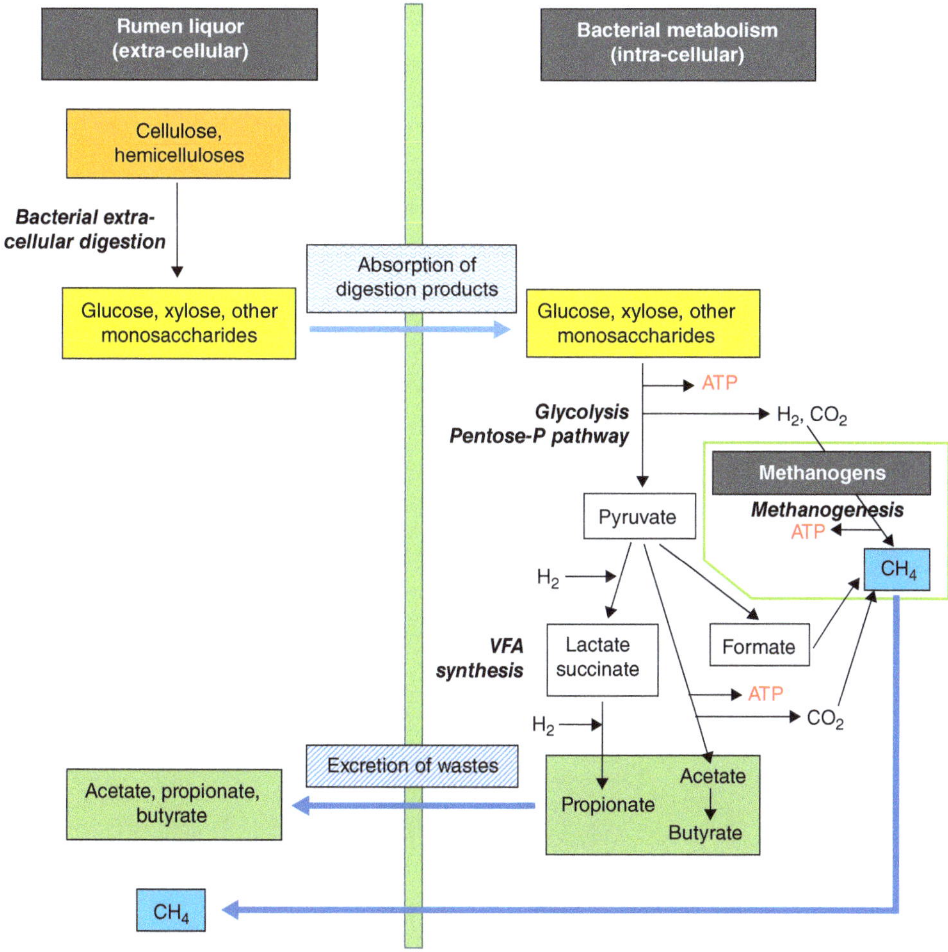

Fig. 3.8. Digestion and metabolism of carbohydrates by rumen bacteria, and methane synthesis by archaea. This is a very simplified view, showing digestion (carried out by a range of cellulases and hemicellulases); the energy-yielding oxidation of monosaccharides through the glycolytic and pentose-P pathways; and removal of H through volatile fatty acid (VFA) synthesis (using acetate, succinate and lactate as intermediates) and methane (CH_4) formation by methanogenic archaea. CO_2 and H are by-products of many of these processes. (Copyright: Gordon McL. Dryden.)

Bacterial fatty acids: Because bacteria use feed fatty acids as H sinks, they become saturated (see Chapter 1). Acetate, propionate and butyrate are also saturated fatty acids. Both the feed fatty acids and the VFA produced by microbial fermentation are used in the animal's metabolism, and so the fats in ruminant body and milk fat are more saturated than that of pigs and poultry. There is concern that a large consumption of this type of fat can have adverse medical consequences in humans.

Bacteria synthesize trans unsaturated fatty acids (see Chapter 1) to use in their cell membranes. Trans fatty acids are not desirable in human diets because they are related to an increased risk of coronary heart disease.

Bacteria produce conjugated linoleic acid (CLA), and much of this is incorporated into milk fat. CLA appears to have anti-cancer properties and may reduce the deposition of body fat.

Wastage of feed protein: Some rumen bacteria use amino acids as energy sources. These 'hyper-ammonia'-producing bacteria break down feed protein and deaminate the released amino acids. They use the carbon skeletons of the amino acids as energy sources but excrete large amounts of NH_3. This has two consequences for the animal, neither of them beneficial:

- The bacteria do not distinguish between essential and non-essential amino acids, and thus can destroy large amounts of essential amino acids which would otherwise be used by the host animal. This either reduces animal productivity, or else the deficient amino acids have to be provided in some form that cannot be destroyed in the rumen.
- The host animal absorbs large amounts of NH_3 from its rumen. This is toxic and must be made safe by being converted into urea, which is excreted in urine.

Protection against feed poisons: As discussed in Chapter 12, some feeds contain potentially poisonous substances. Trypsin inhibitor is an example: if this protein is eaten in large amounts by monogastrics or pre-ruminants, it binds with trypsin and prevents the digestion of other feed proteins. This does not occur in adult ruminants because the trypsin inhibitor protein is destroyed in the rumen.

Connection between feed type and rumen disease: Some bacteria which use starch as a main energy source produce lactic acid as one of their waste products. Lactic acid is a strong acid and rapidly lowers the rumen pH. The consequences of this are discussed in Chapter 13.

Problems associated with rapidly changing the type of feed fed to herbivores: As described above, each bacterial species has its own dietary niche. When we change the diet of a fore-gut fermenter animal, this has to be done at a rate which matches the rate at which the population of specialized micro-organisms are able to grow to use the new feed. We most commonly come across this issue when cattle or sheep are taken off pasture and put into a feedlot and given a grain-rich ration, or when dairy cattle are put on to a concentrate-rich total mixed ration.

Matching the population of bacteria with the feed type is only part of the solution. In some cases, this happens quickly, e.g. *S. bovis* numbers increase when a starch-rich feed is fed. But to safely change feed type we also have to allow enough time for those organisms which serve as rate limiters to increase in numbers. Examples of microbial rate limiters are:

- *Prevotella ruminicola* – determines the amounts of dipeptides available to the cellulolytic (fibre-digesting) bacteria.
- Fibre digesters which limit the amounts of energy substrates and H available to other bacteria and archaea.
- Protozoa limit the amount of starch available to starch-digesting bacteria (e.g. *Lactobacillus*) by ingesting whole starch granules and trapping them within their cells.

The effect of maturity on digestive tract function

The digestive tracts of newborn animals are developed to different degrees, but they are all immature when compared to adults. The digestive tracts of newborn animals mature over 4 to 8 weeks, depending on the species.

When digestive tracts mature, several things occur:

- The digestive tract gets longer and larger (Pluske, 2016). In pigs, the small intestine grows by 80% in length and 30% in diameter, with a doubling of the absorptive area.
- Digestive enzyme production increases: including chymosin, pepsins, amylase, lactase and aminopeptidases. Chymosin (also called rennin) causes milk solids to form clots in the stomach or abomasum of pigs and ruminants, thus retaining these for more extensive digestion. Stomach acid secretion also increases.
- A microbial population develops: newborn animals have a sterile digestive tract, e.g. there are no microbes in the foetal reticulo-rumen or large intestine. Microbes begin to establish in the newborn's digestive tract soon after birth or hatching. The tracts of ruminants begin to get a population of archaea and fibre-digesting bacteria within 20 minutes of the animal's birth but it takes 6 to 8 weeks for the rumen microbial population to fully mature and diversify (Raabis *et al.*, 2019). Bacteria colonize the young pig's digestive tract soon after birth and develop into a stable population. These microbial populations develop through contact with adults and the environment.

Colostrum: Around the time of parturition, breeding females produce a type of milk called colostrum. Colostrum is a source of:

- Readily available energy: colostrum has higher solids and fat contents than ordinary milk (Table 3.1;

Table 3.1. Compositions of domestic animal colostrum. (Data from Wallace *et al.*, 2001; Malacarne *et al.*, 2002; Theil *et al.*, 2014; McGrath *et al.*, 2016; Pecka-Kiełb *et al.*, 2018; Puppel *et al.*, 2019.)

	Colostrum (%)				Milk (%)			
Species	Dry matter	Protein	Fat	Lactose	Dry matter	Protein	Fat	Lactose
Cow	25.8	13.9	7.2	3.1	12.5	3.3	4.2	4.5
Goat	17.9	9.1	8.5	2.2	13.2	4.1	4.5	4.4
Sheep	32.8	18.4	10.1	2.9	15.4	5.7	3.5	5.5
Horse	19.3	17.1	1.2	3.6	10.9	2.1	1.4	6.5
Pig	26.8	17.7	6.9	3.6	19.5	5.1	7.3	5.0

indicative data because breed, time after parturition and feeding all affect colostrum and milk compositions). These characteristics, plus the lactose in colostrum, give the newborn animal a readily available source of energy.

- Essential amino acids and fatty acids, minerals and vitamins: casein has a very high proportion of essential amino acids.
- Bioactive proteins: there are over 600 proteins in colostrum, ranging through enzymes, hormones and other bioactive peptides and proteins. These influence a wide variety of functions in the newborn animal, including growth and immunity.

Passive immunity: Many of the proteins in colostrum are antibody proteins. Breeding females develop antibodies to the diseases they are exposed to and these antibody proteins are transferred to the foetus when it is in the uterus, and through colostrum which the young animal drinks when it first suckles.

Passive immunity means that the newborn does not have to experience the disease itself and develop its own antibodies, but nevertheless it is protected against diseases which the mother has experienced, and which are therefore common in the local environment. The immunoglobulin G (IgG) contents of pig and cow colostrum are about 37 and 101 ng/mL, respectively (Krogh *et al.*, 2016; Jolazadeh *et al.*, 2019). The composition of colostrum changes with time after parturition and between animal species.

Chicks are at risk of diseases for about 2 weeks after hatching, before they are mature enough to begin to develop their own immunity. As in mammals, bird maternal antibodies are provided to the embryonic chick. This happens as the egg forms and protects the hatchling until it is able to make its own immune proteins.

Intestinal closure: For 1 to 2 days after they are born, newborn animals can absorb very large macromolecules from their small intestines. This occurs by pinocytosis, where the epithelial cell membrane wraps around the macromolecule and drags it into the cell. Domestic mammals lose this ability soon after birth, and the colostrum proteins are digested, both by digestive enzymes and by enzymes within the epithelial cells, so that by 2 days after birth the ability to absorb immune proteins is lost. This is called intestinal closure.

In newborn pigs and ruminants closure begins 6 to 12 hours after birth and is completed by 24 to 36 hours. In newborn foals, closure starts by 12 hours after birth and is effectively complete at 24 hours.

Although bioactive proteins cannot be absorbed after closure happens, there are some benefits in keeping on feeding colostrum to older animals, if we have some available (Andrews, 2004). These include beneficial effects on nutrient intake because colostrum is nutrient-rich, and some protection against disease-causing bacteria and viruses.

References

Andrews, A.H. (2004). Colostrum – not just for 24 hours. *Cattle Practice* 12, 121–124.

Blaxter, K.L. (1962). *The Energy Metabolism of Ruminants*. London: Hutchinson.

Clauss, M., Steuer, P., Erlinghagen-Lückerath, K., Kaandorp, J., Fritz, J., Südekum, K-H. and Hummel, J. (2015). Faecal particle size: Digestive physiology meets herbivore diversity. *Comparative Biochemistry and Physiology, Part A: Molecular & Integrative Physiology* 179: 182–191.

Deppenmeier, U., Muller, V. and Gottschalk, G. (1996). Pathways of energy conservation in methanogenic archaea. *Archives of Microbiology* 165: 149–163.

Dryden, G.McL. (2008). *Animal Nutrition Science*. Wallingford, UK: CAB International.

Goff, J.P. (2018). Invited review: Mineral absorption mechanisms, mineral interactions that affect acid–base and antioxidant status, and diet considerations to improve mineral status. *Journal of Dairy Science* 101: 2763–2813.

Jolazadeh, A.R., Mohammadabadi, A.R., Dehghan-banadaky, M., Chaji, M. and Garcia, M. (2019). Effect of supplementing calcium salts of n-3 and n-6 fatty acid to pregnant nonlactating cows on colostrum composition, milk yield, and reproductive performance of dairy cows. *Animal Feed Science and Technology* 247: 127–140.

Krogh, U., Oksbjerg, N., Purup, S., Ramaekers, P. and Theil P.K. (2016). Colostrum and milk production in multiparous sows fed supplementary arginine during gestation and lactation. *Journal of Animal Science* 94(3 Suppl): 22–25.

Lapierre, H. and Lobley, G.E. (2011). Nitrogen recycling in the ruminant: a review. *Journal Dairy Science* 84(E. Suppl.): E223–E236.

McGrath, B.A., Fox, P.F., McSweeney, P.L.H. and Kelly, A.L. (2016). Composition and properties of bovine colostrum: a review. *Dairy Science and Technology* 96:133–158.

Malacarne, M., Martuzzi, F., Summer, A. and Mariani, P. (2002). Protein and fat composition of mare's milk: some nutritional remarks with reference to human and cow's milk. *International Dairy Journal* 12: 869–877.

Pecka-Kiełb, E., Zachwieja, A., Wojtas, E. and Zawadzki, W. (2018). Influence of nutrition on the quality of colostrum and milk of ruminants. *Mljekarstvo* 68(3): 169–181.

Pluske, J.R. (2016). Invited review: Aspects of gastrointestinal tract growth and maturation in the pre- and post-weaning period of pigs. *Journal of Animal Science* 94(3 Suppl): 399–411.

Puppel, K., Gołebiewski, M., Grodkowski, G., Slósarz, J., Kunowska-Slósarz, M., Solarczyk,P., Łukasiewicz, M., Balcerak, M. and Przysucha, T. (2019). Composition and factors affecting quality of bovine colostrum: a review. *Animals* 9, 1070. DOI: 10.3390/ani9121070.

Raabis, S., Li, W. and Cersosimo, L. (2019). Effects and immune responses of probiotic treatment in ruminants. *Veterinary Immunology and Immunopathology* 208: 58–66.

Richard, V., Dodson, G.G. and Mauguen, Y. (1993). Human deoxyhaemoglobin-2,3-diphosphoglycerate complex low-salt structure at 2.5 A resolution. *Journal of Molecular Biology* 233: 270–274. PDB ID: 1B86.

Theil, P.K., Lauridsen, C. and Quesnel, H. (2014). Neonatal piglet survival: impact of sow nutrition around parturition on fetal glycogen deposition and production and composition of colostrum and transient milk. *Animal* 8(7): 1021–1030.

Vasta, V., Daghio, M., Cappucci, A., Buccioni, A., Serra, A., Viti, C. and Mele, M. (2019). Invited review: Plant polyphenols and rumen microbiota responsible for fatty acid biohydrogenation, fiber digestion, and methane emission: Experimental evidence and methodological approaches. *Journal of Dairy Science* 102(5): 3781–3804.

Wallace, J., Bourke, D., Da Silva, P. and Aitken, R. (2001). Nutrient partitioning during adolescent pregnancy. *Reproduction* 122: 347–357.

4 Feed digestibility

Digestibility and nutrient availability

The digestible fraction of feeds is those constituents which can be broken down by digestive enzymes and so provide nutrients to the animal. Feed digestibility is a measure of the proportion of a feed which can be digested. It is important that we know the digestibility of the feeds we use because losses due to indigestibility are the first, and often the largest, reason for nutrients in feeds being unavailable to the animal. Only those nutrients which are released from the feed by digestion contribute to the pool of nutrients absorbed from the digestive tract and available to the animal.

Different types of animal feed – seeds (cereal grains, legume grains, oilseeds), vegetative plant material (leaves, stems) and animal carcase products (fish meals, meat meals) – all have their own limitations to complete digestion.

Factors which limit the digestibility of feeds

Cell wall amount and composition influence the digestibility of plant-origin feeds: The digestibility of plant cell contents is almost complete – about 98%, while that of plant cell walls varies. So, we have the situation which is illustrated in Fig. 4.1: the digestibility of a forage feed is determined by the amount and digestibility of its cell walls.

Plant cell walls are a large, but variable, proportion of forage material; typically, 45–70%, but ranging from 30–85% of the total plant dry matter (DM), depending on the age and species of the plant. The amount of cell wall material increases as the plant matures, as cell walls become thicker.

To understand why the digestibility of plant cell walls falls as the plant matures, we need to know something about plant cell wall composition. Plant cell walls are made from several different polysaccharides. These are carbohydrate macromolecules which are made from combinations of many monosaccharides or their derivatives, such as glucose, xylose, arabinose, rhamnose and galacturonic acid. These are joined together in chains: either long linear (unbranched) or shorter branched chains.

The polysaccharides of plant cell walls are:

- Cellulose: a long, coiled linear chain of glucose sugars joined by β1-4 glycosidic bonds.
- Hemicelluloses: which all have a long backbone and shorter side chains. The backbone is a linear, coiled chain of glucose or xylose molecules joined by β1-4 glycosidic bonds; the side chains are made of predominantly xylose molecules, but also incorporate other simple sugars like arabinose and ribose.
- Pectins: which have a backbone of α1-4-linked rhamnose or galacturonic acid molecules and side chains of α-linked rhamnose and galacturonic acid attached to the backbone. The pectin macromolecule has regions where there are many branched side chains which have both α and β linkages.

Plant cell walls also contain:

- Lignin, a large, highly branched, complex macromolecule (not a polysaccharide) which has many *p*-coumaryl, coniferyl and synapyl alcohols (these are called 'lignin monomers') linked to each other in a variety of ways, by ester and ether bonds. Lignin content in roughages varies with maturity from 5–25%, and is 2–10% in cereal grains.
- An amount of protein – about 10% of the neutral detergent fibre (NDF) content in forages and up to 40% in concentrates.
- External cell walls are covered with a cuticle which is made of various waxes.

Why plant cell walls affect the digestibility of plant-based feeds: The plant cell wall polysaccharides cannot be attacked by the animal's own intrinsic digestive enzymes – the main animal carbohydrate-digesting

DOI: 10.1079/9781786394453.0004

enzyme, α-amylase, can only break α1-4 bonds. However, bacteria, fungi and protozoa have enzymes which can break β bonds, so those animals and birds which have active microbial populations in their digestive tracts can use plant cell wall material as feed.

From the above information, we can work out the potential digestibility of the plant cell wall's constituents:

- Highly digestible: pectins, because most of the bonds are α1-4 bonds which can be broken by both microbial and animal enzymes.
- Moderately digestible: cellulose, hemicelluloses, and cell wall protein. How completely cellulose and hemicelluloses can be digested by microbes depends on how much of these macromolecules is protected by lignin (see below).
- Indigestible: Lignin and waxes. The bonds between the lignin monomers can only be broken by specialized lignases which are found in organisms like termites. Waxes, which make up the cuticle, are resistant to all enzymes and often appear in the faeces so little damaged that they can be used to identify the plants that were in the animal's diet.

Lignin protects potentially digestible cell wall constituents: The main factor which affects the digestibility of plant cell walls is the way that lignin protects cellulose and hemicelluloses. Enzymes which digest cellulose and hemicelluloses cannot attach to their substrates if these are protected by lignin wrapping around cellulose or chemically bonding to hemicelluloses. Figure 4.2 is a model of how lignin protects the rest of the cell wall from digestion.

Cereal grains and other seeds have physical and chemical limits to digestion: Cereal grains are filled with starch, and oilseeds with protein and oil, but while these are potentially digestible by the animal's intrinsic enzymes they are protected from digestion in several ways:

- A seedcoat (hull or husk): this is a fibrous layer which surrounds the interior of the seed (the endosperm of cereal grains and the cotyledons of oilseeds; Fig. 4.3). The cells of the seedcoat

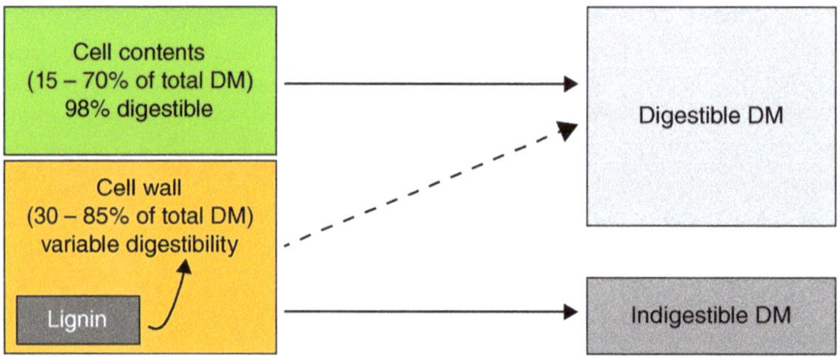

Fig. 4.1. Plant dry matter digestibility – the effects of the amount and chemical composition of the cell wall. Lignin is shown as the cell wall constituent which mainly determines dry matter (DM) digestibility: it is itself indigestible and also protects some of the cellulose and hemicellulose from digestion. (Copyright: Gordon McL. Dryden.)

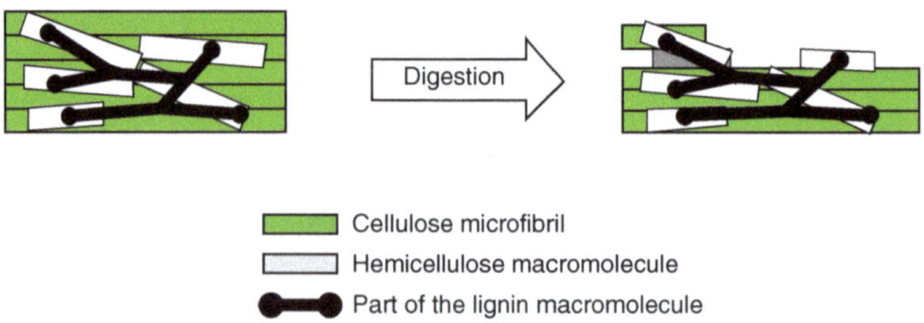

Fig. 4.2. Diagram showing how lignin can protect cellulose and hemicellulose from digestion. (After Chesson, 1988; copyright: Gordon McL. Dryden.)

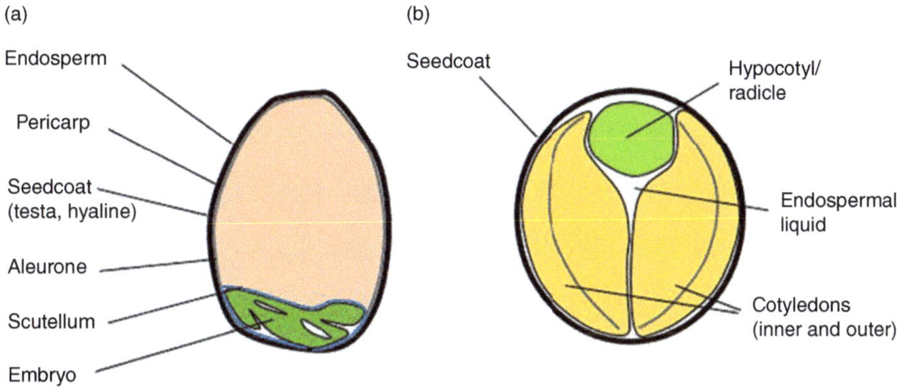

Fig. 4.3. Generalized structures of **(a)** cereal grains and **(b)** oilseeds. (Drawn from data in Rathjen *et al.*, 2009; Borisjuk *et al.*, 2013; Verboven *et al.*, 2013; UK Flour Millers, undated; copyright: Gordon McL. Dryden.)

are lignified and protected by a cuticle. Digestive enzymes cannot attack the interior of a seed unless the seedcoat is broken, either by chewing or by processing such as grinding.

- Tight packing of endosperm cells and a protein network which surrounds starch granules in cereal grains: the cereal grain endosperm contains cells which are tightly packed together. In turn, these cells are filled with starch granules which are surrounded by a network of protein. This arrangement restricts amylase enzymes from digesting all but the starch which is exposed at the surfaces of chewed grain particles. The protein mesh is difficult to digest but it must be disrupted before amylases can contact the starch granules.
- Protease inhibitors: some grain legumes, such as soybeans, contain proteins which interfere with the action of the animal's intrinsic protein-digesting enzymes (proteases). This not only reduces the animal's ability to digest feed protein, but the animal has to use available amino acids to synthesize more proteases and so can be tipped into a negative N balance. The effect of protease inhibitors is important when non-ruminant animals (e.g. pre-ruminant calves, horses, pigs, poultry) are fed untreated (raw) grain legumes.
- β-Glucans: some cereal grains (e.g. barley and oats) contain significant amounts of β-glucans (macromolecules which are made of glucose molecules joined by β1-4 linkages). These cannot be digested by animal amylases, although they can be broken by microbial enzymes.

Feeds made from animal products: Meat meals, meat and bone meals (these include fish products), feather meal and similar products contain large amounts of bone and connective tissue. All of these can be difficult to digest.

Bone is softened by the action of acid. In general, the finer the bone particles the more completely they can be digested because large particles of bone resist the penetration of acid and so are incompletely digested. As a guide, Grain Trade Australia (undated) recommends that 98% of meat meal particles, including bone, should pass a 2 mm screen.

Connective tissue is rich in collagen, which is a protein that makes up about 30% of the total protein in animal tissue. Meat meals contain a great deal of collagen, especially if they contain much skin, tendons or bone. This protein is not easily digested by pepsins or other proteases.

How feed digestibility can be improved

There are several ways that we can increase the digestibility of animal feeds. These methods address both the chemical and physical barriers to digestion.

Chemical treatment: Alkalis such as sodium hydroxide (NaOH, caustic soda) or ammonia (as a gas or an aqueous solution) will break down plant cell wall material and can increase the digestibility by as much as 30%. These reagents can be used with cereal grains and straws. These methods of treating roughages are discussed in Chapter 18.

Conditioning ('tempering'; steeping in water): This process is used with cereal grains (also see Chapter 18). Water is applied by spraying the grain as it is augered into storage to bring the moisture content to about 30%, or by harvesting the grain crop when its moisture content is about 30%. This moisture content promotes germination, which activates the seed's enzymes to begin to break down the starch in the endosperm cells. (Note that this type of conditioning is different to conditioning forage that is to be made into hay, where the cut forage is passed though rollers to crush the stems and promote drying.)

Heat and moisture applied to grains: When these are applied together, as steam, they break down the cereal grain endosperm and can improve digestibility by about 10%. This is the basis of grain processing methods such as pelleting, steam flaking and extrusion (Chapter 18). The dry heat used in micronizing cereal grain also improves digestibility, and when applied to grain legumes heat denatures their anti-protease proteins.

Milling ('grinding'): This is breaking grain or pieces of forage into small fragments by passing through a roller mill (grains and other seeds) or a hammer mill (grains and forages).

Milling (Chapter 18) is the most commonly used method of improving the digestibility of cereal grains; it breaks open the seedcoat and exposes the endosperm. This improves access by digestive enzymes and increases the grain's digestibility. Cattle do not chew grain very well and milled cereal grain fed to cattle is about 10% more digestible than whole grain (Table 4.1). The digestion rate of whole grains is 3–5%/h; this increases to as much as 45%/h if the grains are milled. Some animals, like sheep, pigs and horses, also respond well to milled grain (Vukmirović *et al.*, 2017) even though they are more efficient at chewing.

Milling forages increases the rate at which undigested feed passes through the reticulo-rumen. This is associated with higher feed intake, but lower digestibility. Milling forages is slow and expensive and the cost usually outweighs any financial benefit of milling on animal performance.

Table 4.1. Digestibilities of whole and ground grain by cattle[a] (Adapted from Dryden, 2008; reprinted with permission.)

	Digestibility (%)	
Cereal grain	Whole grain	Ground grain
Barley		
Dry matter	62–75	79–81
Organic matter	53–62	78–85
Protein	64	78–80
Maize		
Dry matter	77	79
Protein	74	72
Oats		
Dry matter	72–75	
Organic matter	52–77	81–83
Sorghum		
Dry matter	48–76	52–94
Protein	42–54	46–65
Wheat		
Dry matter	54–78	
Organic matter	41–63	88
Protein	75	84–90

[a]These values are from several sources and are representative only.

Aspects of digestibility

Potential digestibility is the proportion of the feed which is digested when it is exposed to the digestion process for a long time, e.g. feed held in the rumen in a nylon bag for 72 hours or longer. The resulting digestibility value tells us how much of the feed can be removed by digestive enzymes if they can work for an unlimited length of time.

Potential digestibility is determined by the feed's chemistry (e.g. the type of protein) or the composition of plant cell walls.

Effective digestibility is the digestibility value which is measured under normal physiological conditions: In practice, effective digestibility is less than potential digestibility. If a cow eats a feed which is only slowly digested (e.g. a cereal straw) then the effective digestibility of that feed will be low. If the rate of digestion is high (e.g. milk powder or molasses) then it is likely that digestion will be nearly complete, and similar to the potential digestibility.

Digestion rate and digesta passage rate influence effective digestion. These are independent of each other, but they work together to affect how much of the feed is actually digested.

- Digestion rate: simply, the speed at which a substance is digested, usually given as % per hour (%/h). Some authorities divide the carbohydrate and protein in ruminant feeds into three fractions: fast, medium and slow digesting. Common digestion rates of carbohydrate in the rumen are 200–250%/h for the fast fraction in all feeds (the size of this fraction is greatest in cereal grains and least in forages), the moderate fraction is digested at 15–60%/h and the slow fraction at 2–15%/h (NRC, 2000). These rates are general estimates, and digestion rates become faster if grains are ground or the feed is processed in other ways.

- Digesta passage rate: undigested feed moves through the digestive tract at a rate which is influenced by rumen movements (contractions of muscles in the rumen wall) and peristalsis (waves of muscular contractions in the intestines). In ruminants, the particle size of the undigested feed influences how quickly it moves from the reticulo-rumen; particles larger than 1–2 mm tend to be held in the rumen before being chewed into smaller particles as the animal ruminates. However, particle size has little effect on passage rates in non-ruminants. Diarrhoea, constipation and impaction also alter the flow of digesta.

Associative digestibility is the outcome of how feeds affect the activity of rumen microbes: These organisms have their own nutrient requirements, and if we do not provide for these then the digestion of fibre, in particular, will be impaired. If we give a feedstuff which is deficient in ruminally available N (RAN) or P, or another nutrient required by fibre-digesting bacteria or protozoa, then the digestibility of fibre will be low. If we mix this feed with another which provides RAN or other required nutrients, then the microbial population increases and fibre digestion improves. This effect, of how individual feeds in a mixture influence the digestion of the whole mixture, is called associative digestibility.

True and apparent digestibilities are different measurements: A digestibility measurement gives us a digestibility coefficient which is either:

- Apparent: if we use the total amount of nutrient excreted in faeces; or
- True (also called 'standardized'): if we base our calculation only on the amount of undigested feed material excreted in the faeces. To do this we have to separately measure the amount of excreted endogenous material.

Faeces do not consist only of undigested feed residues. They also contain materials which have been secreted during digestion (e.g. digestive enzymes) and the passage of digesta through the tract (e.g. intestinal cells and mucus). This endogenous material affects the calculated digestibility coefficient.

Figure 4.4 is a schematic of digestion in the pig; the concepts shown here hold true for all animals (also see Chapter 3).

An example: We feed a growing pig 2.75 kg per day of air-dry feed (defined in Chapter 1), and the total amount of protein in this is 467.5 g (17% protein, air-dry basis). The total amount of protein excreted in the faeces is 51.4 g per day, and 12 g per day of this is endogenous.

Apparent digestibility of protein in the feed =
(467.5 – 51.4) / 467.5 = 0.89 or 89%

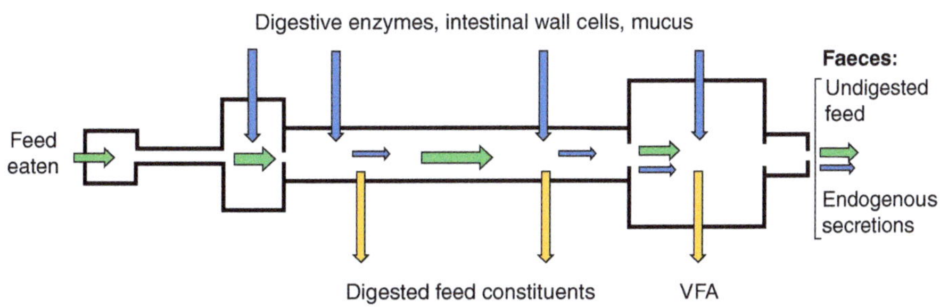

Fig. 4.4. A schematic diagram of the flow of digesta through the digestive tract of a pig showing the absorption of digested nutrient and the secretion of endogenous material into the tract. (Copyright: Gordon McL. Dryden.)

True digestibility of protein in the feed = [467.5 - (51.4 - 12)] / 467.5 = 0.915 or 91.5%

There is not much difference in this example between the apparent and true protein digestibilities, but in other situations, particularly with ruminants, and when protein intake is low, the difference can be quite large.

Measuring digestibility

To calculate a digestibility coefficient, we express the amount of nutrient digested and absorbed as a proportion of the total amount of that nutrient in the feed.

Digestibility is most accurately measured in live animals: In an *in vivo* digestibility trial, animals are given the feed under investigation for an adaptation period of about 14 days, then feed intake and faecal output data and samples are collected for 7 days. The digestibilities of the nutrients or feed constituents under consideration are calculated from this information.

First, we need to know the amount of nutrient that is eaten. It is impossible (in an intact animal) to measure this directly, so we calculate it as the difference between the amount fed and the amount not eaten; the uneaten feed is called the 'refusals' or 'orts':

Amount eaten = (amount fed) - (amount refused)

Animals eat selectively, so we have to determine the concentrations of nutrients in the refusals separately from measurements made on the feed offered.

It is obviously impossible to directly measure the amounts of nutrient digested and absorbed, so we find this by difference:

Amount digested and absorbed = (amount eaten) - (amount excreted in the faeces)

Once we have this data, we calculate the nutrient digestibility as follows:

$$\text{Digestibility} = \frac{[(\text{amount fed}) - (\text{amount refused})] - (\text{amount excreted in the faeces})}{(\text{amount fed}) - (\text{amount refused})}$$

This formula gives us the digestibility as a decimal. We can multiply by 100 to get the digestibility as a percentage.

Ileal ('pre-caecal') digestion: Amino acids are absorbed from the small intestine but not the large intestine. 'Pre-caecal' or 'ileal' digestibility, which is based on measurements of how extensively proteins are digested in the stomach, duodenum, jejunum and ileum, gives a better indication of amino acid availability in monogastric animals than measurements of total tract digestibility. To measure ileal digestibility we use an animal equipped with a T cannula at the end of the ileum so that digesta can be removed there, or with the ileum surgically anastomosed to the rectum so that the digesta does not pass through the large intestine. Alternatively, we can use the mobile nylon bag method (see below).

The digestibility calculation is the same as is given in the equation shown above.

Digestibility can be estimated by laboratory methods: Gas production, *in vitro*, *in sacco* and cellulase incubation methods can be used when:

- A rapid estimate is needed.
- We need to screen a large number of feeds.
- When a feed can be fed as part of a feed mixture, but not as the sole ingredient. The feed may be unpalatable, deficient in important nutrients or likely to cause digestive problems if fed alone. Examples are protein meals, dried distillers' grains and solubles, molasses, and cereal grains in some circumstances.
- We want to measure the rate of digestion and/or potential digestibility – this involves measuring the amount of feed or feed constituent (e.g. protein, starch or fibre) digested at various times, e.g. in the rumen after 6, 12, 18, 24 and 36 hours.

Gas production: When feeds are digested in the rumen, CO_2 and methane (CH_4) are produced as the feed organic matter is fermented. By measuring the amount or rate of gas produced we can estimate the feed digestibility (Menke *et al.*, 1979). Milled feed samples are incubated with buffered, strained rumen liquor at 37°C and the gas produced is trapped and measured.

***In sacco* digestion:** The extent and rate of the digestion of feeds or their constituents in the rumen can be measured by incubating samples in the rumen (Mehrez and Ørskov, 1977). The sample is milled to pass a 1 mm screen and placed into a small bag (about 3 × 10 cm) made of a woven polyester fabric. The sample is incubated for the required time – 48 hours if we just want an estimate of apparent digestibility, or for pre-determined periods if we want to measure the rate of digestion (see above). At the end of the incubation time the bags are removed, washed and the contents analysed for the constituents of interest.

Mobile bags can be used to measure intestinal digestion in pigs (Graham *et al.*, 1985; Steiner *et al.*, 2011). The sample is secured in a synthetic fabric bag which is then introduced via a cannula into the duodenum, and later collected in the faeces or from another cannula at the terminal ileum.

These methods are reliable but do require that we have ruminally fistulated or ileal cannulated animals on hand, and that they are properly cared for and maintained.

***In vitro* digestion:** This method (Tilley and Terry, 1963) mimics the ruminal and intestinal digestion of ruminants. The sample is milled and incubated in buffered, strained rumen liquor at 37°C for 48 hours. The residue is recovered by centrifuging, and then incubated for another 48 hours at 37°C in an acid pepsin solution. It is important to carry out the rumen digestion under anaerobic conditions (flush the incubation tubes with CO_2) because rumen micro-organisms are anaerobic and die in the presence of oxygen.

Incubation with cellulase: This is a two-stage incubation where the milled sample is incubated first in acid pepsin for 24 hours at 40°C, then for 48 hours with a fungal cellulase (a cellulose-digesting enzyme), again at 40°C (Iowerth *et al.*, 1975).

Prediction of digestibility by near infrared reflectance spectroscopy (NIRS): If we know the *in vivo* digestibility of a variety of feeds similar to the one that we want to analyse, then we can construct reasonably precise equations to predict digestibility by NIRS (see Dryden, 2003). This method is non-destructive and very quick, but there is considerable effort involved in developing the prediction equations.

Indicator methods: Sometimes it is not possible to measure feed intake or to completely collect faeces, for example if we want to know the digestibility of pasture eaten by a grazing animal or of a feed given to group-housed pigs. In these situations, we can use the indicator method. This involves measuring the content of an indigestible substance in the feed (e.g. lignin or one of the naturally occurring alkanes) and the content of the same substance in a sample of faeces. The digestibility of any constituent (DM in this example) is calculated in this way:

$$\text{DM digestibility} = 1 - \left[\frac{(\text{feed indicator content}) \times (\text{faeces DM content})}{(\text{faeces indicator content}) \times (\text{feed DM content})}\right]$$

References

Borisjuk, L., Neuberger, T., Schwender, J., Nicolas, N., Sunderhaus, S., Fuchs, J., Hay, J.O, Tschiersch, H., Braun, H.-P., Denolf, P., Lambert, B., Jakob, P.M. and Rolletschek, H. (2013). Seed architecture shapes embryo metabolism in oilseed rape. *Plant Cell* 25(5): 1625–1640.

Chesson, A. (1988). Lignin polysaccharide complexes of the plant-cell wall and their effect on microbial degradation in the rumen. *Animal Feed Science and Technology* 21(2-4): 219–228.

Dryden, G.McL. (2003). *Near Infrared Reflectance Spectroscopy: Applications in Deer Nutrition*. RIRDC Publication No. W03/007. Canberra: Rural Industries Research and Development Corporation. Available at: www.researchgate.net/profile/G_Dryden/publication/37629601_Near_infrared_reflectance_spectroscopy_applications_in_deer_nutrition/links/55beb31308aed621de121439/Near-infrared-reflectance-spectroscopy-applications-in-deer-nutrition.pdf (accessed 27 December 2020).

Dryden, G.McL. (2008). *Animal Nutrition Science*. Wallingford, UK: CAB International.

Graham, H., Aman, P., Newman, R.K. and Newman, C.W. (1985). Use of a nylon-bag technique for pig feed digestibility studies. *British Journal of Nutrition* 54: 719–726.

Grain Trade Australia (undated). *Animal Protein Standards 2015/16*. Available at: www.graintrade.org.au/commodity_standards (accessed 27 December 2020).

Iowerth, D., Jones, H. and Hayward, M.V. (1975). The effect of pepsin pretreatment of herbage on the prediction of dry matter digestibility from solubility in fungal cellulase solutions. *Journal of the Science of Food and Agriculture* 26: 711–718.

Menke, K.H., Raab, L., Salewski, A., Steingass, H., Fritz, D. and Schneider, W. (1979). The estimation of the digestibility and metabolizable energy content of ruminant feedstuffs from the gas production when they are incubated with rumen liquor *in vitro*. *Journal of Agricultural Science* 92: 217–222.

Mehrez, A.Z. and Ørskov, E.R. (1977). A study of artificial fibre bag technique for determining the digestibility of feeds in the rumen. *Journal of Agricultural Science* 88: 645–650.

National Research Council (NRC) (2000). *Nutrient Requirements of Beef Cattle*, 7th rev. edn. Update 2000. Washington, DC: The National Academies Press. Available at: www.nap.edu/catalog/9791/nutrient-requirements-of-beef-cattle-seventh-revised-edition-update-2000 (accessed 27 December 2020).

Rathjen, J.R., Strounina, E.V. and Mares, D.J. (2009). Water movement into dormant and non-dormant wheat (*Triticum aestivum* L.) grains. *Journal of Experimental Botany* 60(6):1619–1631.

Steiner, T., Bornholdt, U., Sauer, W.C., Ahrens, F., Jørgensen, H. and Mosenthin, R. (2011). Use of the mobile nylon bag technique for determination of apparent ileal digestibilities of crude protein and amino acids in feedstuffs for pigs. *Czech Journal of Animal Science* 56, (10): 451–464.

Tilley, J.M.A. and Terry, R.A. (1963). A two stage technique for the *in vitro* digestion of forage crops. *Journal of the British Grasslands Society* 18: 104–111.

UK Flour Millers (undated). *Wheat Structure*. Available at: www.ukflourmillers.org/wheatstructure (accessed 3 March 2021).

Verboven, P., Herremans, E., Borisjuk, L., Helfen, L., Ho, Q.T., Tschiersch, H., Fuchs, J., Nicolaï, B.M. and Rolletschek, H. (2013). Void space inside the developing seed of *Brassica napus* and the modelling of its function. *New Phytologist* 119(4): 936–947.

Vukmirović, Đ., Čolović, R., Rakita, S., Brlek, T., Đuragić, O. and Solà-Oriol, D. (2017). Importance of feed structure (particle size) and feed form (mash vs. pellets) in pig nutrition – A review. *Animal Feed Science and Technology* 233: 133–144.

5 Feed nutritive value

The nutritive value of animal feeds

Nutritive value is a concept which combines information on:

- the chemical composition of feeds, i.e. their nutrient content;
- the availability of the nutrients in a feedstuff;
- characteristic levels of intake;
- palatability;
- the effects of the feed on animal health; and
- the effects of the feed on the quality of animal products.

All tables of feed nutritional data give information on the first two points (see Chapters 1 and 6), and the INRAE (2017–2020) and CVB tables (Blok and Spek, 2016) report 'fill units' or 'satiety values' (Chapter 7) which can be used to predict dry matter (DM) intakes. These are additive and so can be used in ration formulation. However, they are only estimates because in practice feed intake varies – influenced by the animal's physiological state, environment, previous experience with that feed, how the feed has been processed and presented, and the range of other feeds available to them at that time (see Chapter 7 for more information). Feed tables may include information on secondary substances such as tannins, alkaloids, etc., which affect health, and this information is very valuable. Guidance on how a feed might affect product quality is not commonly given.

Nutrient availability

It is relatively easy to measure the total nutrient contents in a feed, but this data does not indicate how well the feed supplies nutrients which are available to the animal. For this, we need to know something about nutrient availability, or better still, the available nutrient contents. For example, we can think about the contents in a feed of:

- digestible or metabolizable or net energy;
- digestible or metabolizable or net protein; or
- available minerals.

Energy and protein digestibilities are quite easily measured (Chapter 4), and we can use digestibility as the reference and base assessments of feed nutritive value on 'digestible' nutrient contents. But there are other losses of nutrients (especially of energy and amino acids) which occur as they are metabolized that should be taken into account. For example, some feed energy is lost as CH_4, in the heat of microbial fermentation when feeds are metabolized in the rumen, and some of the energy of digested and absorbed nutrients is lost as heat when ATP is used to fuel maintenance or production. Excess amino acids cannot be used or stored in the animal's tissues and so they are deaminated. The N removed from these amino acids is excreted in the urine and so the animal loses some of the amino acid-N which was absorbed from the digestive tract.

To understand the amount of available nutrients which a feed can supply we need to know:

- How digestible are the energy sources (carbohydrates, fats, proteins) in the feed?
- To what extent can the animal digest mineral sources and absorb the minerals in the feed?
- How digestible are the amino acid sources (proteins), and how well does an animal retain in its body the amino acids which are supplied by the feed?
- How digestible are the fatty acid sources (fats) in the feed?
- What happens to the absorbed nutrients as they are metabolized within the animal's cells?
- How readily available to rumen micro-organisms are the nutrients that are needed to support active rumen function?

DOI: 10.1079/9781786394453.0005

How the available energy in feeds is measured and expressed

Chemical energy (usually in the form of ATP) is obtained when amino acids, fatty acids, carbohydrates and other substances are oxidized within the body's cells (see Chapter 1). The energy content of feeds is expressed in megajoules (MJ) or megacalories (Mcal) per kilogram; 1 MJ = 0.239 Mcal. These contents can be expressed on either a DM or as-fed basis.

Losses of energy as feed is digested and metabolized: There are three routes of energy loss, as shown in Fig. 5.1. As we go from digestible energy (DE) through metabolizable energy (ME) to the feed's net energy (NE) content, we get increasing accuracy in predicting the amount of usable energy that animals get from their feed.

Total (gross) energy (GE): To find the total energy content of a feed, we measure the heat emitted when the feed organic matter (OM) is completely burnt in a calorimeter. This heat represents the chemical energy of the feed's carbohydrates, proteins, fat, and minor organic constituents such as vitamins and secondary substances (Chapter 1).

The total energy content, measured as heat when the feed is burnt, is approximately 18.4 MJ/kg DM and 20 MJ/kg OM. The total energy content of any particular feed depends on the amounts of minerals and fat in the DM. As the mineral (ash) content increases, the total energy content of DM decreases; and as the fat content increases, the total energy contents of DM and OM also increase.

Digestible energy: This is the energy of the sugars, amino acids and fatty acids absorbed from the small intestine, and of the volatile fatty acids (VFA) produced by microbial fermentation and absorbed from the rumen or large intestine.

DE content is measured by carrying out a digestibility trial (Chapter 4) and measuring the total energy contents of feed and faeces. From this data we can calculate:

DE eaten = (total feed energy eaten) − (faecal energy voided)

or

DE content = (total feed energy content) × (energy digestibility)

Example: For a horse grazing immature ryegrass (*Lolium* spp.) pasture, a digestibility coefficient of 0.65 or 65% for the DM in this feed is a reasonable estimate:

Total energy content of ryegrass DM = 18.4 MJ/kg

Energy digestibility = 0.65

DE content = 18.4 × 0.65 = 11.9 MJ/kg DM

This method of assessing the DE content of feeds can be used for all domestic species except for birds (see below).

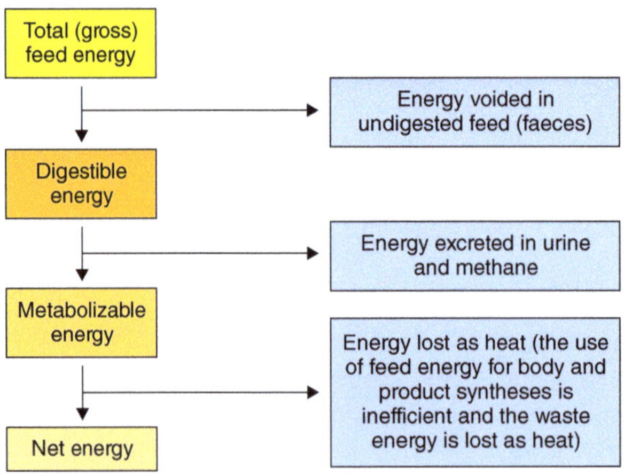

Fig. 5.1. Routes of energy loss during digestion and the metabolism of absorbed energy precursors. (Copyright: Gordon McL. Dryden.)

Digestible dry matter (DDM) and digestible organic matter (DOM): If energy digestibility cannot be measured directly, an alternative is to measure the digestibilities of those feed constituents which contain the carbohydrates, proteins and fats which provide energy. Thus we can find the digestibilities of OM, giving the DOM content; or of DM, giving the DDM content (these are expressed as % of the feed or feed DM). However, DOM and DDM contents are approximations of the DE content because of the effects of varying mineral and fat contents, and as energy is conveniently measured with a calorimeter it is best to measure DE directly rather than to rely on estimates based on OM or DM.

Total digestible nutrients (TDN): This method of expressing the available energy content of feeds was developed by Haecker in the early 1900s (Corbett and Freer, 2003) and popularized by Morrison (who wrote the standard American nutrition textbook *Feeds and Feeding*). TDN contents are expressed as % in the feed or feed DM. TDN is similar to DOM except that it recognizes the extra energy available from fat (or 'ether extract', EE; Chapter 1) which is approximately 2.25 times more than in carbohydrates or proteins.

$$\text{TDN } (\%) = (\text{DOM}, \%) + [1.25 \times (\text{digestible EE}, \%)]$$

Roughages and cereal grains have less than 3–5% fat (Chapter 6) so their TDN values are similar to their DOM contents.

More accurate TDN prediction equations have been developed to allow for the differences between different feed types, e.g. for cool-season grasses, warm-season grasses, and legumes and legume/grass mixtures (NRC, 2001).

DE, DDM, DOM and TDN are not accurate measures of usable feed energy: These units are less accurate than ME or NE because they do not take into account the energy lost during rumen fermentation (in ruminants), or when absorbed sugars, amino acids, long-chain fatty acids and volatile fatty acids are metabolized prior to their incorporation into animal products or used for maintenance.

With better understanding of nutrition and better data, DE (and estimates of this) have been replaced by ME and NE in animal feeding standards.

Metabolizable energy: This is the energy of absorbed sugars, amino acids and fatty acids less the energy of CH_4 produced in the rumen and large intestine by microbial fermentation, and the energy of organic substances excreted in the urine.

Micro-organisms in the rumen and large intestine use the animal's feed as a source of energy and other nutrients, and the principal products of their metabolism are microbial cells, VFA; mainly acetate, propionate and butyrate) and methane (CH_4). Microbial cells which are formed in the rumen are digested in the small intestine and their constituents (nucleic acids, amino acids, fatty acids, vitamins and minerals) are absorbed and used by the animal. The VFA produced in the rumen and large intestine are absorbed and used as an energy source for the host animal. The gases produced by bacteria are excreted by eructation (belching) and from the anus.

Urine contains substances which are the end-products of a variety of metabolic process. These include:

- Urea or uric acid: in animals, urea is made by the deamination of excess dietary amino acids and the detoxification of NH_3 absorbed from the rumen or made when excess absorbed amino acids are deaminated. Uric acid is the nitrogenous excretion product of birds' kidneys, analogous to urinary urea in mammals. Most avian species void excess nitrogenous material, after appropriate metabolism, as uric acid rather than urea, as this helps them to conserve water.
- Creatinine: the dehydration product of creatine, which is an energy storage molecule found in all cells.
- Purine derivatives: residues of nucleic acid metabolism.
- Ketones (especially in ruminants): products of fatty acid metabolism.
- Other constituents: water, mineral salts, amino acids, (small amounts of) protein and glucose.

● Because the energy lost in CH_4 and the organic substances excreted in urine are taken into account in measuring the ME content of feeds, ME is a more accurate measure of available energy than DE.

Feed ME contents can be determined directly by measuring feed intake and collecting faeces, CH_4 and urine. However, it is technically difficult to measure CH_4 production and so ME is usually estimated from the feed's DE content.

For ruminants: ME = 0.82 × DE

For pigs: ME = 0.96 × DE

For horses: ME = 0.9 × DE

We should note that many different datasets have been used to calculate the relationships between DE, ME and NE, and the values reported by different authorities vary a little, even for the same type of animal.

ME is a preferred measure of available energy for poultry: The ME contents of poultry feeds are easier to measure than their DE contents because birds void a mixture of urine and faeces.

The available energy of poultry feeds is expressed as either true ME (TME) or apparent ME (AME or ME). 'True' and 'apparent' have the same meanings here as they have for true and apparent digestibilities (Chapter 4). Values for AME and TME become more similar as the bird's feed intake increases (Fig. 5.2).

N-corrected AME and TME (AME_n and TME_n): Poultry feeds are fed to a variety of different types of bird, e.g. laying hens, broilers, roosters, turkeys, quail, etc., and all of these retain N (i.e. grow and produce muscle tissue) with different efficiencies. The N correction allows AME_n and TME_n values to be used for all of these different types of birds.

AME_n and TME_n values are calculated by adding to the energy excreted in the bird's droppings (the combined faeces and urine), an amount which represents the energy content of the uric acid which would have been excreted had the bird not retained any feed N (Lopez and Leeson, 2007). This would have happened if the bird was not growing. N correction reduces the AME values by 4–5% at usual levels of feed intake (Fig. 5.2).

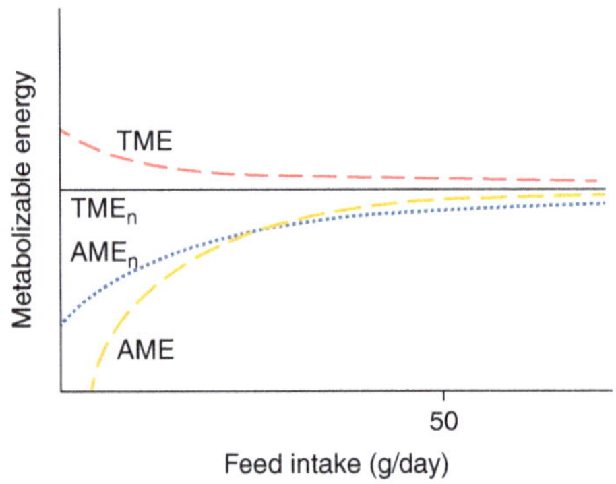

Fig. 5.2. Relationships between true and apparent metabolizable energy, either corrected for N retention or not, in the diet of adult poultry. (Adapted from Wolynetz and Sibbald, 1984; reproduced with permission).

Efficiency of use of ME by pigs, ruminants and horses: The relationship between ME and NE is given the symbol k, and we have:

- k_m, for maintenance;
- k_g, for growth;
- k_y, for pregnancy; and
- k_{milk} for milk production.

The conversion of ME to NE by growing pigs is highly efficient, 75–80% for pigs fed conventional diets. Efficiency is highest for oil-rich feeds (80–90%), moderate for starch (about 80%) and least for fibrous feeds (about 60%). However, efficiencies also vary with the animal's growth stage – growers which are depositing mainly lean tissue use ME with lower efficiency than finishers which are depositing more fat (Kil *et al.*, 2013).

When ME is used for maintenance, ruminants convert it to NE with an efficiency of about 65%, although this varies a little between different feeds. However, ruminants use ME for growth with very different efficiencies depending on the ME concentration in the feed. An equation to predict k_m for ruminants is (CSIRO, 2007):

$$k_m = [0.02 \times (\text{ME content, MJ/kg DM})] + 0.5$$

And equations to predict k_g are (CSIRO, 2007):

For concentrates and very digestible early-growth temperate forages: $k_g = [0.042 \times (\text{ME content, MJ/kg DM})] + 0.006$

For all other forages: $k_g = [0.063 \times (\text{ME content, MJ/kg DM})] - 0.308$

Indicative k_m and k_g for fibrous, low-quality roughages, medium-quality roughages, and low-fibre feeds (concentrates) are:

Cereal straw:	maintenance (k_m)	62%
	growth (k_g)	26%
Grass hay:	maintenance (k_m)	68%
	growth (k_g)	31%
Cereal grain:	maintenance (k_m)	77%
	growth (k_g)	45%

The efficiencies of use of ME in conventional dairy diets for maintenance (k_m) and milk production (k_{milk}) are very similar: k_m = 0.62 and k_{milk} = 0.64. Because of this, and because lactating cows usually do not gain much body weight during their lactation, it is possible to merge these two requirements into a single unit and to cite the dairy cow's total NE requirements as NE_l (NE for the lactating cow) (NRC, 2001; INRAE, 2017–2020). Likewise, the NE requirements for the combined requirements for maintenance, pregnancy and growth of breeding beef cows can be expressed as equivalent amounts of NE_m (NRC, 2000).

There is less information on the efficiency of converting ME to NE for horses, than for ruminants. As a guide, k is between 65% and 85%, with the lower value appropriate for roughages and the higher for cereal grains.

Net energy: This is the amount of energy that can be extracted from a feed and used:

- for maintenance (basic life processes; and wool and hair production, control of core body temperature, and voluntary activity);
- for product synthesis (e.g. the total energy contained in eggs, fibre, meat, milk, foetus); and
- to produce work (non-voluntary activities such as racing and draught work).

The NE available from a feed depends on:

- the animal species that uses the feed;
- the mix and amount of nutrients that the animal has available after the digestion of feed and the absorption of nutrients from its digestive tract; and
- the purposes for which these nutrients will be used in the animal's metabolism, e.g. maintenance, growth, milk production (Chapter 8).

Ruminant feed tables give NE content values for maintenance (NE_m), growth (NE_g) and lactation (NE_l). These may be derived for different feeding levels, e.g. daily DM intakes equivalent to an amount which will meet the animal's maintenance requirement or various multiples of that, or percentages of live weight.

NE values for pig feeds are generally quoted as a single value which encompasses all the animal's physiological functions, i.e. different values are not given for maintenance, growth, or reproduction. The NRC (2012) standards give only one NE value for each feed. INRAE (2017–2020) takes a similar approach, although in this case they quote separate feed NE contents for growing and finishing pigs.

Other ways of expressing the available energy content of feeds: Because energy was the first nutrient to be investigated and quantified, several energy units were developed in the 1800s and early 1900s and are still used (after refinement and updating) in several countries.

The starch equivalent (SE) was devised by Kellner in the 1800s. SE values were derived by comparing the animal's response (e.g. fat deposition) to the test feed with the response when starch was fed. The French feeding standards (INRAE, 2017–2020) use the Unité Fourragère Lait (UFL), Unité Fourragère Viande (UFV) and Unité Fourragère Cheval (UFC) to describe the NE requirements for maintenance, moderate growth and lactation of ruminants (UFL), for fast-growing ruminants (UFV) and for horses (UFC). These forage units use barley grain as the standard for comparison. A similar approach is used in the Scandinavian Feed Unit (SFU), and the Dutch Feed Unit Milk (VEM) and Feed Unit Beef Cattle (VEVI). Other units, such as the net energy for fattening and net energy for lactation, were developed from measurements of energy retention obtained in feeding experiments. Derived energy units are expressed as % (e.g. SE, TDN and SFU) or as units per kg (e.g. UFL, UFV and UFC).

Sundstøl (1993) and Corbett and Freer (2003) have described these ways of expressing feed energy contents and compared them with the ME and NE systems.

The availability of feed energy can be predicted from feed composition: There are now enough measurements of the available energy contents of animal feeds to predict these values from the feed's chemical composition, as shown in these examples:

(a) AME_n content of soybean meal fed to poultry (Alvarenga *et al.*, 2013):

$$AME_n = 0.004184 \times [-822.33 + (69.54 \times CP) - (45.26 \times ADF) + (90.81 \times EE)]$$

(b) DE content of all conventional pig feeds (INRAE, 2017–2020):

$$DE = (0.2247 \times CP) + (0.3171 \times EE) + (0.1720 \times Starch) + (0.0318 \times NDF) + (0.1632 \times Residue)$$

(c) DE content of horse feeds (Pagan, 1998):

$$DE = 0.0041855 \times [2118 + (12.81 \times CP) - (9.37 \times ADF) - (3.83 \times Hemicellulose) + (47.18 \times Fat) + (20.35 \times NSC) - (23.6 \times Ash)]$$

(d) ME content of dairy cattle feeds predicted for production levels of feed intake (NRC, 2001):

$$ME = 4.184 \times [1.01 \times (DE) - 0.45] + [0.0046 \times (EE - 3)]$$

In these equations: ADF = acid detergent fibre (% DM); AME_n = metabolizable energy (N corrected) (MJ/kg DM); Ash = material remaining after complete burning of the feed (% DM); CP = crude protein content (% DM); DE = digestible energy (MJ/kg DM); EE = Fat = ether extract (fat) content (% DM); Hemicellulose = (NDF content – ADF content) (% DM); ME = metabolizable energy (MJ/kg DM); NDF = neutral detergent fibre (% DM); NFE = N-free extract (% DM); NSC = non-structural carbohydrate (% DM); Starch = starch (% DM); Residue = [OM – (CP + EE + Starch + NDF)] (% DM); and TDN = total digestible nutrients (decimal).

We can see from these equations that energy availability (both metabolizability and digestibility) is influenced by the proportions of readily digestible feed constituents such as protein, fat and non-fibre (also called non-structural) carbohydrates. The positive coefficient for NDF (plant fibre, Chapters 1 and 4) in the pig DE equation may seem puzzling, because the pig (in fact, no mammal) has intrinsic enzymes which can digest this feed component. The NDF coefficient is much smaller than the others in the equation, indicating that NDF contributes less digestible energy than starch or protein. Nevertheless, the coefficient is positive. This indicates that the micro-organisms in the pig's digestive tract ferment plant fibre, and that the VFA they produce contribute to the pig's available energy. Note the negative coefficient for ash in the horse equation – this is because minerals do not contribute any energy.

Indexes which combine energy availability and feed intake: Relative Feed Value (RFV), Quality Index and Relative Feed Quality (RFQ) are indexes for forages which combine information on the digestible energy content with the expected DM intake (Moore and Undersander, 2002). These indexes rank forage feeds relative to full bloom lucerne (alfalfa) hay.

$$RFV = (DM\ intake, kg/day) \times (DDM\ content, \%DM) / 1.29$$

DM intake and the DDM content are estimated from the feed's ADF and NDF contents, respectively.

The RFQ index is similar, but uses TDN instead of DDM (Undersander *et al.*, 2010):

$$RFQ = (DM\ intake, \%\ live\ weight\ per\ day) \times (TDN, \%DM) / 1.23$$

DM intake is predicted from the forage's protein, ADF or NDF, and TDN contents; and TDN is predicted from non-fibre carbohydrate, fat, NDF and crude protein contents (see Chapter 1 for information about these) and the *in vitro* digestibility of NDF (see Chapter 4).

Protein

The protein and amino acid contents of feeds are expressed as % or g/kg; 1% = 10 g/kg. Both units can be expressed on either a DM or an as-fed basis.

Feed protein is a source of amino acids. The nutritional value of proteins is determined by their amino acid composition, because it is these that are released during digestion, absorbed into the blood vessels draining the small intestine, and then become available for use in the synthesis of the animal's own body proteins.

Amino acids are either essential or non-essential. Whether an amino acid is essential or not depends on the animal's species, age and physiological status. The list for pigs (Table 1.3 in Chapter 1) gives a good indication of those amino acids which are required in the diets of all animals.

Absorption and retention of dietary amino acids: In a healthy animal fed conventional protein sources, about 90% of the protein in the feed is digested. The amino acids released from the digested protein are absorbed from the intestine and then metabolized in the animal's body cells.

Not all of the absorbed amino acids are used for protein synthesis. Some are in excess of immediate requirements and as the animal has limited ability to store amino acids for later use this excess is deaminated in the liver and the N which is removed from the amino acid molecule is excreted.

$$\text{amino acids} \rightarrow \text{keto acids} + NH_3$$

The N removed from these amino acids forms NH_3, which is poisonous and must be detoxified. The NH_3 is converted to a non-toxic form by using it for urea synthesis in the mammal (Krebs, 1973), or uric acid synthesis in the bird. Urea and uric acid are excreted via the kidneys.

This chain of events is illustrated in Fig. 5.3.

Feed protein and amino acid analysis: Protein in feeds is commonly measured by determining the feed's total N content and multiplying this value by 6.25; many proteins contain 16% N, and 100/16 = 6.25. There are some proteins, e.g. those in milk, maize, wheat and soybean, which have different N contents and we should use different factors, but this is often ignored.

The result is called crude protein because of the approximation involved in using this universal conversion factor, and also because some of the N in feeds is not amino acid-N and total N analysis does not distinguish between the different sources of N in feeds.

Digestible protein contents of feeds are calculated from data on feed intake and faecal output (see Chapter 4). This methodology measures the effects of all those processes which remove feed constituents as they pass from the mouth to the anus.

Amino acid analyses of feeds for pigs and poultry are routine and are increasingly done for dairy cattle and horse feeds. At the least, the concentrations of the probably limiting amino acids (see Chapter 1 and below) should always be determined.

There are several ways that we can evaluate amino acid availability for pigs and birds:

- standardized (true) ileal digestibility (Chapter 4) – a commonly-used index, and data on the ileal digestibilities of the essential amino acids is widely available;
- retention in the body;
- slope ratio assay – the 'gold standard' evaluation method (see Dryden, 2008); and
- indicator amino acid oxidation.

Using protein and amino acid information for pigs and poultry: When we formulate diets for these species, we:

- Formulate a ration which will meet the requirements for the essential amino acids. Lysine is usually the first limiting (see Chapter 1) amino acid in pig feeds, and methionine, glycine, serine or lysine in poultry feeds, although the actual limiting amino acid depends on the diet (Baker, 2009). Threonine, valine and tyrosine + phenylalanine can also be limiting amino acids in pig and poultry diets. Where possible, it is best to use information on available, rather than total, amino acid contents.
- Formulate diets using information on 'ideal amino acid ratios' (Chapter 8). These are ratios of digestible amino acid to digestible lysine which exactly meet the animal's or bird's requirements for maintenance and production. Lysine is used as the reference amino acid because it is often the first limiting amino acid, is used only for protein synthesis, and is easily measured in feeds.
- Assess the total protein content of the formulated ration to make sure that this will cover the requirements for the non-essential amino acids. This method works when pigs and poultry are fed commercial diets that are made up from conventional ingredients. However, it does assume that all feeds have similar protein digestibilities; if there is doubt about this it is best to use digestible protein values if these are available.

Describing the available protein in horse feeds: The horse initially digests feed in its stomach and small intestine with its intrinsic enzymes (see Chapter 3)

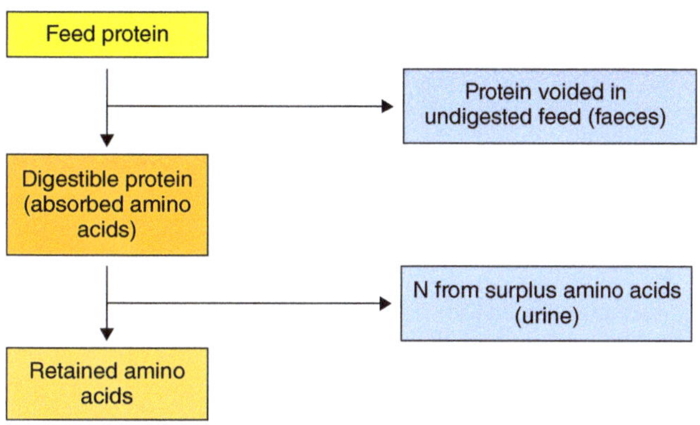

Fig. 5.3. Pathways of amino acid absorption and retention. (Copyright: Gordon McL. Dryden.)

and then by microbial digestion in the large intestine. Only digestion in the small intestine provides amino acids which can be absorbed from the digestive tract, so we need to know the 'pre-caecal' or 'ileal' digestibility of feed protein. There are two ways we can do this – either by measuring ileal amino acid digestibility with surgically altered animals (Chapter 4) as is also done in pigs; or by feed analysis (NRC, 2007a) where the available protein (AP) can be calculated from:

$$\text{Available protein} = [(\text{total N}) - (\text{NPN} + \text{ADIN})] \times 6.25$$

where: NPN = non-protein N (e.g. the N of nitrates, urea or ammonium salts) and ADIN = acid detergent insoluble N (the N of plant cell wall proteins – see Chapters 1 and 4).

AP is about 60% of the measured whole-tract digestible protein (NRC, 2007a).

INRAE (2017–2020) provide data on whole-tract digestible true protein contents. True protein is measured by subtracting the contributions of non-protein-N (e.g. urea-N, nitrate-N and nucleic acid-N) in the feed from its content of crude protein. Note the difference between 'true protein' and 'truly digestible' protein (Chapter 4).

The ideal amino acid ratio concept (see above and Chapter 8) also applies in horse nutrition, but there is limited information on ideal ratios for equines. However, lysine is likely to be important, and so data on total lysine contents is provided in both NRC (2007a) and INRAE (2017–2020) nutritive value tables.

Measures of feed protein quality for ruminants: Older ruminant feeding standards may cite requirements for digestible protein, but these are of little practical use – the concept of whole-tract protein digestibility is not useful with ruminants. Instead, we measure:

- the amount of feed protein which is degraded by micro-organisms in the rumen;
- the amounts of microbial and undegraded feed protein which flow to the small intestine; and
- the digestibilities of the microbial and undegraded feed protein in the small intestine.

As well as considering the animal's amino acid requirements, we have to take into account the N requirements of the rumen micro-organisms. This is because the rumen microbes are responsible for the fermentation of fibrous OM in the feed and this has implications for:

- the availability of energy from the usually fibre-rich feed that these animals eat and which cannot be digested by the animal's intrinsic abomasal or small intestinal enzymes;
- the animal's ability to consume adequate amounts of roughage feed; and
- the supply of essential and non-essential amino acids from digested microbial protein.

Animals eating low-quality pasture or forage can be deficient in ruminally available N, while highly productive animals can be deficient in the amino acids which are often supplied by ruminally undegradable protein (RDP). Consequently, we need to know these things about ruminant feed protein:

- The degradability (dg) of feed protein. This is determined by its chemistry and thus its susceptibility to digestion in the rumen. Protein chemistry establishes its potential degradability. However, this is not usually achieved in practice because the digesta does not remain in the reticulo-rumen for long enough for the potentially degradable protein to be completely degraded. A much better measure of degradability is the effective degradability (Edg), which allows for the effect of the rate of passage of undigested protein through the rumen (Ørskov and McDonald, 1979). Rumen degradability determines the amount of feed protein which will provide a N source for rumen micro-organisms.
- The concentration in the feed of RDP (also called degradable intake protein, DIP). This consists of two parts: the 'quickly degraded' fraction (which is water-soluble protein plus non-protein N such as nitrates, urea and free amino acids) and a 'slowly degraded' protein fraction.

  $$\text{RDP} = (\text{quickly degraded protein}) + [(\text{slowly degraded protein}) \times \text{Edg}]$$

  There is a third, small fraction consisting of some protein associated with plant cell walls or bound to tannins, which cannot be degraded at all. This fraction is insoluble in acid detergent.

- Most bacteria require NH_3-N as their source of N. They get this by deaminating feed amino acids, and also from non-protein N (e.g. urea). RAN is another useful measure of the N available to rumen micro-organisms.

RAN = [(feed protein) × Edg / 6.25] + NPN

or = RDP / 6.25

- Undegradable dietary protein (UDP) (also called bypass protein; or undegradable intake protein, UIP; or ruminally undegradable protein, RUP):

  UDP = (total protein) – RDP

- The amino acid composition and digestibility of UDP: lysine, histidine and methionine can be limiting amino acids in dairy cattle diets, and S-amino acids (cysteine and methionine) in feeds for wool-producing sheep. These amino acids can be supplied from UDP which is digested in the small intestine.

Metabolizable protein (MP; also called protein digestible in the small intestine, PDI, in the INRAE system) is the preferred measure for ruminants of available protein. MP is derived from the UDP, microbial crude protein (MCP) and endogenous protein (EP) which flow from the rumen into the small intestine (Fig. 5.4). RDP and UDP are the most important determinants of the MP available from a feed: RDP serves as a source of the NH_3-N, amino acids and small peptides required for microbial protein synthesis, and both the UDP and MCP are sources of amino acids which can be absorbed by the animal after these proteins have been digested in the abomasum and small intestine.

Because MP is the source of the amino acids needed for maintenance and production, we need to know the concentrations of essential amino acids in the MP derived from individual feeds. These values are provided by INRAE (2017–2020), and NRC (2001) reports a representative essential amino acid profile of rumen bacteria and protozoa.

The MP available from feeds can be calculated in these ways:

- From the amounts of digestible MCP and digestible UDP passing into the small intestine (Jarrige, 1989), and ignoring the small amount of digestible EP produced by the passage of undigested feed:

  MP = (UDP × 0.8) + (MCP × 0.8 × 0.8)

  In this equation the digestibility of UDP is assumed to be 80% (although it can vary from 55 to 95%), and that MCP is 80% true protein which is 80% digestible. We can predict the amount of

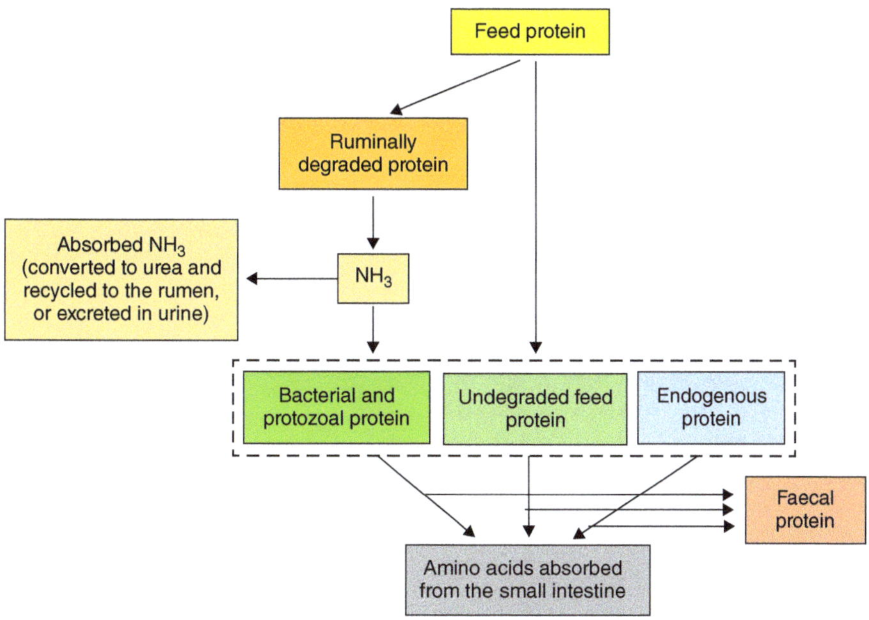

Fig. 5.4. Pathways of feed protein digestion in the ruminant. The digestible parts of the protein fractions in the dashed box make up metabolizable protein. (Copyright: Gordon McL. Dryden.)

MCP flowing to the small intestine either from the amount of RDP the animal has eaten or from the amount of ruminally fermentable OM (FOM) which is available to the rumen micro-organisms (FOM is the DOM less digestible fat, silage fermentation products, and UDP).

- From the feed's apparently digestible protein content (NRC, 2007b):

MP (%) = (apparently digestible feed protein, %) × 0.7

= [(feed protein, %) × 0.9) – 3] × 0.7

or = (feed protein, %) × {[64 + (0.16 × UDP, %)] /100}

Net protein (NP) is the amount of feed amino acids which are used to synthesize the protein and other nitrogenous materials which are retained in the animal's own tissues (including lean body tissue and fibre) or produced in milk or in a foetus.

MP is not converted to NP with complete efficiency because there is usually not an exact match between the amino acid composition of MP compared to the amino acid profile of the product being synthesized, and also because there is an inherent inefficiency of use of an 'ideal' feed protein. The efficiencies of use (kp) of MP are:

kp_m, maintenance = 0.7 to 1.0
kp_g, live weight gain = 0.83 – (0.0008 × W, kg); a range of 0.4 to 0.75 decreasing with increasing live weight
kp_y, pregnancy = 0.33 to 0.7, because the conceptus includes the foetus plus the placenta and growing uterus
kp_{milk}, lactation = 0.4 to 0.6
kp_{fibre}, wool or mohair growth = 0.54 to 0.6, because MP is usually deficient in S-amino acids compared to the amino acids in wool and mohair protein.

These indicative values are from Jarrige (1989), CSIRO (2007) and NRC (2007b). There are very large differences in the published values for some efficiencies – this area of ruminant nutrition is still developing.

Fatty acids

The fatty acid content of feeds is expressed as g/kg or %, either on a DM or as-fed basis.

The essential fatty acids (Chapter 1) include linoleic acid (LA), an 18-carbon molecule with two double bonds; and α-linolenic acid (ALA), an 18-carbon molecule with three double bonds. The LA and ALA contents of feeds are reported as total amounts. No allowance is made for availability.

Minerals

The contents of the major minerals in feeds are given in either g/kg or %, and those of the trace or ultra-trace minerals are expressed as mg/kg, parts per million (ppm) or μg/kg. Concentrations are quoted on either a DM or as-fed basis. Conversions for these units are: 10 mg/kg = 1%; 1 mg/kg = 1 ppm; 1000 μg/kg = 1 mg/kg.

The value of feeds as mineral sources: This depends on the concentrations of each mineral, and the availability of the mineral to animals. There are two complementary concepts:

- Digestible mineral: this is the proportion of the feed mineral in question which is digested. We can use either apparent total tract digestibility (ATTD), which is simply based on the amount of mineral eaten and the amount excreted in faeces; or better, the standardized (or 'true') total tract digestibility (STTD), which involves correcting for any endogenous mineral which might be secreted into the intestine.
- Absorption and retention of digested mineral: not all of the digested mineral is retained in the animal's body or products. Some may be excreted as endogenous mineral in the faeces or urine.

Minerals have varying availabilities, e.g. for cattle the coefficients of absorption of Mn, Ca and I are about 1%, 50–60%, and 90%, respectively (NRC, 2001). Mineral availabilities are affected by:

- The mineral source and its chemical form: e.g. ferrous Fe is better absorbed than the ferric form, phytate-P is largely unavailable to monogastric animals, and Ca in limestone is less available to cattle than Ca in pure $CaCO_3$.
- Other diet constituents: e.g. Cu absorption is affected by the diet Mo and S contents (see below); P by the diet Ca content (the optimal ratio for pigs and poultry is between 1 Ca:1 P and 2 Ca:1 P); competition for absorption from the digestive tract between Cu and Zn and between K and Mg; oxalate binds Ca and makes it unavailable, and phytate binds Ca, Mg and

other minerals. Vitamin D is needed for adequate Ca, P and Mg absorption.
- The animal's age: e.g. young animals absorb Ca and P more effectively than adults.
- Animal species: different species absorb minerals differently, e.g. the absorption of Mn by pigs (30–100%), horses (10–30%), and cattle (1%). The animal's demand for the mineral in question compared to the amount supplied by the feed. For example, growing pigs absorb 95% of STTD Ca but this figure drops to about 80% if more Ca is fed; horses fed a Ca-deficient diet absorb a greater proportion of Ca and exercising horses increase their absorption of Na; and P-deficient poultry absorb feed P much more efficiently than birds which are given their P requirement.

Any cited availability coefficient can only be an estimate, because for many minerals, particularly the trace and ultra-trace minerals, there are so many factors which influence availability and retention that it is very difficult indeed to get a value which applies in most situations. This is discussed more fully by Dryden (2008) and Goff (2018). Tables of feed nutritive values usually report just the total amounts of each mineral in the feed, e.g. total Mg, total Ca, etc. However, mineral sources fed as feed supplements may be treated differently: data on total contents of the primary minerals in these ingredients are published, with some authorities giving estimates of the bio-availabilities or digestibilities of Ca and P.

Quoting just the total mineral content of feeds does not mean that the problem of availability is ignored. Recommended mineral requirements are adjusted to take account of their expected availabilities.

Phosphorus: Much of the P in cereal grains and legume seeds occurs as phytic acid (Fig. 5.5). This plant storage form of P generally accounts for 50–80% of the total P in these feeds, although there are strains of some grains which have been bred to have a low phytic acid content. Phytate-P is largely unavailable to non-ruminant animals and poultry. Most of the P in vegetative plant material is in nucleic acids, phospholipids and ATP, although there is also some P stored as phytic acid.

P in animal-derived feeds such as meat meal and fish meal is present as nucleic acids, phospholipids and ATP. If the feed contains substantial amounts of bone, then most of the P will be in the form of

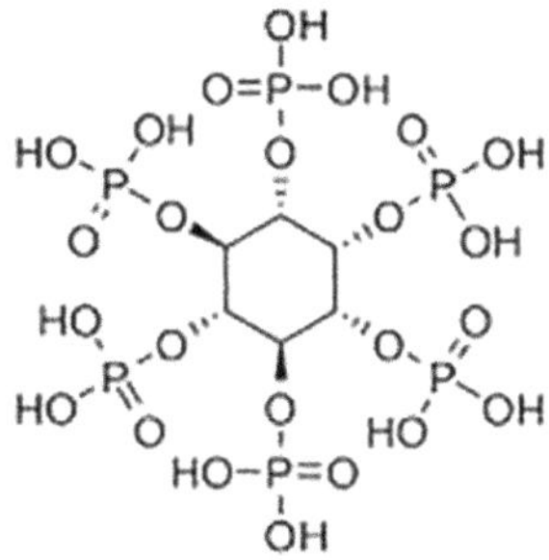

Fig. 5.5. Phytic acid. The structure in the middle of the molecule is a 6 C ring. (From Wikipedia, reproduced under the terms of CC BY SA 3.0.)

bone mineral (hydroxyapatite). P in these feeds is readily available.

Inorganic sources of P – mainly bone meal, phosphate rock and the salts of phosphoric acid – are often used as P supplements. In most cases, between 75% and 90% of the P in these substances is available to animals and birds.

Because of differences in their compositions, the availability of P (the available phosphorus, avP, content) in animal feeds is quite variable. Availability to horses is reviewed by Fowler *et al.* (2013), to cattle by NRC (2001, 2016) and to poultry by Li *et al.* (2016).

In summary, there are three types of information about P in feeds which help to predict animal performance:

- Total P content: this data is usually given for ruminant and horse feeds. It is also reported for pig and poultry feeds but for these species measures of non-phytate (i.e. available) P are much more useful, as explained below.
- Standardized (true) total tract digestible P content: data on the proportion of feed P which is digested in the small intestine is very useful because it indicates the absorbable P contents of the commercial diets which pigs and poultry are fed. The World Poultry Science Association has a standard method for measuring the STTD of feed P, although the method's reliability has been questioned. The NRC (2012) pig feeding standards report both STTD and ATTD measures for P for those feeds where there is published information.
- Phytate-P content: some authorities (e.g. NRC, 1994, 2012; INRAE, 2017–2020) report the phytate-P or non-phytate-P contents of feeds, especially of those seeds and grains which are

fed to pigs and poultry. The availability of phytate-P to pigs and poultry is usually very low (with some exceptions, because the activity of plant phytase in grains influences this) so the P available to monogastric animals in plant-based feeds can be approximated as the non-phytate-P. Ruminants are able to extract almost all of the P from phytate because microbial digestion in the rumen destroys phytate. Phytate-P is about 35% available for horses.

Phytase is an enzyme which breaks down phytic acid and releases its P atoms (see Chapter 11). If we add phytase to pig and poultry feeds (also sometimes in feeds given to cattle and sheep), this increases the availability of P in phytate-rich feeds. This means that avP data obtained without feeding phytase will underestimate the amount of P absorbed if phytase is included in the diet. In addition, phytase added to pig and poultry diets can increase the availability of other minerals (e.g. Ca, Zn, Cu), amino acids and energy. Because it has these wide-ranging effects, the amounts of nutrients released by added (exogenous) phytase to the diet (called the 'phytase matrix values') are taken into account when formulating rations.

Calcium: All nutritive value tables report the total Ca contents of feeds. There is some data for available Ca (avCa), especially for inorganic Ca sources fed to cattle.

Lucerne (alfalfa; *Medicago sativa*) is the most Ca-rich forage, with contents of 1.5–2.5% (DM basis). The content of Ca in most other forages is about 0.45–0.6% (DM basis). The Ca in forages is either ionized or is bound to phytic acid or to oxalic acid. The phytate- and oxalate-Ca is not readily available.

Almost all the Ca in meat meals and meat and bone meals is in the bone fraction of the meal. This Ca is in the form of hydroxyapatite, with absorption coefficients of up to 100% for all animals.

The Ca in mineral Ca sources, such as limestone and dicalcium phosphate, is also readily absorbed.

Much of the Ca in cereal grains is bound to phytate and is not very available. Pigs and poultry, dairy cattle fed a total mixed ration or a concentrate supplement, and lot-fed cattle fed grain-rich diets, are all given diets which have high cereal grain contents – usually 75–80% for pigs and poultry, and 50% or more for dairy cattle and lot-fed beef cattle. The amount of Ca supplied to the total feed from the cereal grains in these diets is very small in relation to animal requirements (cereal grains have between 0.03% and 0.09% Ca, DM basis) and so an inorganic Ca supplement has to be included. Consequently, in these diets, the availability of the Ca in cereal grains is not of much importance.

Copper: The factors which affect Cu availability include:

- The amount of Cu that the animal is currently storing in its liver and kidneys. Although 40–60% of dietary Cu is absorbed, much of this is excreted via the bile and is voided in the faeces. The amount of Cu excreted in this way depends on the amount of Cu stored in the liver (where it is mainly stored after absorption).
- Other minerals in the feed: Zn interferes with Cu absorption, and Fe with either absorption or release of Cu from the liver. Mo and SO_4 form an insoluble complex with Cu in the digestive tract, thus making Cu unavailable.
- Silicates and clay minerals in the soil ingested by grazing animals can bind Cu. It is interesting to note that grazing cattle can eat an amount of soil equivalent to 10% of their DM intake when grazing short pasture.
- Lignin and other plant fibre constituents can trap Cu, although this has probably a very small effect on Cu availability.
- Binding to microbial cells: Cu atoms may attach to microbial cells and thus become unavailable for absorption from the digestive tract.
- Animal genotype: there are species and individual differences in the ability to absorb Cu and to excrete excess Cu. Sheep are much more likely than other ruminants or monogastric animals to suffer from Cu poisoning.

Vitamins

Vitamins were originally identified by a number or letter, but their chemistries have been worked out and most are now referred to by their chemical name (see Table 1.4 in Chapter 1). Exceptions are the fat-soluble vitamins which have several provitamins and/or active chemical forms.

The contents of vitamins in feeds are expressed as mg/kg or µg/kg for the B group vitamins and vitamin C (1 mg/kg = 1000 µg/kg), and as mg/kg or international units of vitamin activity per kg (IU/kg) for the fat-soluble vitamins and/or their precursors.

Water-soluble vitamins: These are the B group vitamins and vitamin C (ascorbic acid) as listed in Table 1.4 in Chapter 1. They are present in feeds in their active form. The concentrations of these vitamins are given as the total amounts of each vitamin.

Note that we need to know the concentration in the feed of each individual B group vitamin. There is no such thing as 'vitamin B'!

Fat-soluble vitamins: The situation with the fat-soluble vitamins is more complicated. This is because they occur in feeds as different forms which have different vitamin activities, or as inactive precursors. Rather than stating the concentration of each of these differing forms or precursors, we state the potential concentration of active vitamin.

The contents of vitamins A, D and E in feeds are given as international units (IU) which is the unit which measures vitamin activity; the definition of an IU is different for each vitamin. In addition, different animal species convert precursors into active vitamins with differing efficiencies (see Dryden, 2008).

Vitamins E and K are present in feeds as the active vitamin. These vitamins exist in several different forms: vitamin E as a group of tocopherols and tocotrienols, and vitamin K as phylloquinone, menaquinone and menadione. Because each of these compounds has a different vitamin activity, we simply state the 'vitamin E' or 'vitamin K' activity in the feed. Vitamin E and K concentrations are given as mg/kg in some publications.

Vitamin A (retinol) is usually present as the inactive precursors α-, β- and γ-carotenes. Different animal species convert provitamins A to the active form with differing efficiencies. That means that the vitamin A activity content of a feed is different for each of the animal species that might be given that feed.

Cholecalciferol (vitamin D3) is the main form of vitamin D used by animals, and it is formed in the animal's skin by the action of ultraviolet light on cholesterol. Ergocalciferol (vitamin D2) is another active form, also formed by the action of ultraviolet light on its precursor, ergosterol. There are small amounts of ergosterol in animal feeds.

Feed nutritive value tables report either the total amount of vitamin, or the amount of active vitamin for a specified animal type. Do not mix active vitamin values between animal species.

Sources of feed nutritive value information

Most countries and regions publish their own feed quality data but as well as domestic data, we can use international nutritive value information in many cases. This applies especially when we are looking at the nutritive value of concentrates – e.g. cereal grains and their by-products, oilseeds and the meals made from them, and mineral sources. This is because there is surprisingly little difference between the nutritive values of these ingredients in different regions. This is not to say, though, that the effects of environment – weather, altitude, fertilization practices, etc. – do not affect feeds. Nevertheless, the averages that we find in most feed nutritive value tables give a reasonable indication of the expected nutritive value of a particular feed type. However, we should modify them to cater for particular growing and processing conditions (see below).

These three compendia provide information for a wide range of animal types and feeds, and animal managers in most places in the world will find useful information here:

- INRAE/CIRAD/AFZ/FAO (2012–2019), *Feedipedia, The Feed Resources Information System*: this resource has descriptive, nutritional and nutrient content information on 770 feeds. The data encompass pigs, poultry, horses and ruminants.
- INRAE (2017–2020), *INRAE-CIRAD-AFZ Feed Tables*: a large compendium of nutritive values of feeds for cattle, sheep, goats, pigs, poultry, rabbits, horses and salmonids.
- National Research Council (NRC, various dates): the *Nutrient Requirements of Domestic Animals* series is an up-to-date set of compilations published by the US National Academies Press. Although they are essentially North American, the values do apply to concentrate feeds found in other regions.

Other useful data are available from:

- Kyntäjä (2014), *Tables of Composition and Nutritional Values of Organically Produced Feed Materials for Pigs and Poultry*: this publication provides data on new feed sources such as insects and by-products in the different European feed evaluation systems.
- Preston (2018), *2018 Feed Composition Tables: Use this to mix your cattle feed rations*: this compilation of information on 280 cattle feeds is published by *BEEF* magazine.

- Evans (1985), *Nutrient Composition of Feedstuffs for Pigs and Poultry*: Michael Evans compiled this collection of nutritive value data for pig and poultry feeds. It includes valuable comments on the non-nutritive aspects of these feeds, e.g. toxicities, and effects of processing methods on nutritive value.
- International Livestock Research Institute (undated), *Sub-Saharan Africa Feed Composition Database*: listings of feed chemical composition, mostly derived from Ethiopian feeds.
- CABI (2019), *AHPC The Animal Health & Production Compendium*: a subscription database which has links to NRC, FAO and other databases.
- Blok and Spek (2016), *CVB Feed Table 2016*: a wide variety of information on feeds for ruminants, pigs, horses and poultry for Dutch feeds.

Variation from published nutritive values: Individual samples of feeds will have different nutritive values than the averages given in the tables (see Chapter 6). In particular:

- Roughage nutritive values vary with the stage of maturity of the plant when it was harvested, e.g. vegetative, early bloom, mid-bloom, etc. Choose a description which matches as closely as possible the sample that you have.
- Oilseed processing, especially the way that oil was extracted (e.g. expeller versus solvent extraction; Chapter 6), affects the composition of oilseed meals.
- The nutritive value of cereal grains varies according to the conditions under which they are grown, e.g. drought-affected grain has less starch and more protein than grain grown under better rainfall conditions.

Characteristics of feed nutritive value libraries

Information that is provided in most feed nutritive value tables: The types of data provided in feed libraries for pigs, birds, equines and ruminants are described below. The data is limited to what is available to the compilers; do not expect to find complete sets of data for all feeds.

In almost all cases, the values are displayed as means (averages), with a standard deviation (an indication of the variability in the original data used to compile the table) and a record of the number of samples contributing to the mean. How we can use this information is discussed in Chapter 9.

In general, all tables provide information on:

- The feed's 'proximate composition', i.e. its DM, CP, EE (crude fat), (crude) fibre (CF), and ash contents. The CF analysis has been superseded by the NDF and ADF analyses (for the reasons see Chapter 1), but CF is still often included for historical or legal reasons. Data on lignin and hemicellulose contents may also be included.
- Measures of available energy, protein and amino acids.
- The total contents of the major (e.g. Ca, P, Mg, Cl, K, Na and S) and trace (e.g. Co, Cu, I, Fe, Se, Mo, Mn and Zn) minerals. Some data sets have information on mineral availability, including phytate-P contents, and whole-tract apparent and true digestibilities.
- Contents in feeds of selected vitamins, especially vitamins A and D.

Feed libraries may use different names for the same feed (see Chapter 6). We can resolve this by referring to the NRC (1982) definitions of names of feeds and feed parts, and the INRAE/CIRAD/AFZ/FAO (2012–2019) *Feedipedia* also describes feeds in detail. Libraries may also use different methods of expressing feed constituent data. Usually, the nutrient contents of pig feeds are expressed on an 'as-fed' or 'whole feed' or '90% DM' basis, while the nutrient contents of horse and ruminant feeds are usually given on a DM basis. The reasons for this are discussed in Chapter 9.

Available energy contents are given as DE, ME and/or NE contents in most libraries; but other national or regional units such as TDN, UFV or UFL, and SFU are used in some data sets. If we want to combine data from different publications, e.g. use feed NE contents to formulate a diet to provide a given ME requirement, note that NE values are not directly translatable to ME because we have NE_m, NE_l and NE_g, i.e. values for maintenance, lactation and growth, and the efficiencies with which ME is used to meet these NE requirements all are different. In addition, these feed NE content values are quoted as though maintenance, milk production or growth is the only physiological function that the feed is used for.

The typical layout and content of feed nutritive value libraries is illustrated in the INRAE (2017–2020) tables. We should note that these data cover an unusually wide variety of animal species: ruminants (with an emphasis on beef and dairy cattle), pigs, poultry, horses, rabbits and salmonids. This is unusual – many libraries are compiled with a particular species or animal type in mind. The included data are selected for appropriateness, e.g. blood meal is not fed to ruminants because of the risk of transmitting bovine spongiform encephalopathy (mad cow disease), and the entry for this feed does not include any ruminant data. As well, there is information for feeds which have recently come into use in animal feeding, e.g. insect meals.

This web-based library allows the user to roll the cursor over each entry and get a definition of the nutrient and a brief description of how it was measured. It is also possible to replace the default values with custom analytical values by using the Feedinamics program. The table automatically updates certain constituent contents, e.g. NDF if the ADF value is changed, or NE content if the ME content is varied. Also, there are options to display nutrient contents on DM or as-fed bases, or both.

Horse, pig and poultry feed libraries provide:

- Comprehensive information on both essential and non-essential amino acids, including total amounts and apparent and/or true (standardized) ileal digestibilities. Particularly important are data on the most often limiting amino acids – lysine, methionine, threonine and tryptophan for pigs; lysine, glycine and serine for poultry; and lysine for horses.
- Data on individual fatty acids, especially linoleic acid, is useful because of the effect of dietary fat composition on pig meat quality. This can be provided either as concentrations in the total feed or in the feed fat (ether extract). As well as data for each fatty acid, values for the total contents of short-chain fatty acids, monounsaturated fatty acids (MUFA) and polyunsaturated fatty acids (PUFA) can be provided, and/or the overall iodine value (IV; an index of the degree of unsaturation; see Fig. 1.2 in Chapter 1). It is best if the individual fatty acids are cited by name, but they can be referenced by the number of carbon atoms and number of double bonds. To interpret this: 18:2 is linoleic acid, 18:3 is α-linolenic acid and 20:4 is arachidonic acid.
- Values for all vitamins. This includes the water-soluble vitamins (see Chapter 1) – vitamin C and the nine B group vitamins, and the fat-soluble vitamins – A, D, E and K. In some libraries, β-carotene concentrations are given, either as well as or instead of active vitamin A. β-Carotene data may have to be converted to the equivalent active vitamin A contents (IU/kg) as some nutrient requirement tables cite the vitamin A requirement rather than a β-carotene requirement.

Data for ruminant feeds reflect the special effects of rumen metabolism on feed intake and the supply of nutrients. Ruminant feed data includes:

- Measures of available energy include contents of ME, NE_m and NE_g (NE for maintenance and growth) and NE_l (NE for lactating cows); some libraries may include DE. TDN is retained in the NRC (2000, 2001, 2007b) tables because it is still widely used in North American cattle and sheep feeding. Also, the ME and NE values published in the beef cattle tables (NRC, 2000) are derived from calculated TDN values. Feed digestibility falls slightly as the feeding level increases, and this is reflected in the feed's available energy content. The NRC (2001) dairy standards include a refinement of TDN, DE, ME and NE data (see their Table 15-1) where they cite 'DE-1X', 'NE_l-4X', etc. values. The X values indicate the feeding level – 1X means that the available energy contents were measured when cows were fed a maintenance level of feed, and 3X and 4X indicate that these values for ME and NE were determined or predicted for cows fed 3 and 4 times their maintenance requirement.
- Effective NDF (eNDF; Chapter 1) is a useful indicator of the potential effects of the feed on rumen health, and milk fat content for dairy cattle.
- Information on the rumen degradability of feed protein is essential for the accurate feeding of ruminants. This is given either as protein degradability (% RDP in the feed or feed protein), or as measures of the undegradable protein (UDP, % of feed or feed protein). The concentrations of protein insoluble in neutral detergent (NDFIP, NDIN or NDICP) and in acid detergent (ADFIP, ADIN or ADICP) give additional information about the feed protein's probable rumen degradability. Some libraries provide estimates of the rates at which feed proteins are degraded in the rumen (K_d, %/hour) and this allows us to calculate their effective degradabilities (Edg). In addition, it is useful to have estimates of the digestibility of UDP in the small intestine. These data are useful to predict the amount of MP likely to flow to the duodenum.
- Some libraries also have data on metabolizable protein contents.

- Essential amino acids (see Table 1.3 in Chapter 1) contents are useful data, even though they may not be routinely considered in ruminant feed formulations other than those for dairy cattle. Amino acid contents can be reported as % of the total protein or, more usefully, as % of the UDP (e.g. Appendix Table 1 in the NRC (2000) beef standards), or truly digestible amino acid as a % of MP (INRAE, 2017–2020).

What feed composition information is most useful? The libraries discussed above have information that is useful for commercial feed milling companies or animal science consultants who will use the mathematical models built on these feeding standards. But if we simply want some guidance on how to make up a feed for our animals, we need to identify which of this mass of information is likely to be the most useful.

In brief, we will most usefully use information on:

- Energy: we must match the feed energy supply with the animal's energy requirement. Identify the available energy unit used in the nutrient requirements table (e.g. TDN, SFU, DE, ME, NE, etc.). If several are given, then choose the one which we are comfortable with.
- Amino acids and protein: lysine is usually the first limiting amino acid, although others might be limiting as well (see above and Chapters 1 and 8). Also check the total protein content, as meeting this requirement will help to ensure that the requirements for non-essential amino acids are met. Remember that ruminants need adequate RDP and UDP and that these have to be considered separately.
- Minerals: Table 1.5 in Chapter 1 has a list of the most important minerals, i.e. those that are most likely to be limiting in normal animal management. Be aware of needs for Ca, especially if we are dealing with laying poultry, pigs, dairy cattle fed a total mixed ration based on cereal grains, and lot-fed beef cattle. Grazing animals are much less likely to need a Ca supplement, although they may need P and trace minerals supplements depending on soil and pasture type, and season. Available Ca, and available or non-phytate-P, are preferred to total Ca and P if this information is provided in the library.
- Vitamins: monogastric animals must be provided with B vitamins as these are likely to be deficient in cereal-based diets. Poultry and domestic animals (but not guinea pigs or primates) are able to synthesize vitamin C themselves, but heat-stressed poultry may respond well to a supplement. Check the vitamin A status of pigs and poultry. Grazing animals are not likely to be vitamin A deficient. Animals and birds make vitamin D3 in their skin when they are exposed to ultraviolet light, and we can assume that grazing ruminants and horses, grazing pigs and free-range poultry do not need a vitamin D supplement. However, animals kept outdoors in high latitudes in winter, and housed animals, may become deficient. But note that excess vitamin D is toxic and causes calcification of soft tissues (e.g. heart and blood vessels), kidney damage, and brittle and deformed bones.

References

Alvarenga, R.R., Rodrigues, P.B., Zangeronimo, M.G., Makiyama, L., Oliveira, E.C., Freitas, R.T.F., Lima, E.M.C. and Bernardino, V.M.P. (2013). Validation of prediction equations to estimate the energy values of feedstuffs for broilers: performance and carcass yield. *Asian-Australasian Journal of Animal Science* 26(10): 1474–1483.

Baker, D.H. (2009). Advances in protein–amino acid nutrition of poultry. *Amino Acids* 37: 29–41.

Blok, M.C. and Spek, J.W. (2016). *CVB Feed Table 2016. Chemical Composition and Nutritional Values of Feedstuffs*. Zoetermeer, The Netherlands: Federatie Nederlandse Diervoederketen.

CABI (2019). *AHPC. The Animal Health & Production Compendium.* Available at: www.cabi.org/ahpc (accessed 26 December 2020).

Commonwealth Scientific and Industrial Research Organisation (CSIRO) (2007). *Nutrient Requirements of Domesticated Ruminants*. Collingwood, Vic., Australia: CSIRO Publishing.

Corbett, J.L. and Freer, M. (2003). Past and present definitions of the energy and protein requirements of ruminants. *Asian-Australasian Journal of Animal Science* 16(4): 609–624.

Dryden, G.McL. (2008). *Animal Nutrition Science*. Wallingford, UK: CAB International.

Evans, M. (1985). *Nutrient Composition of Feedstuffs for Pigs and Poultry*. Brisbane: Queensland Department of Primary Industries.

Fowler, A.L., Strasinger, L.A., Hansen, T.L., Davis, B.E., Hayes, S.H. and Lawrence L.M. (2013). The availability of dietary phosphorus to long yearlings and mature horses. *Journal of Equine Veterinary Science* 33(5): 342–343.

Goff, J.P. (2018). Invited review: Mineral absorption mechanisms, mineral interactions that affect acid–base and antioxidant status, and diet considerations to improve mineral status. *Journal of Dairy Science* 101: 2763–2813.

INRAE (2017–2020). *INRAE-CIRAD-AFZ Feed Tables*. Available at: www.feedtables.com/ (accessed 26 December 2020).

INRAE/CIRAD/AFZ/FAO (2012–2019). *Feedipedia, The Feed Resources Information System*. Available at: www.feedipedia.org (accessed 26 December 2020).

International Livestock Research Institute (undated). *Sub-Saharan Africa Feed Composition Database*. Available at: https://feedsdatabase.ilri.org/ (accessed 18 March 2021).

Jarrige, R. (1989). *Ruminant Nutrition. Recommended Allowances and Feed Tables*. Paris: INRA and Paris-London-Rome: John Libbey Eurotext.

Kil, D.Y., Kim, B.G. and Stein, H.H. (2013). Feed energy evaluation for growing pigs. *Asian-Australasian Journal of Animal Science* 26(9): 1205–1217.

Krebs, H.A. (1973). The discovery of the ornithine cycle of urea synthesis. *Biochemical Education* 1: 19–23.

Kyntäjä, S. (2014). *Tables of Composition and Nutritional Values of Organically Produced Feed Materials for Pigs and Poultry*. Available at: www.orgprints.org/28116 (accessed 26 December 2020).

Li, X., Zhang, D., Yang, T.Y. and Bryden, W.L. (2016). Phosphorus bioavailability: a key aspect for conserving this critical animal feed resource with reference to broiler nutrition. *Agriculture* 6, 25. DOI: 10.3390/agriculture6020025.

Lopez, G. and Leeson, S. (2007). Relevance of nitrogen correction for assessment of metabolizable energy with broilers to forty-nine days of age. *Poultry Science* 86: 1696–1704.

Moore, J.E. and Undersander, D.J. (2002). Relative Forage Quality: An Alternative to Relative Feed Value and Quality Index. *Proceedings of the 13th Annual Florida Ruminant Nutrition Symposium*, pp 16-32. Available at: www.researchgate.net/publication/268354500_Relative_Forage_Quality_An_Alternative_to_Relative_Feed_Value_and_Quality_Index (accessed 26 December 2020).

National Research Council (NRC) (1982). *Feed Composition: Nutritional Data for United States and Canadian Feeds*, 3rd rev. edn. Washington, DC: National Academies Press. Available at: www.nap.edu/catalog/1713/united-states-canadian-tables-of-feed-composition-nutritional-data-for (accessed 26 December 2020).

National Research Council (NRC) (1994). *Nutrient Requirements of Poultry*, 9th rev. edn. Washington, DC: National Academies Press. Available at: https://www.nap.edu/catalog/2114/nutrient-requirements-of-poultry-ninth-revised-edition-1994 (accessed 11 March 2021).

National Research Council (NRC) (2000). *Nutrient Requirements of Beef Cattle*, 7th rev. edn. Update 2000. Washington, DC: National Academies Press. Available at: www.nap.edu/catalog/9791/nutrient-requirements-of-beef-cattle-seventh-revised-edition-update-2000 (accessed 26 December 2020).

National Research Council (NRC) (2001). *Nutrient Requirements of Dairy Cattle*, 7th rev. edn. Washington, DC: National Academies Press Available at: www.nap.edu/catalog/9825/nutrient-requirements-of-dairy-cattle-seventh-revised-edition-2001 (accessed 26 December 2020).

National Research Council (NRC) (2007a). *Nutrient Requirements of Horses*, 6th rev. edn. Washington, DC: National Academies Press. Available at: www.nap.edu/catalog/11653/nutrient-requirements-of-horses-sixth-revised-edition (accessed 26 December 2020).

National Research Council (NRC) (2007b). *Nutrient Requirements of Small Ruminants*. Washington, DC: National Academies Press. Available at: www.nap.edu/catalog/11654/nutrient-requirements-of-small-ruminants-sheep-goats-cervids-and-new (accessed 26 December 2020).

National Research Council (NRC) (2012). *Nutrient Requirements of Swine*, 11th rev. edn. Washington, DC: National Academies Press. Available at: www.nap.edu/catalog/13298/nutrient-requirements-of-swine-eleventh-revised-edition (accessed 26 December 2020).

National Research Council (NRC) (2016). *Nutrient Requirements of Beef Cattle*, 8th rev. edn. Washington, DC: National Academies Press. Available at: www.nap.edu/catalog/19014/nutrient-requirements-of-beef-cattle-eighth-revised-edition (accessed 26 December 2020).

Ørskov, E.R. and McDonald, I. (1979). The estimation of protein degradability in the rumen from incubation measurements weighted according to rate of passage. *Journal of Agricultural Science* 92(2): 499–503.

Pagan, J.D. (1998). Measuring the digestible energy content of horse feeds. In J.D. Pagan (ed.). *Advances in Equine Nutrition*. Nottingham: Nottingham University Press, pp. 71–76.

Preston, R.L. (2018). *2018 Feed Composition Tables: Use this to mix your cattle feed rations*. Available at: www.beefmagazine.com/nutrition/2018-feed-composition-tables-use-mix-your-cattle-feed-rations (accessed 8 January 2021).

Sundstøl, F. (1993). Energy systems for ruminants. *Búvísindi Iceland Agricultural Science* 7: 11–19.

Undersander, D., Moore, J.E. and Schneider, N. (2010). Relative forage quality. *Focus on Forage* 12(No. 6): 1–3. Available at: www.foragelab.com/Media/Relative_Forage_Quality.pdf (accessed 26 December 2020).

Wolynetz, M.S. and Sibbald, I.R. (1984). Relationships between apparent and true metabolizable energy and the effects of a nitrogen correction. *Poultry Science* 63: 1386–1399.

6 Animal feeds

Animal feed classification

We often find that we are unable to get supplies of the feeds that we have been using. Seasonal and market factors may mean that particular feeds are unavailable or expensive. This means that we have to change the feeds we use, but the question is how to choose new feeds that are similar to the old, and which will do the job that we want them to do – i.e. to provide the required amounts of nutrients, to be accepted and eaten readily, and to avoid causing digestive or other problems. The answer lies in feed classification.

Feed classification is the grouping together of feeds in classes, so that within a class, feeds have similar nutritive values and can be used in similar ways. Animal feeds can be grouped into several different categories, or classes, based on:

- their available nutrient content;
- the types and amounts of constituents such as fibre and starch;
- the feed's origin, e.g. animal or plant or processing by-product;
- the part of the original material which makes up the feed;
- any processing that the feed has been subjected to; and
- the feed's physical characteristics.

Using feed classification to select feeds and feed replacements/alternatives: Feeds in the same class have similar nutritive values, are likely to have similar effects on animal health and product quality and can be used in similar ways to make up rations. On the other hand, feeds in different classes are relatively dissimilar.

Feed classification will help to predict the quality and potential use of a novel feed if we know what feed class it belongs to. In addition, we can use classification to choose alternatives for a feed which is no longer available.

A caution: always be cautious in using feed classifications – do not assume that all of the feeds in a particular class are similar enough to be substituted for each other without appropriate care.

Feed names: All animal feeds have common, or local, names, but this can cause confusion. For example, 'corn' can mean maize (*Zea mays*) or wheat (*Triticum aestivum*) or oats (*Avena sativa*), or indeed any cereal grain depending on where we are. 'Meat meal' can mean a meal made by drying, rendering and grinding either the soft tissues of an animal carcase, or more loosely the whole carcase residues including bone; and 'wheat middlings' can mean the same thing as 'millrun'.

So, we need a naming system which removes this ambiguity. Protocols developed by the International Network of Feed Information Centres (INFIC), and later adopted by other national and international authorities, name feeds according to their:

- Origin: either plant, animal, mineral, vitamin, etc. In the case of plant and animal origins, we might indicate the taxonomic name (e.g. *Medicago sativa* for lucerne (alfalfa)) and also the variety or strain.
- Part fed to animals as affected by processing: this may be 'grain' or 'gluten meal' or 'by-product' or 'meal without hulls'.
- Processing or treatment: if the plant material is cut and cured then the name would include terms such as 'dry' or 'sun-cured', while meals made from oilseeds would include 'solvent extracted' or 'mechanically extracted'.
- Stage of maturity: terms used for plant material include 'early bloom' or 'mid-bloom'.
- Cutting: e.g. '4 weeks'; this nomenclature is not often used, but it may help to describe a particular class of forage crop.
- Grade: the nutrient content of some feeds can vary widely according to how they are made; an example is the protein content of oilseed meals.

DOI: 10.1079/9781786394453.0006

This method gives unambiguous names, and they are used in some feed libraries. But they are complex and long and are not really suited to everyday use. Local or common names are generally used.

Feed classification systems: there are several ways to classify animal feeds, some are more satisfactory than others. The system described here is based on that suggested by INFIC (Alderman *et al.*, 1983), which identifies eight classes of feeds. These are:

- dry forages and roughages;
- pasture, range plants, and forages which have not been cut and cured;
- silages;
- energy feeds;
- protein supplements;
- mineral sources;
- vitamin sources; and
- additives.

Although the INFIC system includes categories for minerals, vitamins and additives, feed classification is usually applied only to so-called 'whole feeds', i.e. those materials which we recognize as animal feeds and which each provide a range of nutrients. Sources of minerals and vitamins, and additives such as rumen modifiers, pellet binders, feed flavours and so on are not generally included in feed classifications.

Although adequate, the INFIC classification is relatively simple. A more detailed list is the 19 classes used in *Feedipedia* (INRAE/CIRAD/AFZ/FAO, 2012–2019).

Concentrates and roughages: The main classification is based on the feed's plant fibre content. Fibre-rich feeds, i.e. those with more than 18% crude fibre (equivalent to about 24% acid detergent fibre (ADF)) on a dry matter (DM) basis, are referred to as roughages. These are feeds such as silages, hays and straws. They contain large amounts of the vegetative parts of plants, for example stems, leaves and seed heads. The threshold value of 18% crude fibre is used in this discussion, but this is quite arbitrary and we are free to use whatever value we feel is appropriate.

Low-fibre feeds are referred to as concentrates because they have relatively high concentrations of available energy, protein and other nutrients. Concentrate feeds include cereal grains, animal and plant protein meals, and feeds rich in fats or soluble sugars.

Feed nutritive values: The following discussion outlines the nutrient content of feeds in the major feed classes. These data are summaries of published information. More detailed data on feed nutrient content is in the list of sources in Chapter 5 and the references in this chapter.

Where possible, always check the nutritive value of the actual sample before using it.

Nutritive value of concentrates

Concentrates are separated into two main classes – energy concentrates with less than 20% protein, and protein concentrates with 20% or more protein. The different types and their sub-classes are shown in Fig. 6.1.

In most cases the placement of concentrate feeds is straightforward, but legume grains (also called 'pulses') have protein contents which are not much higher than the 20% threshold. These feeds are in the 'Plant protein meals' group because of their protein content but they could also be placed in the 'Energy-rich concentrates' category. Cereal by-products have a wide range of fibre and starch contents, but we can distinguish between milling by-products and the by-products of brewing and ethanol production. Generally, the protein contents of milling by-products are less than the 20% threshold and are classed as 'Energy-rich concentrates', while distillers' and brewers' grains have quite high protein contents and are classed as 'Protein-rich concentrates'.

Nutritive value of energy-rich concentrates

Cereal grains: These are the seeds of barley, maize (corn), millet, oats, rice, rye, sorghum, triticale and wheat, as well as several other less common grains including 'pseudo-cereals' such as buckwheat and quinoa.

Cereal grains are essentially energy feeds as their main constituent is starch, which is an energy reserve for the growing plant embryo. Most grains have 60% or more starch: barley and rye have 60–62%, triticale and wheat have 68–69%, maize and sorghum 73–75%, and rice (brown) has 87% starch. Oats are an outlier as they have only 40% starch, the lowest level of the cereal grains, and a comparatively high fibre content. Grains with higher bulk densities have more starch and higher available energy contents.

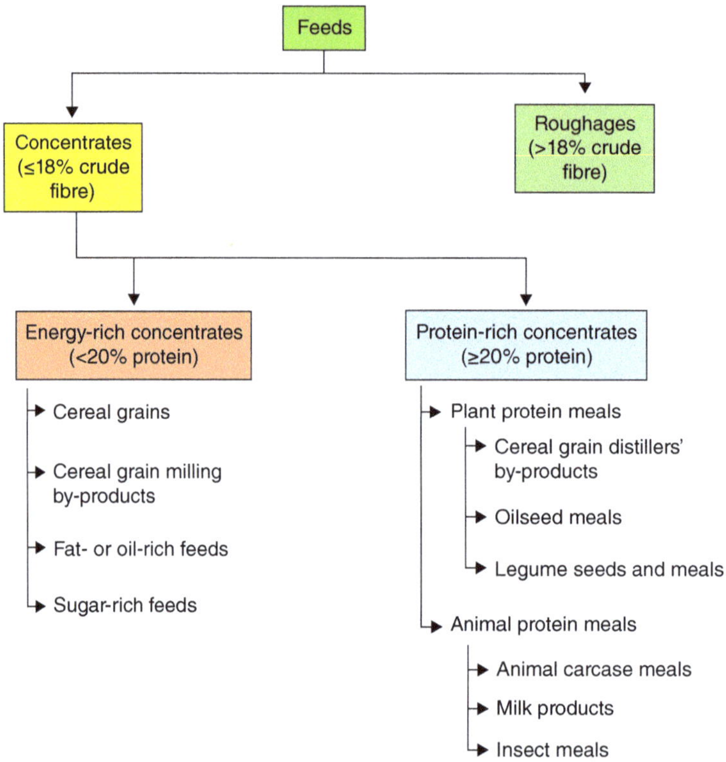

Fig. 6.1. Classification of 'concentrate' feeds according to their nutrient contents and origins. (Copyright: Gordon McL. Dryden.)

Starch is potentially readily digested by both micro-organisms in the reticulo-rumen and large intestine, and the animal's own intrinsic digestive enzymes in the small intestine. However, the way that the starch granules are packed in the endosperm cells, the nature of the protein network which enmeshes these granules, and the proportions of amylose and amylopectin in the starch itself all influence the susceptibility of starch to digestion (Chapter 4). Barley, triticale and wheat starch is readily fermented in the rumen with degradabilities of 89–94%, brown rice starch is 74% degradable, while maize and sorghum starches are less degradable at 60% and 62%, respectively (INRAE/CIRAD/AFZ, 2017–2020).

Cereal grains have modest protein contents, between about 8% and 16%, depending on grain type and growing conditions. N fertilization increases the protein content, as does water stress, although this occurs because droughted (or 'pinched') grain has less starch. Cereal grain protein is not an excellent source of essential amino acids, with lysine contents of about 3% of the grain protein compared to grain legumes and oilseed meals which have up to 6%. Cereal grain protein is degraded in the rumen to different extents: the potential degradabilities of sorghum and maize protein are 43–47%, brown rice 69%, and barley, triticale and wheat 71–77%.

Other characteristics of cereal grains are:

- They are very palatable, and most are accepted readily by all animals. 'Bird-resistant' sorghum is an exception because of its high tannin content.
- They are not good sources of minerals. Most of the phosphorus (P) in these feeds is phytate P and so is essentially unavailable to pigs and poultry unless we use an added phytase enzyme, and they have very low calcium (Ca) contents (see also Chapter 5).

- Barley, rye, oats, wheat and triticale contain arabinoxylans and β-glucans which impair the action of digestive enzymes (see Chapter 11).
- Sorghum contains tannins between about 0.3% in low-tannin varieties to 5% or 6% in older varieties and up to 10% in bird-resistant types. These tannins reduce the availably of protein and digestibility of the grain DM.
- Cereal grains are good habitats for moulds and *Salmonella* if they become damp in storage.

While the high starch contents, and their palatability, make these feeds potentially very useful energy sources, unwise feeding practices such as allowing horses and ruminants access to quantities of this starch-rich feed can cause severe rumen disorders and laminitis (see Chapter 13). To reduce this risk, we must carefully adapt animals to grain-rich diets. In addition, but less effectively, we can use information on starch and dietary protein degradabilities to choose grain types which are less likely to cause rumen acidosis or which are more likely to contribute ruminally undegradable dietary protein (UDP) to the diet; sorghum and maize fit both these categories.

Nutrient content data for cereal grains are summarized in Table 6.1. Use these data with caution: variety and growing conditions have significant effects on the nutrient content of cereal grains.

Cereal processing by-products: These are an important sub-group of energy-rich concentrate feeds. They are derived from the milling of mainly barley, maize (corn) and wheat, although sorghum, oats and rye products are also used.

This feed class includes (see also INRAE/CIRAD/AFZ/FOA 2012–2019):

- milling by-products: bran, middlings or millrun, pollard or shorts, hominy feed and several other fractions; or
- starch and germ oil extraction residues: gluten meal and gluten feed.

The composition of cereal milling by-products varies, affected by the type of milling that is used, sieving methods, and how different milling fractions are re-combined after separation. Commonly used flour milling by-products are:

- Wheat middlings: which contain varying proportions of endosperm, embryo (germ) and bran. The 'average' starch, protein and crude fibre contents are 27%, 18% and 6% (DM basis), respectively.
- Wheat bran: this is the pericarp and seedcoat (see Fig. 4.3, Chapter 4) which are removed from the

Table 6.1. Nutritive value of selected cereal grains (dry matter (DM) basis). (Data from INRAE/CIRAD/AFZ/FAO, 2012–2019; INRAE/ CIRAD/AFZ, 2017–2020.)

	Barley[a]	Maize[b]	Sorghum[c]	Wheat[d]
ME (ruminants) (MJ/kg DM)	12.4	13.5	13.5	13.1
ME (pigs) (MJ/kg)	14.6	15.9	16.1	15.5
AME_n (poultry) (MJ/kg DM)	11.3	15.1	15.7	13.8
DE (horses) (MJ/kg DM)	14.6	16.0	16.1	15.6
Protein (% DM)	12	9	11	13
Lysine (% protein)	3.7	3.1	2.2	2.9
Methionine (% protein)	1.7	2.1	1.7	1.6
NDF (% DM)	22	12	11	14
Fat (% DM)	2	4	3	2
Linoleic acid (% DM)	0.8	2.1	1.0	0.76
Ca (% DM)	0.08	0.05	0.03	0.07
Non-phytate P (% DM)	0.18	0.06	0.11	0.13

[a]*Hordeum vulgare*,
[b]*Zea mays*
[c]*Sorghum bicolor*
[d]*Triticum* spp.

grain at the first break milling. In practice, bran also includes fragments of endosperm. The 'average' starch, protein and crude fibre contents are 23%, 16% and 12% (DM basis), respectively.

- Shorts (also called pollard): contain the embryo, fine particles of bran and small amounts of endosperm. In some mills shorts and bran are distinguished by their particle size rather than by how they are generated during milling.
- Millrun: is a by-product which has different origins and thus different compositions. Millrun can be the same as 'middlings', or it can be either the whole non-endosperm fractions separated during milling, or a re-mixture of bran and pollard.

The fibre and starch contents of the by-products of flour milling vary inversely: feed flour has 69% starch and 1% fibre, while bran has 23% starch and 10% fibre. On the other hand, their protein contents (except for maize gluten meal which has about 65% protein, DM basis) are all similar (Fig. 6.2).

Milling by-products retain the grain's bran (pericarp and seedcoat), but they also contain varying amounts of endosperm and embryo (germ). Consequently, their protein and fibre contents are higher than those of the cereal grain parent material, but less than the concentrations found in brewers' or distillers' grain (see protein concentrates, below). The nutrient contents of milling by-products are summarized in Table 6.2.

In summary, cereal milling by-products:

- are used as sources of available energy and protein, and to improve feed palatability;
- can have laxative properties for non-ruminants;
- are bulky because of their fibre content; this can make them difficult to handle and can make feed mixtures 'bridge' (become stuck and not flow through openings; Chapter 17) in bins and silos;
- should be generally limited to 15% of feed mixtures because of their bulk, and the effect of their fibre diluting the available energy in pig and poultry rations; and
- may become rancid in storage if they have high fat contents.

Sugar-rich feeds: This group includes several feeds. Molasses (cane and beet) has large amounts of soluble sugars such as sucrose, glucose and fructose. Other sugar-rich feeds include some bakery wastes (e.g. biscuit and bun waste), which have high sucrose contents, and whey and milk permeate, which have high lactose contents.

Molasses is widely used in animal feeding, either as a ration component or as a major ingredient (as in molasses-based beef cattle lot feeding). Molasses has these nutritional characteristics:

- The high soluble sugar content of molasses makes it a good source of available energy (Table 6.3), but it is not a good source of amino acids, fibre or fatty acids.

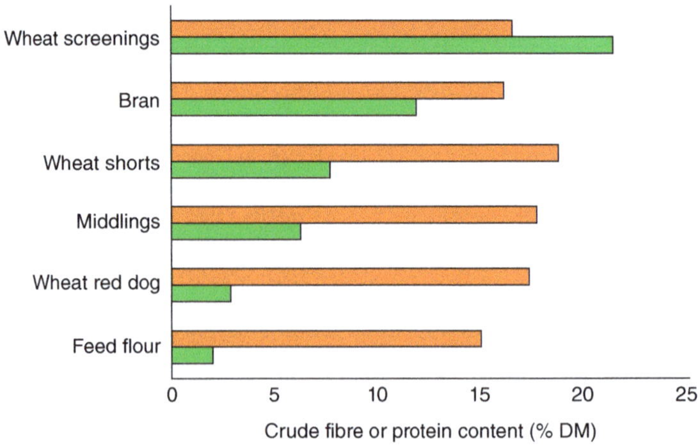

Fig. 6.2. Crude fibre (green) and protein (orange) contents of selected wheat milling by-products. (Copyright: Gordon McL. Dryden. Data are averages from INRAE/CIRAD/AFZ/FAO, 2012–2019; INRAE/CIRAD/AFZ, 2017–2020; NRC, 1982, 2001, 2012.)

Table 6.2. Indicative data on the nutritive value of cereal grain milling by-products (dry matter (DM) basis). (Data from Evans, 1985; NRC, 2007, 2012; INRAE/CIRAD/AFZ/FAO, 2012–2019; INRAE/CIRAD/AFZ, 2017–2020.)

	Rice bran[a]	Wheat bran[b]	Wheat middlings[b]	Wheat millrun[b]
ME (ruminants) (MJ/kg DM)	10.1	11.0	11.7	11.0
ME (pigs) (MJ/kg DM)	11.3	11.0	12.9	10.8[c]
AME_n (poultry) (MJ/kg DM)	10.3	7.4	9.5	7.4
DE (horses) (MJ/kg DM)	11.8	12.6	13.8	14.2
Protein (% DM)	13	17	18	17
Lysine (% protein)	4.4	4	0.7	4
Methionine (% protein)	1.9	1.5	0.3	1.5
NDF (% DM)	33	45	35	45
Fat (% DM)	14	4	4	4
Linoleic acid (% DM)	4.0	1.7	2.0	1.9
Ca (% DM)	0.09	0.14	0.13	0.14
Non-phytate P (% DM)	0.18	0.22	0.19	0.11

[a]'Full-fat' rice bran, 11–20% crude fibre.
[b]See the text for descriptions of these products.
[c]Estimated.

Table 6.3. Indicative nutrient contents for selected sugar-rich feeds (dry matter (DM) basis). (Data from NRC, 2001, 2007, 2012; INRAE/CIRAD/AFZ/FAO, 2012–2019, INRAE/CIRAD/AFZ, 2017–2020.)

	Bakery waste[a]	Molasses[b]	Molasses[c]	Whey (dried)
ME (ruminants) (MJ/kg DM)	15.5	12.0	11.6	12.3
ME (pigs) (MJ/kg)	18.5	13.3	13.2	14.7
AME_n (poultry) MJ/kg	13.2	9.3	9.8	8.2
DE (horses) (MJ/kg DM)	16.3[d]	17.0	17.0	–
Protein (% DM)	11	8.5	5.5	13
Total sugars (% DM)	14	63	63	71
Lysine (% protein)	3.3	1.0	0.1	7.6
Methionine (% protein)	1.5	0.3	0.3	1.4
NDF (% DM)	9	0.1	0.4	0
Fat (% DM)	12.3	0.2	0.2	1
Linoleic acid (% DM)	0.63	0.1	0.1	Trace
Ca (% DM)	0.1	0.15	0.9	0.5
Non-phytate P (% DM)	0.2	0.03	0.1	0.6

[a]This is a very variable product; biscuit wastes can contain 30% or 40% sugars.
[b]Molasses from sugar beet (*Beta vulgaris*).
[c]Molasses from sugar cane (*Saccharum officinarum*).
[d]Estimated.

- Beet and sugarcane molasses are palatable (although citrus molasses is bitter and may be rejected initially by pigs) and can be used to mask unpalatable ingredients such as urea.
- Molasses as a major ration ingredient must be used carefully. Its sugars are rapidly and completely digested and excesses could cause rumen disorders and laminitis. When used in molasses

lot feeding it should be fed with urea to provide ruminally available N and to control intake, and with a good quality roughage and a source of UDP to provide fibre and glucogenic amino acids.

Molasses has a high DM content – typically 76% for sugarcane molasses. Nevertheless, the product is a liquid, although sugarcane molasses is very viscous especially in cold weather when it may need to be heated to make it easy to handle. Its viscosity makes it difficult to mix into dry ingredients but helps to stabilize feed mixtures once it has been adequately incorporated. Sugar beet molasses is less viscous than cane molasses.

Molasses is stable in storage at less than 38°C provided that no water has been added. During storage, CO_2 gas is generated from chemical reactions between amino acids and sugars, and from microbial fermentation. The gas dissolves in the molasses and temporarily increases its volume by up to 20%.

Whey and milk permeate are by-products of cheese and butter manufacture. During cheese-making, whey separates from the curd produced when casein is acted upon by chymosin (also called rennin). Permeate is produced when milk intended for cheese- or butter-making is passed through an ultrafilter to remove some of the non-fat and non-casein components.

Whey and milk permeate have similar compositions. They have high water contents, and their DM fraction includes lactose, the whey proteins and minerals (Table 6.3). They are good energy sources, provide a reasonable amount of protein (which is almost completely degraded in the rumen), and are good sources of lysine, Ca and P.

Whey powder is often a major ingredient in milk replacers (feeds for unweaned animals), although whey proteins do not form a fat/protein clot in the same way that casein does.

Starch-rich feeds include:

- Cassava meal: made from the roots of the cassava plant. It is a starch-rich feed (65–75% starch) and a useful energy source, although the content of other nutrients is low. Bitter and sweet cassava varieties both contain poisonous cyanogenic glucosides which must be removed before they are fed.
- Bakery products: have starch contents of 52–75%. Some products, e.g. biscuits and buns, can have as much as 30–40% sugars, although commercial white and wholemeal breads have much less – only about 3%. A hidden problem with bread and similar products is that they are often contaminated with plastic wrappers and unless care is taken to remove these, the product will contain plastic residues.

Starch-rich feeds are used as cheap sources of available energy and can replace some of the cereal grain in cattle and pig feeds.

Fat or oil-rich feeds: examples include tallow and lard, and vegetable oils. Tallow and lard are both derived from the rendering of animal tissue – tallow from ruminants and lard from pigs. Ruminant carcase fat is more saturated (Chapter 1) than fat from pigs or poultry and this affects their melting points – tallow is solid at up to 40°C while lard melts at temperatures above 20°C. Oils are liquid at usual ambient temperatures. Although the fat content of most fats and oils is nearly 100%, some commercial grades contain up to 5% moisture and substances other than fatty acids.

The energy content and fatty acid composition of some commonly used fats are summarized in Table 6.4. Fats and oils have very high total energy contents, typically 39 MJ/kg DM, or 2.25 times more than other feeds. However, they contain no protein, starch, fibre, minerals or B vitamins, and only small amounts of fat-soluble vitamins. They are rich sources of energy and fatty acids, but their contribution to the supply of other nutrients is minimal.

Some conventional feeds are rich in fat, e.g. meat meals made from some animal carcasses, and raw or un-extracted oilseeds (e.g. full-fat soybean meal) which have between 30% and 50% vegetable oil.

Oils and unsaturated fats may oxidize in storage and become rancid. Do not allow fats or oils to come into contact with brass, copper or galvanized fittings as Cu and Zn catalyse the oxidation reactions. Added water also promotes rancidity.

Fats and oils are used to:

- Increase the available energy content in feeds such as milk replacers where the main ingredients are skim milk and whey, and in feeds for performance horses.
- Bind the ingredients in a mash mixture and reduce de-mixing during handling.

Nutritive value of protein-rich concentrates

By-products from the use of cereal grains for brewing and ethanol distillation, and starch and germ oil extraction: This feed class derives from a range of different processing methods, but they all have in common the fact that starch is removed from the grain and we are left with the bran (pericarp and seedcoat), germ (embryo) and endosperm residues. This group includes brewers' grains, distillers' grains, distillers' grains and solubles, germ meal (the residue after oil has been removed from the embryo) and gluten meal.

Because the bran and endosperm residues are protein-rich, these feeds have fairly high protein contents. However, their amino acid composition is unchanged from the original grain and so they are not especially good sources of essential amino acids (Table 6.5). They have variable fibre contents – between 5% and 60% neutral detergent fibre (NDF), and generally low Ca contents.

These feeds are used as palatable protein and fibre sources in ruminant diets, with recommended maximum inclusions of up to 40%.

Brewers' and distillers' by-products can be fed to adult breeding pigs (they are not suitable for young or growing pigs) but limited to 30 to 40% of the diet (on a DM basis) because of their poor amino acid profiles and high fibre contents. For a useful list of maximum inclusion rates of brewers' and

Table 6.4. Nutrient contents of selected fats and oils (DM basis). (Data from NRC 2001; INRAE 2017–2020.)

	Tallow	Lard	Palm oil	Sunflower oil
ME (ruminants) (MJ/kg DM)	23.7	24*	29.6	29.6
ME (pigs) (MJ/kg)	33.2	33.2	33.2	33.2
AME_n (poultry) MJ/kg	30.2	34.5	29.4	37.7
DE (horses) (MJ/kg DM)	34.6	34.6	34.6	34.6
Fat (% DM)	100	99	100	100
Linoleic acid (% DM)	2.8	9.5	10.0	6.5

*estimated

Table 6.5. Indicative nutritive values of selected brewing and distillation by-products (dry matter (DM) basis). (Data from NRC, 2007, 2012; INRAE/CIRAD/AFZ/FAO, 2012–2019; INRAE/CIRAD/AFZ, 2017–2020.)

	Brewers' grains[a]	Brewers' grains[b]	Dried distillers' grains and solubles[c]	Maize gluten meal[d]	Maize gluten feed[d]
ME (ruminants) (MJ/kg DM)	9.9	11.8	15.1	16.6	12.2
ME (pigs) (MJ/kg DM)	10.9	–	15.2	17.4	13
AME_n (poultry) (MJ/kg DM)	9.2	–	12.1	16.6	8.5
DE (horses) (MJ/kg DM)	11.8	–	14.5	15.1	12.6
Protein (% DM)	26	26	30	67	22
Lysine (% protein)	3.1	3.8	0.9	1.7	2.9
Methionine (% protein)	1.5	2.3	0.6	2.4	1.7
NDF (% DM)	56	40	36	4	40
Fat (% DM)	7	–	12	3	3
Linoleic acid (% DM)	1.7	–	6.2	1.4	1.5
Ca (% DM)	0.03	0.8	0.07	0.03	0.16
Non-phytate P (% DM)	0.02	–	0.64	0.6[e]	0.34

[a]From barley.
[b]From sorghum.
[c]By-products from maize distillation for ethanol.
[d]Maize gluten meal is the residue after removing the bran and germ (embryo) and extracting the starch; maize gluten feed is a mixture of maize bran and the germ (embryo) after the germ oil has been extracted.
[e]Estimated.

distillers' by-products in pig feeds, see Westendorf and Wohlt (2002).

Similarly, these feeds can be fed to adult poultry, at about 20% of the diet, but are unsuitable for young or growing birds.

Oilseed meals: These feeds are the residues left after the extraction of vegetable oil from oilseeds, e.g. cottonseed, soybean, canola (rapeseed), sunflower and safflower meals. They are sometimes called 'cakes'.

The main factor which affects the nutritive value of these protein meals is the way in which the oil has been extracted. Expeller and solvent extraction are the two main processes:

- Expeller extraction: in the simplest method, the seed is dehulled if necessary, crushed and heated to up to 130°C for several minutes, and then the oil is removed by compressing the mash through a screw press. A refinement introduced by Nelson *et al.* (1987) includes a preliminary extrusion step which generates similar temperatures but only for 30 seconds, then the material is passed through the screw press. Expeller extraction leaves 15% or more oil in the residual meal. Because these meals are heated, most of the trypsin inhibitor (in soybeans) is deactivated and the protein in expeller-extracted meals is somewhat resistant to rumen degradation. These meals are used in a niche market in the production of 'organic' animal products; EU regulations prohibit the use of hexane-processed meals in the feeding of these animals.
- Solvent extraction: hexane is used to dissolve the oil after the seed has been cleaned, crushed and gently heated to about 70°C. This method can be combined with mechanical extraction before the hexane is applied, in a process called 'pre-press' solvent extraction. Solvent extraction removes more oil than expeller extraction – only about 1% oil remains in the feed. Because of this, and because solvent extraction involves heating the seed at a lower temperature than the temperatures generated during expeller extraction, solvent-extracted meals have higher protein contents, higher rumen protein degradabilities and lower metabolizable energy (ME) contents than expeller-extracted meals.
- Aqueous enzymatic extraction is a new technique where the seed is milled and then reacted with protease or pectinase enzymes. The processing temperature is low – about 35°C – which means that amino acids are readily available but that, unless heated, the meal is likely to still retain active secondary substances and have a low UDP content.

Many oilseeds have a very robust seedcoat (see Chapter 4), and this is usually removed before oil extraction, giving 'decorticated' ('dehulled') meal. In some cases it is allowed to remain (or may be partially added back), giving 'undecorticated' ('undehulled') meal. Cottonseed meal usually contains small pieces of seedcoat (distinguished by their black colour in the brown meal). Safflower and sunflower seed meals can be sold as either undecorticated or decorticated meals.

Oilseed meals are generally palatable, although animals may take a week or two to accept palm kernel meal. Their ME contents are similar to those of cereal grains and are good sources of protein and some essential amino acids (Table 6.6).

Solvent-extracted meals are stable in storage, while the unsaturated fats in expeller-extracted meals may oxidize and become rancid. Water-damaged meals are good habitats for micro-organisms, including *Salmonella*.

Legume grains are the seeds of the Fabaceae family – field peas, lupins, mung beans, navy beans, vetch, and others.

Soybeans and peanuts are legume seeds, but they are classed as oilseeds because their main industrial use is as sources of vegetable oil.

Grain legumes have 25–35% protein, and this is 60–95% degradable in the rumen. Most grain legumes are rich in lysine but have low levels of methionine and available P (Table 6.7). Lupins have only 4 to 6% starch (DM basis), but many, e.g. faba beans, lentils, field peas and cowpeas, have between 45% and 50% starch (DM basis). This is enough to make it prudent to introduce these feeds carefully into ruminant and equine diets.

Many grain legumes contain secondary substances (lectins, proteinase inhibitors, non-protein amino acids, tannins, cyanogens, saponins, alkaloids, phytates, non-starch polysaccharide gums; Table 6.8; and see Chapter 12). These can be poisonous or interfere with digestion. This problem can be managed in two ways: first, by washing and/or heating the grains, or removing the hull, to destroy or remove the secondary substance; and second, by limiting the inclusion levels in pig and other monogastric animal diets. For example, navy beans and cowpeas should be heat-treated before feeding to pigs; they should not be included in weaner pig diets and comprise no more than 15% in diets for older stock. Other recommendations are in Table 6.8.

Table 6.6. Indicative data on the nutritive value of oilseed meals (dry matter (DM) basis). (Data from NRC, 2001, 2007, 2012; INRAE/CIRAD/AFZ/FAO, 2012–2019.)

	Canola meal[a]	Cottonseed meal[b]	Palm kernel meal[c]	Soybean meal[d]	Soybean meal[e]
ME (ruminants) (MJ/kg DM)	11.2	11.3	10.7	14.7	13.6
ME (pigs) (MJ/kg)	13.8	12.2	13.3	15.9	15
AME_n (poultry) MJ/kg	9.6	10.6	10.1	10.7	10.7
DE (horses) (MJ/kg DM)	12[f]	12.5	–	14.6	15.6
Protein (% DM)	38	47	19	49	52
Lysine (% protein)	5.5	4	3.2	6.3	6.1
Methionine (% protein)	2	1.4	1.7	1.4	1.4
NDF (% DM)	31	27	73	11	14
Fat (% DM)	3	3	3	8	2
Linoleic acid (% DM)	0.5	1.4	trace	3.2	0.8
Ca (% DM)	0.1	0.2	0.3	0.5	0.4
Non-phytate P (% DM)	0.4	–	0.2	0.3	–

[a]*Brassica* spp. (00 type with low erucic acid and glucosinolates); solvent extraction.
[b]*Gossypium* spp.; solvent extraction, dehulled.
[c]*Elaeis guineensis*; solvent extraction.
[d]*Glycine max*; expeller extraction, non-dehulled.
[e]*Glycine max*; solvent extraction, non-dehulled.
[f]Estimated.

Table 6.7. Indicative data on the nutritive value of grain legumes (pulses) (dry matter (DM) basis). (Data from Hawthorne, 2006; NRC, 2012; INRAE/CIRAD/AFZ/FAO, 2012–2019; INRAE/CIRAD/AFZ, 2017–2020.)

	Field pea[a]	Faba bean[b]	Lupin (blue)[c]	Mung bean[d]
ME (ruminants) (MJ/kg DM)	12.5	14.5	13.4	12.7
ME (pigs) (MJ/kg DM)	15.5	14.2	14.6	15.7
AME_n (poultry) MJ/kg	13.4	10.9	9.5	14.7
Protein (% DM)	26	25	32	27
Lysine (% protein)	6.5	6.2	5	6.9
Methionine (% protein)	1.4	0.8	0.6	1.3
NDF (% DM)	17	16	24	16
Fat (% DM)	1.6	1	6	2
Linoleic acid (% DM)	0.5	0.6	2.8	–
Ca (% DM)	0.1	0.15	0.3	0.16
Non-phytate P (% DM)	0.24	0.22	0.1	–

[a]*Pisum sativum*.
[b]*Vicia faba*.
[c]*Lupinus angustifolius* (also called narrow-leafed lupin).
[d]*Vigna radiata*.

Legume grains are usually fed after milling and heating. Field peas and lupins are sometimes processed to remove their hull (seedcoat). This improves their nutritive value for monogastric animals.

Animal carcase meals are the dried and milled residues of meat and fish processing. Animal and fish meals include meat meal, meat and bone meal, and blood meal made from the residues of sheep, goat

Table 6.8. Secondary substances in selected grain legumes and recommended inclusion limits. (Data from Evans, 1985; Hawthorne, 2006; INRAE/CIRAD/AFZ/FAO, 2012–2019.)

Legume grain	Secondary substances	Recommended maximum inclusion[a]
Chickpea[b]	trypsin inhibitors, tannins	Ruminants: 25% Pigs: 20 to 30% Poultry: 10% (processed)
Field pea[c]	tannins, trypsin inhibitors, hemagglutinin, lectins (all in low quantities)	Ruminants: no limit other than that imposed by the low UDP content Pigs: 20 to 40% Poultry: 25%
Faba bean[d]	tannins, vicine and convicine, protease inhibitors, lectins, phytic acid	Ruminants: no practical limit, possibly use no more than 50% Pigs: 30%, limit to 15% for breeding sows Poultry: 20% for low vicine and convicine cultivars, otherwise 5%
Lupins[e]	alkaloids (in bitter lupins), raffinose oligosaccharides, saponins, phytic acid	Ruminants: no limit except that imposed by the very low UDP content; in practice 15 to 20% Pigs: 15% for weaner pigs, 40% for growers Poultry: 10%
Mung bean[f]	trypsin inhibitors, tannins, lectins	Ruminants: limited information Pigs: 15% Poultry: 30%

[a]These inclusion rates are based on published data which, in some cases, is quite variable. It is best to be conservative and to use legume grains which have been treated to remove poisonous secondary substances. The low cystine and methionine contents, and high rumen degradation rates, also limit the use of these legume grains.
[b]*Cicer arietinum*.
[c]*Pisum sativum*.
[d]*Vicia faba*.
[e]*Lupinus angustifolius*.
[f]*Vigna radiata*.

and cattle processing; fish meal or fish and bone meal made from whole fish or the residues from fish processing; and poultry, poultry offal and feather meals from poultry processing.

Animal carcases are made into meals by first being skinned and eviscerated, then heated to dry the tissue and help remove the fat, and then milled. The nutritive values of these products depend on the relative proportions of lean tissue, fat and bone in meat meals and meat and bone meals, the part of the fish (e.g. whole fish or heads and tails) that is used in producing fish meals, and on the degree of heating that has been used during processing.

All of these products can have variable amounts of Ca, P and other minerals, and of protein, and this applies especially to meat meals and meat and bone meals. Carcase meals with more than 5% P (DM basis) are classed as meat and bone meals. The specifications for Australian meat and bone meals are given in Table 6.9; the 50% meat and bone meal contains 10.3% Ca and 5.1% P. The amino acid composition of carcase meal proteins is also variable, with some, e.g. fish meals, having high levels of essential amino acids, and others, e.g. low-quality meat and bone meals, having less.

The protein and other nutrient contents given in Table 6.10 should be taken as indications only. It is best to get an analysis of the particular batch of meat and fish meals that we intend to use.

Table 6.9. Specifications for selected Australian meat and bone meals (as-fed basis).[a] (From Grain Trade Australia, 2015; reproduced with permission).

Meal class (crude protein content)	45%	48%	50%	55%
Fat (%)	15	15	15	15
Moisture (%)	10	10	10	10
Ash (total mineral) (%)	38	37	32	30

[a]Maximum levels for fat, moisture and ash; minimum levels for protein; all meals must have at least 86% protein digestibility.

Table 6.10. Indicative data on the nutritive value of selected animal and fish meals (dry matter (DM) basis). (Data from Evans, 1985; NRC, 2012; INRAE/CIRAD/AFZ/FAO, 2012–2019; INRAE/CIRAD/AFZ, 2017–2020.)

	Meat meal[a,b]	Meat and bone meal[a,b]	Poultry offal meal[b,c]	Fish meal[b,d]
ME (pigs) (MJ/kg)	13.4	13.0	12.1	15.8
AME_n (poultry) MJ/kg	11.3	10.5[e]	14.0	14.2
Protein (% DM)	58.2	48.6	62.7	71.7
Lysine (% protein)	5.7	5.2	6.7	7.5
Methionine (% protein)	1.1	1.1	1.2	2.7
Fat (% DM)	10.9	11.7	15.5	8.3
Linoleic acid (% DM)	0.4	0.4	1.1	0.2
Ca (% DM)	9.9	13.7	2.1	4.3
Non-phytate P (% DM)	4.9	6.6	1.1	3.1

[a]Feed made from animal carcasses less hide and digestive tract contents.
[b]The energy, protein, Ca and P contents of these meals vary with the type of raw material used to produce the meal and with the amount of bone included in the meal – see text. Meat and bone meal has 5% or more P.
[c]Viscera, feet and heads.
[d]Mid-quality fish meal (66–68% protein as-fed).
[e]Estimated.

If the heating and drying processes are not carried out properly, and if the animal tissue was carrying the prions which cause bovine spongiform encephalopathy (BSE or mad cow disease; Chapter 12), then there is a risk of transmitting prions to animals which eat the meal.

Animal carcase meals MUST NOT be fed to ruminants because of this risk. That is why there are no ruminant nutritive value data in Table 6.10. Many countries ban feeding animal protein meals to ruminants: Australia bans the feeding of meals made from all vertebrate animals (including birds and fish), the European Union bans meals made from all mammals, New Zealand bans the feeding of ruminant protein in all forms; other jurisdictions have similar regulations.

Feeds which contain animal carcase meals will have a label similar to this:

This product contains restricted animal material – DO NOT FEED TO CATTLE, SHEEP, GOATS, DEER OR OTHER RUMINANTS

Milk by-products: Skim milk is the main representative in this feed class. Dried whole milk and casein (an important milk protein) are also included although they are not often used in animal feeding because of competition from human food manufacture. Whey and milk permeate are not included in this list of milk by-products as their high lactose and low protein contents makes them more appropriately members of the 'Sugar-rich feeds' class.

Skim milk is dried and marketed as a powder. It has 35% protein (DM basis; which includes casein and the whey proteins) which is rich in essential amino acids (7.8% lysine and 2.2% methionine in the protein), 56% lactose, 0.02% linoleic acid, 1.2% Ca and 0.9% P (DM basis) and quantities of B vitamins. Its available energy contents are 13.7 MJ ME/kg DM (ruminants), 16.3 MJ ME/kg DM (adult pig) and 11 MJ AME_n/kg DM (broiler) (data from NRC, 2012; INRAE/CIRAD/AFZ, 2017–2020).

Skim milk can be fed as a dry powder mixed with other ingredients or as a suspension in water and fed as a liquid feed. It is an expensive ingredient (although not as dear as whole milk powder) and is mainly used to make milk replacers. The ability of casein (about 80% of the skim milk proteins) to form a clot with milk fat when the outer layer of the casein micelle is removed by pepsin digestion (an intrinsic animal enzyme secreted in the abomasum or gastric stomach; Chapter 3) is a key element in making this ingredient an essential component of an effective milk replacer for calves, lambs and baby pigs. Its excellent essential amino acid composition makes it a useful ingredient in feeds for young, rapidly growing animals.

Insect meals: Relatively new products made from processing purposely grown larvae, pupae and adults of insects such as mealworms, houseflies, darkling beetles, silkworms, or adult grasshoppers, locusts and crickets. The insects can be fed whole or dried and milled.

Insect meals are accepted by pigs and poultry, and animal performance is usually similar to that obtained from soybean meal and similar plant protein sources.

The DM is mostly protein (45–60%) and fat (25–45%), with a low mineral content. They tend to have low cystine and methionine contents, and variable Ca – some have very low Ca while others such as the soldier fly larvae are Ca-rich. However, insects can be loaded with Ca if they are fed a Ca-rich feed before processing.

The nutrient contents of representative insect meals are shown in Table 6.11.

Roughages

Roughages can be divided into several different classes, based on:

- the type of plant material which forms the majority of the feed, e.g. legumes versus grasses versus fodder trees; or plant material with the seedhead retained versus plants without the seedhead or grain;
- photosynthesis type (C3 versus C4) of grasses, because this is associated with large differences in leaf anatomy, plant fibre content, and digestibility (see Chapter 15);
- forage processing method: e.g. hays versus silages. Particle size after processing is important because this affects the rate of passage through the rumen and thus the feed's digestibility, metabolizability and eNDF content (see Chapter 4); and
- industrial processing, e.g. the residues of sugar refining and fruit canning.

The INFIC system (Harris *et al.*, 1968) identifies three classes of roughages (dry forages and roughages; pasture, range plants and forages fed green; silages) but we should add other classes (Fig. 6.3) to expand and modify this group to cater for the factors listed above.

Green pasture and forage crops: These are forages which are fed fresh, i.e. they are either grazed *in situ*, or are cut and immediately fed to penned animals. This class includes:

- Pasture grasses, including those which are grown in conventional pasture, e.g. ryegrasses (*Lolium*

Table 6.11. Indicative data on the nutritive value of selected insect meals (dry matter (DM) basis). (From Makkar *et al.*, 2014; De Marco *et al.*, 2015; Jayanegara, *et al.*, 2017.)

	House cricket[a]	Black soldier fly larvae[b]	Meal worm[c]	Silkworm pupae meal[d]
ME (ruminants) (MJ/kg DM)	–	12.6[e]	13.8[e]	–
AME_n (poultry) MJ/kg DM	12[e]	–	16	10.2
Protein (% DM)	57	42	53	61
Lysine (% protein)	5.4	6.6	5.4	7
Methionine (% protein)	1.4	2.1	1.5	3.5
NDF (% DM)	18	7[f]	12	4[f]
Fat (% DM)	17	26	36	26
Linoleic acid (% DM)	6.5	1	10	–
Ca (% DM)	1	7.6	0.3	0.4
non-phytate P (% DM)	0.8	0.9	0.8	0.6

[a]*Acheta domestica*, whole body (undefatted).
[b]*Hermetia illucens.*
[c]*Tenebrio molitor.*
[d]*Bombyx mori* and other species.
[e]Estimated.
[f]These values are for crude fibre. Insects have a cuticle which is made from chitin and protein and this is presumably the residue which remains after extraction by detergents or the acid/alkali reagents used in crude fibre determination. However, the chemical composition of insect 'fibre' is not fully known, and it is difficult to compare crude fibre and NDF values.

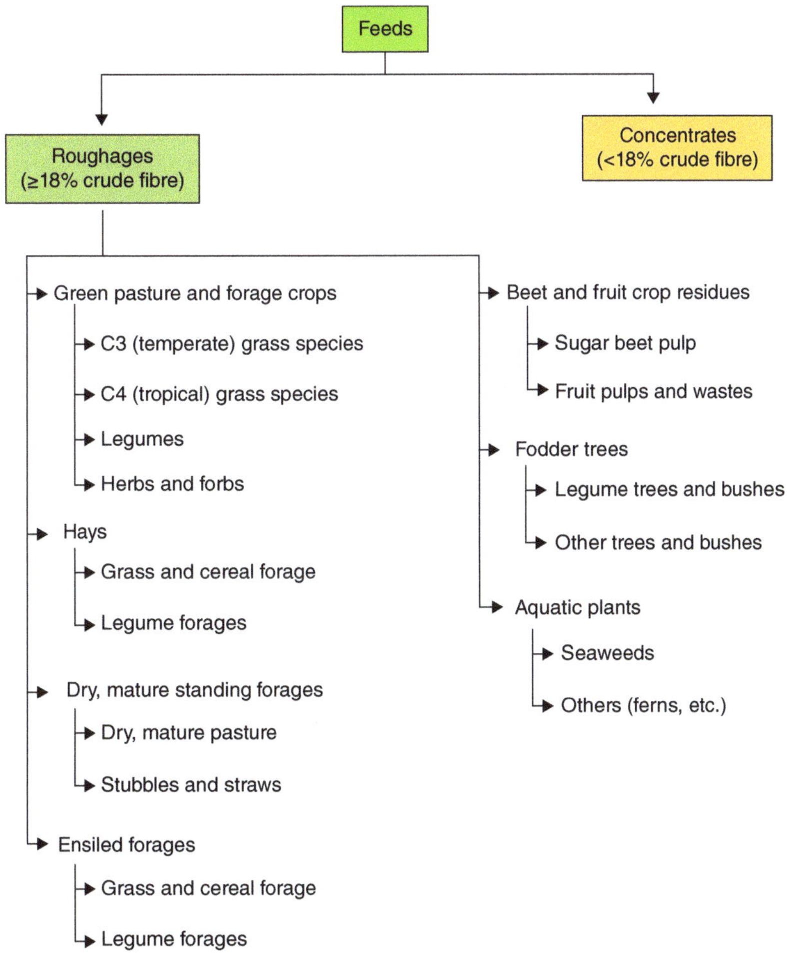

Fig. 6.3. Classification of 'roughage' feeds according to their origins and nutrient contents. (Copyright: Gordon McL. Dryden.)

spp.) and guinea grass/green panic (*Megathyrsus maximus*), rangeland grasses such as black speargrass (*Heteropogon contortus*) and Mitchell grasses (*Astrebla* spp.), and grasses which grow in wetlands or as ponded pastures, e.g. para grass (*Urochloa/Brachiaria mutica*) and marsh grasses (*Hymenachne* spp.). Grasses are divided into C3 (temperate) and C4 (tropical) species (Chapter 15) because these have different fibre contents, and thus different available energy contents and potential intakes.

- Cereal forages: these are crops which are harvested at dough stage before their seed fully ripens, and cereal grain crops which have been grazed before forming a seedhead, or which have failed due to drought or have lodged under high winds or heavy rain.
- Forage legumes: these typically have higher protein and Ca contents than grasses and cereals. They are palatable and may be lost from a mixed pasture because of preferential grazing.
- Herbs and forbs (herbaceous plants other than grasses) which are found in both sown and natural pastures.
- The leaves of fodder root crops.

Factors which influence the nutritive value of pasture grasses: The nutritive value of pasture and forage crops changes consistently through the plant's life cycle, affected by:

- temperature, soil moisture and day length. These change with season and influence the initiation of growth and pasture or crop productivity;
- plant maturity stage (e.g. early growth, dough stage, over ripe);
- grass species, especially the differences between the C3 and C4 photosynthesis types; and
- fertilization used to improve pasture growth, and pasture mineral and protein contents.

These aspects of pasture quality, and indicative data on the nutritive value of pastures, are discussed in Chapter 15.

Hays: These are green cereal, grass or legume forages which have been harvested before their seed has ripened, e.g. cereal forages cut for hay at the dough stage. There are many similarities between green forages and the hays that are made from them, but these classes are separated because:

- There is always some loss of nutrients as the forage dries during the curing process.
- The moisture contents of these materials are very different – green forage has between 55 and 90% water while hay has only 10 to 15%; these differences mean that green forages and hays must be handled, stored, combined with other feeds, and fed out, in different ways.

Not all hays can be substituted for others. In general, legume hays (e.g. from lucerne, alfalfa) have 15–25% protein (DM basis) while the protein contents of grass and cereal forage hays are often between 5% and 15%, although some C3 grasses can have protein contents above 25%. Substituting grass hay for legume hay will usually reduce the animal's ME and protein intakes.

Not all hays in the same sub-class have similar nutritive values. To assess the quality of a hay sample, we should look at:

- Leaf:stem ratio and stem thickness: the stems of cereal and legume forages become thicker as they mature, and their appearance is a good indicator of nutritive value. The effect of increasing maturity is illustrated by the two lucerne (alfalfa) hay samples in Table 6.12.
- Presence and stage of development of any seed-head: grain at the dough stage of development should be present in cereal forage hays because

Table 6.12. Indicative nutrient contents for selected hay types (DM basis). (Data from NRC, 2001; Martinson *et al.*, 2012; INRAE/CIRAD/AFZ, 2017–2020.)

	Lucerne[a] (immature)	Lucerne[a] (mature)	Lucerne[a] meal (20% protein)	Orchard grass[b] (vegetative)	Orchard grass[b] (flowering)
ME (ruminants) (MJ/kg DM)	9.1	8.3	9.3	–	9.8
ME (pigs) (MJ/kg)	–	–	9.0	–	–
AME_n (poultry) (MJ/kg DM)	–	–	5.2	–	–
DE (horses) (MJ/kg DM)	10.3	9.0	–	9.2	8.8
Protein (% DM)	20	17	20.1	14	12
Lysine (% protein)	–	–	4.6	2.8[c]	2.8[c]
Methionine (% protein)	–	–	1.3	0.7[c]	0.7[c]
NDF (% DM)	39	49	43	58	60
Fat (% DM)	–	–	3	3	3
Linoleic acid (% DM)	–	–	0.3	–	–
Ca (% DM)	1.6	1.2	2.5	0.5	0.4
Non-phytate P	–	–	0.3	–	–
Total P (% DM)	0.2	0.2	0.3	0.4	0.3

[a]*Medicago sativa.*
[b]*Dactylis glomerata* (also called 'cocksfoot').
[c] % of ruminally undegraded protein.

this increases the hay's ME content. On the other hand, ripe seed heads in grass or legume hays indicate that the crop is mature and has lower energy digestibility and protein and P contents.

- Loss of leaf from lucerne (alfalfa) hay: dry lucerne loses its nutrient-rich leaves easily during tedding, raking and baling because during field drying, water is lost from leaves much more rapidly than from the stem, and these very dry leaves 'shatter' and are lost as dust. Most lucerne hay is 'conditioned' by being passed between heavy rollers as it is cut. This breaks the outer cells of the stem and allows water to escape more readily, so that the moisture content of the whole crop can be reduced for baling without over-drying, and losing, the leaves. Application of a K_2CO_3 solution also damages the cuticle of these cells and has a similar effect to roller conditioning.
- Colour: well-made hay is green, although not as bright as the original forage. A pale colour indicates that the material has lain in the windrow for some time and has been exposed to ultraviolet light, with probable loss of much of the vitamin A activity – in some cases only 10% of the amount in the fresh material remains in the hay. Brown hay may have been water-damaged by rain or possibly by a heavy dew. Water in contact with damaged plant cells leaches water-soluble constituents such as protein, water-soluble carbohydrates, and B group vitamins. Hay which was baled without adequate drying will have heated due to microbial action. This changes the colour, can damage proteins, and reduce the activity of heat-labile vitamins, e.g. vitamin A and thiamine (vitamin B1).
- Odour: look for a smell similar to newly mown grass; off-smells indicate possible mould growth. Damp hay is a good substrate for mould growth.

Indicative nutritive values (and that is all they can be) are given for selected hays in Table 6.12. Obviously, there are many other types of hay than those mentioned in Table 6.12 and many grades of hay within each forage type. It is clear from the data in this table and in Chapter 15 how variable forage nutritive values can be. The data are collected from several sources and while the nominated protein and NDF contents relate to the stage of maturity descriptions, each value in the table relates to the particular sample on which the analysis was done.

Lucerne meal is also fed to pigs and poultry. Its carotene and xanthophyll contents help to ensure that egg yolks have a rich orange colour.

Dry, mature standing forages: There are two subgroups in this feed class:

- Pasture or cereal forage which has matured, developed seeds and the ripened seed has been lost from the seedhead. This growth stage is called 'over ripe' or 'stem cured'. The fibre in this material is very lignified and therefore not readily digested. In addition, these feeds have little protein and are deficient in some minerals, especially P. This material is sometimes called 'standing hay', but its nutritional value is similar to cereal straw.
- Straw: cereal forage from which the grain has been harvested and therefore consists mainly of mature stem and leaf. 'Straw' usually refers to fine-stemmed crops such as wheat, barley and oats. When a maize, sorghum or soybean crop is harvested the residue can be called 'stover'.

Over-ripe forages and straws have:

- ME contents between 6 and 8 MJ ME/kg DM;
- between 3% and 6% protein (DM basis); this protein is less ruminally degradable (60–75%) than the protein in less mature forages;
- low P contents, between 0.02% and 0.07% P (DM basis); and
- low potential intakes: these feeds are not palatable; and their low ruminally degradable protein (RDP) content limits rumen microbial activity, and slow carbohydrate digestion rates limit the rate at which these feeds can leave the rumen.

When given as the only feed ingredient, these feeds do not satisfy any animal's nutrient requirements, except for the maintenance requirements for energy of mature cattle and sheep provided that the animal can eat the required amount. They do not meet maintenance protein requirements and should be supplemented with a protein or non-protein N source. They are good sources of fibre (although much of this is not digestible) and can help to maintain digestive tract health when included in rations that have a large proportion of cereal grain. There is a risk of rumen or omasal impaction when cattle eat this type of feed (see 'Fodder trees' below and Chapter 13).

Ensiled forage

Ensiled forage (silage or ensilage) is plant material which has been preserved by the action of microorganisms which partly digest (ferment) the material and produce lactic acid which makes the pH fall to a level which prevents any further microbial action and thus preserves the forage. Silages can be subdivided into maize (corn), grass and legume silages. 'Silage' also includes haylage and baleage, two products which are made slightly differently to stack or pit silage, but which also rely on microbial fermentation to preserve the ensiled material. Coblentz and Akins (2018) have reviewed this method of making silage.

Well-made silage ferments rapidly and the pH falls quickly to less than 5. To get good fermentation the forage has to contain readily fermentable carbohydrates, enough water to allow microbial growth, and it should be chopped finely and well compacted to exclude oxygen. 'Lactic acid' silage will keep in storage indefinitely. Silage that is badly made and affected by oxygen entering the stack will contain butyric acid which gives it an unpleasant smell, and it may be contaminated by mould and other organisms.

Well-made silage loses water-soluble carbohydrates and protein, and thus has less ME and protein than the original material. The ensiling process does not improve the quality of the feed over that of the original forage. Ensiling is a way of preserving forage, not of improving it.

Silage is accepted by most herbivores. It is most commonly fed to dairy and beef cattle, but it can be fed to sheep and horses.

This feed class does not include ensiled cereal grains. These retain most of the nutritional features of dry cereal grain and are classed as energy concentrates.

Fodder trees: These are trees and shrubs which are used as feed for sheep, goats, cattle and buffalo. They include a wide variety of species, but some of the more important, depending on the locality, are calliandra (*Calliandra calothyrsus*), leucaena (*Leucaena leucocephala*), gliricidia (*Gliricidia sepium*), mulga (*Acacia aneura*), willow (*Salix* spp.), *Desmanthus* spp. and oil palm (*Elaeis guineensis*). They are a valuable feed resource, but they have many other uses, for example timber, for shelter, for soil stabilization and hedges.

Most fodder trees are slow growing and some are not very productive, although calliandra, leucaena, sesbania, desmanthus, tagasaste and willow are exceptions to this generalization.

Fodder trees are managed in several different ways: planted in plots where they may be managed to have a shrub-like form with either continuous or controlled animal browsing; occur in a natural tree/pasture ecosystem with continuous access; used in a cut-and-carry or cut-and-browse system; and by feeding prunings to animals on pasture. Leaves and edible twigs can be pelleted or dried, and some species (e.g. *Salix*) can be preserved by ensiling.

Because of their protein contents, leguminous trees are usually used as protein supplements to sheep, goats and cattle grazing grass pastures, and they often give substantial improvements in animal performance. Non-leguminous trees are used to supplement the animal's total feed intake, and to alleviate shortages of pasture in dry times. Some of these trees tolerate low rainfall and thus contribute to the enterprise's drought resistance.

The leaves of these trees have moderate to high NDF contents (30–75% DM basis) depending on species, and modest ME contents (6–10.5 MJ/kg DM). The leguminous tree leaves are protein-rich (20–30%, DM basis) and can be useful protein sources while non-leguminous tree leaves have less protein (10–25%, DM basis). However, most tree leaves contain significant amounts of condensed tannins which make the feed astringent and unpalatable and combine with proteins and reduce their rumen degradability. Consequently, fodder trees are not good sources of RDP, although they contribute UDP. Condensed tannins can also help to control internal parasites.

Fodder trees can cause rumen or omasal compaction. Impaction can occur with both browsing and cut-and-carry feeding. It is more likely to happen if animals are hungry and eat larger twigs (more than about 3 mm in diameter) and small branches, and the risk is exacerbated if they are hand-fed and have limited ability to select their diet.

Some leguminous trees have deleterious secondary substances. The popular leucaena (*Leucaena leucocephala*) tree contains mimosine, an amino acid which poisons the hair follicle cells which produce the emerging fibre, and which is metabolized in the rumen to the goitrogenic 3-hydroxy-4-(1H)-pyridone (3,4-DHP) (see Chapter 12).

The nutritional characteristics of some representative fodder trees and shrubs are listed in Table 6.13.

Fruit and beet crop residues: This is a varied class but the members have in common moderate fibre contents (40% and quite high available energy contents. They have little starch (0–8%, DM basis) but they have water-soluble fibre (pectins)

Table 6.13. Nutritional characteristics of selected fodder tree leaves. (Data from ACIAR/Bioversity International/CIAT, undated; Smith, 1991; Karda, 2000; Kemp *et al.*, 2001; O'Reagain and McMeniman, 2002; Clem, 2009; Wiley, 2009; INRAE/CIRAD/AFZ/FAO, 2012–2019; Revell *et al.*, 2013; Vandermeulen *et al.*, 2018.)

Name/species	DM digestibility (%)	Protein (% DM)	Tannins (% DM)	Characteristics
Wet/dry subtropics				
Calliandra calothyrsus	24–60	12–24	1.5–19.4	No known toxicities to ruminants. The condensed tannin content makes it unsuitable for non-ruminants
Gliricidia sepium	60–65	18–30	2.6–7.8	Inexperienced animals refuse gliricidia leaves (possibly because of their dihydrocoumarin content) but with experience will accept them, some cultivars (e.g. Retalhuleu) are more acceptable. Wilting leaves for 12–24 hours before feeding increases intake
Leucaena leucocephala	42–70	17–28	2–13	Very palatable, although the tannin content in young leaf can be as high as 12%. The edible fraction commonly contains 1–6% mimosine (see Chapter 12)
Sesbania grandiflora	75	25–30	–	Highly palatable to ruminants, accepted by pigs. No evidence of toxicity to grazing animals but leaf and seed meal are poisonous to poultry
Sesbania sesban	79–80	25–30	0.2	Moderately well accepted by ruminants after an introductory period (up to 3 months). No tannins but has saponins. Poisonous for poultry
Dry subtropics				
Albizia lebbeck	45–70	16–23	0.1	Well accepted by sheep and cattle which eat fresh and fallen leaves. Cattle but not sheep will eat seedpods (these contain saponins). Leaves have little tannin, and are low in other phenolic compounds
Desmanthus virgatus	60–65	16–24	2–3	Accepted by sheep and cattle, giving good to high growth rates. There are no toxins although it has some tannins. The shrub tolerates heavy grazing
Mulga (*Acacia aneura*)	50–62	9–14	5–24	A commonly used feed for sheep and cattle in semiarid and arid Australia. Contains high levels of tannins which impair protein availability (35–40%). Sheep feeding solely on mulga suffer from S and P deficiencies

Continued

Table 6.13. Continued.

Name/species	DM digestibility (%)	Protein (% DM)	Tannins (% DM)	Characteristics
Wet/dry temperate				
Willow (*Salix* spp.)[a]	40–70	12–22	2–10	Used as a supplement to pasture and gives good animal performance (lambing %), the tannin content varies between cultivars
Tagasaste (*Cytisus proliferus*)	57–73	14–33	0–2.6	Yields of 5–16 tonnes DM/ha have been reported. Nutritive value varies widely between growth and dormancy, and acceptability is best when actively growing. 'Tagasaste staggers' can occur when dormant plant material is fed but animals recover quickly (<30 minutes) and there is no permanent injury
Poplar (*Populus* spp.)[a]	56–70	11–18	0.1–3	Leaves are a feed source of moderate quality, they contain tannins and may contain a glucoside which reduces their palatability
Dry temperate				
Saltbush (*Atriplex* spp.)[a]	46–56	12–22		High Na (3.5–8% DM) and S contents (0.2–0.8% DM), low P. Can make a useful contribution to nutrient intake by sheep

[a]Non-leguminous trees.

which is readily digested in the rumen. This makes them rich in available energy but not prone to causing rumen disorders or laminitis. Their protein contents are quite low and they are, in general, not good sources of essential amino acids (Table 6.14). Some of these feeds have less than 18% crude fibre but are classed here because of their origins and general characteristics.

Sugar beet pulp is mainly used as an ingredient in cattle and horse feeds but it can also be fed to growing pigs and breeding sows.

The feeds in this class are usually used in a dried form as they have a limited storage life when stored wet.

Minerals, vitamin sources, 'synthetic' amino acids, non-protein N sources and additives

It was noted above that feed classification usually deals only with 'whole feeds', i.e. those materials which animals use as sources of a wide variety of nutrients, especially energy and protein. However, for completeness we will add three other classes.

Contrary to the situation with 'whole feeds' where we can substitute one feed for another (within the same feed class), this does not apply to minerals or vitamins, where each of these nutrients has its own specialized metabolic function which cannot (in almost every case) be performed by another mineral or vitamin, although some essential amino acids can substitute for others, either wholly or partially (Chapter 1).

Minerals: Sources of the major minerals include feeds like limestone, shell grit or crushed coral for Ca, salt for Na, and dicalcium phosphate for both Ca and P.

Trace minerals are provided as mineral salts such as Zn carbonate, K iodide, Cu carbonate and sulphate, etc., and as chelates. Amino acid complexes are examples of chelates where a trace mineral ion (e.g. Cu, Fe, Mn, Se, Zn, etc.) is complexed with an amino acid (e.g. glycine or methionine).

Vitamins: These are provided either as the pure chemical or from a vitamin-rich source (e.g. yeast as a source of B group vitamins. Each vitamin has its own role in animal metabolism and cannot be

Table 6.14. Indicative nutritive value of selected feeds made from the residues of sugar beet and fruit processing (DM basis). (Data from NRC, 1982; INRAE/CIRAD/AFZ/FAO, 2012–2019; INRAE/CIRAD/AFZ, 2017–2020.)

	Sugar beet pulp (dried)[a]	Citrus pulp (dried)[b]	Apple pomace (dried)[c]	Pineapple waste (dried)[b,d]
ME (ruminants) (MJ/kg DM)	11.2	12.4	8.9	10.8
ME (pigs) (MJ/kg)	12.6	13.6	9.2	10.6
AME_n (poultry) MJ/kg	–	5.6	4.7	–
DE (horses) (MJ/kg DM)	12.6	12.2	10.7	–
Protein (% DM)	9	7	8	5
Lysine (% protein)	6.6	0.2	4.9	2
Methionine (% protein)	1.8	0.1	2.0	0.5
NDF (% DM)	50	22	60.5	42
Fat (% DM)	0.5	2.5	3	1
Linoleic acid (% DM)	0.3	5.3	–	–
Ca (% DM)	1.4	1.8	0.1	0.5
Non-phytate P (% DM)	0.1	0.06	–	–

[a]*Beta vulgaris*.
[b]The fibre and protein contents of citrus pulp (14% crude fibre and 7% protein, DM basis) and pineapple waste (18% crude fibre and 5% protein, DM basis) qualify them as energy concentrates, but they are included here because of their similarity in other respects to these crop residues.
[c]The dried residue produced after juice extraction, includes skins, cores, seeds and stems.
[d]*Ananas comosus*; residues from the canning process, includes skins, tops and cores; may include pomace.

substituted by any other nutrient. This applies to all vitamins, including each of the B group vitamins.

Non-protein N ingredients: this is a 'catch-all' class with two important members:

- Amino acids, e.g. 'synthetic' lysine, tryptophan and threonine which are harvested from micro-organisms, and methionine hydroxy analogue. These amino acids are included in pig and poultry diets, and increasingly in lactating dairy cow and horse feeds, to improve the amino acid profile of feeds which are based on cereal grains and other energy concentrates which are deficient in essential amino acids.
- N-rich substances such as ammonium salts and urea. Urea is used as a supplement to ruminant feeds which are low in RAN (Chapter 16). Urea contains 46% N; it can be poisonous if fed in excess.

Miscellaneous additives: This class contains a wide variety of substances which can be added to animal feeds, e.g. antibiotics, anabolic agents, rumen modifiers, flavours and pellet binders.

Feeds that should not be used

One of the less obvious consequences of unwisely using some potential feeds is that they can be vehicles for the transmission of animal diseases (see Chapter 12) or chemical residues which can affect animal products. As well as animal carcase meals (see above), swill (human food wastes), poultry litter (or poultry manure), and cotton trash are examples of at-risk feeds.

Poultry litter: This is a mixture of chicken manure, feathers, spilled feed and straw or other bedding used in free-range or barn housing, and it may contain dead birds. At first sight, this feed could be a source of physically effective fibre (peNDF) (from the straw) and protein (from the droppings). What is not apparent is the load of pathogenic micro-organisms that it is likely to contain (Chapter 12). Poultry litter will also contain residues of antibiotics and coccidiostats if these were given as part of the birds' feed. Litter can also be contaminated with soil, and possibly scrap metal, glass and other contaminants.

The main risk of feeding this material is that, unless it has been sterilized, it will carry disease organisms. Several ways have been suggested to reduce (but not eliminate) the risk of bacterial diseases transmitted in fresh litter; e.g. it should be artificially dried to at least 85% DM. Other methods of treating poultry litter, including ensiling and deep stacking, are described by Daniel and Olson (2005).

Feeding poultry litter to cattle is legal in the US but prohibited in the EU and Australia because of the risk that it will transmit diseases such as botulism and salmonellosis, and the risk that it may contain poultry feed which in turn contains restricted animal material which should not be fed to ruminants because of the risk of transmitting prions which cause BSE. Badly processed poultry litter has been responsible for the deaths of feedlot cattle in Australia and Mexico.

Human food wastes (swill): This is meat and meat products which have been part of human food, and anything which has been in contact with these things. It does not include bakery waste, provided that this has not been obtained from table scraps. 'Swill' can encompass all or any of these things:

- Any product derived from a mammal or bird, including meat, feathers, milk and milk products, and faeces (note the comment above about poultry litter).
- Human food waste which has come into contact with meat or meat by-products. 'Human food waste' includes plant material such as salads and other vegetables and also cheese; 'into contact with' includes being on the same plate or in a container which has been used to carry meat or meat products; and 'by-products' includes pies and pasties, hamburgers, bacon, etc.
- Cooking oil which has not been rendered in accordance with biosecurity rules.

Swill feeding is prohibited in many jurisdictions, e.g. the EU, the UK and Australia, because of the risk that meat products in waste food may carry food-borne pathogens. Biosecurity agencies in countries which are free of specific diseases, such as foot-and-mouth disease and African swine fever, are especially concerned about the risk from illegally imported meat products. This risk is not trivial – the foot-and-mouth disease outbreak in the UK in 2001, which cost the country's economy about £8 billion, was traced to 'unprocessed or inadequately processed waste food' fed to pigs.

Feeds contaminated with insecticides and other chemicals: Some roughage and concentrate feeds are protected from insect damage by treatment with insecticides (e.g. cereal grains are sometimes treated like this in storage). Cotton trash is an example of this type of feed; it has been used in times of high demand for roughages for feeding to drought-affected cattle. Cotton plants are treated with insecticides while they grow, and with defoliants just before harvesting. These chemicals remain in the plant material and are absorbed into the animal's tissues and can be present in meat or milk (Australian Pesticides Map, 1996). It is essential that we observe the withholding periods that are mandated for insecticides and other chemicals used to treat plant material (see also Chapter 11).

References

ACIAR/Bioversity International/CIAT (undated). *Tropical Forages*. Available at: www.tropicalforages.info/text/intro/index.html (accessed 26 December 2020).

Alderman, G., Barber, W.P. and Stranks, M.H. (1983). Databases for the composition and nutritive value of animal feeds. In Haresign, W. (ed.) *Recent Advances in Animal Nutrition – 1982*. London: Butterworths.

Australian Pesticides Map (1996). *1996 May: Cotton Insecticides Contaminates Calves. Pesticides: Chlorfluazuron, Endosulfan*. Available at: www.pesticides.australianmap.net/1996-may-cotton-insecticides-contaminates-calves-pesticides-chlorfluazuron-endosulfan/ (accessed 26 December 2020).

Clem, B. (2009). Desmanthus. In *Pastures Australia*. Available at: www.keys.lucidcentral.org/keys/v3/pastures/Html/Desmanthus.htm (accessed 26 December 2020).

Coblentz, W.K. and Akins, M.S. (2018). Silage review: Recent advances and future technologies for baled silages. *Journal of Dairy Science* 101: 4075–4092.

Daniel, J. and Olson, K.C. (2005). *Feeding Poultry Litter to Beef Cattle*. University of Missouri Extension. Available at: www.mospace.umsystem.edu/xmlui/handle/10355/3354 (accessed 26 December 2020).

De Marco, M., Martinez, S., Hernandez, F., Madrid, J., Gai, F., Rotolo, L., Belforti, M., Bergero, D., Katz, H., Dabbou, S., Kovitvadhi, A., Ivo, Z., Gasco, L. and Schiavone, A. (2015). Nutritional value of two insect larval meals (*Tenebrio molitor* and *Hermetia illucens*) for broiler chickens: Apparent nutrient digestibility, apparent ileal amino acid digestibility and apparent metabolizable energy. *Animal Feed Science and Technology* 209: 211–218.

Evans, M. (1985). *Nutrient Composition of Feedstuffs for Pigs and Poultry*. Brisbane: QDPI.

Grain Trade Australia (2015). *Trading Standards. Animal Protein Standards 2015/16*. Available at: www.graintrade.org.au/commodity_standards (accessed 26 December 2020).

Harris, L.E., Asplund, M.J. and Crampton, E.W. (1968). *An International Feed Nomenclature and Methods for Summarizing and Using Feed Data to Calculate Diets*. Bulletin 479, Agricultural Experiment Station, Utah State University.

Hawthorne, W. (2006). *Pulses nutritional value and their role in the feed industry*. Edgecliff, NSW: Pulse Australia Pty Ltd. Available at: www.pulseaus.com.au/storage/app/media/using_pulses/2006_Pulses-Feed-value-livestock.pdf (accessed 26 December 2020).

Jayanegara, A., Yantina, N., Novandri, B., Laconi, E.B., Nahrowi, R. and Ridla, M. (2017). Evaluation of some insects as potential feed ingredients for ruminants: chemical composition, in vitro rumen fermentation and methane emissions. *Journal of Indonesian Tropical Animal Agriculture* 42(4): 247–254.

Karda, W.I. (2000). *Feeding Value for Sheep of the Leaf of Gliricidia sepium and Leucaena leucocephala cv Tarramba*. PhD thesis, University of Queensland.

Kemp, P.D., Mackay, A.D., Matheson, L.A. and Timmins, M.E. (2001). The forage value of poplars and willows. *Proceedings of the New Zealand Grassland Association* 63: 115–119.

INRAE/CIRAD/AFZ (2017–2020). *Feed Tables*. Available at: www.feedtables.com/ (accessed 26 December 2020).

INRAE/CIRAD/AFZ/FAO (2012–2019). *Feedipedia – Animal Feed Resources Information System*. Available at: www.feedipedia.org/ (accessed 26 December 2020).

Makkar, H.P.S., Tran, G., Heuzé, V. and Ankers, P. (2014). State-of-the-art on use of insects as animal feed. *Animal Feed Science and Technology* 197: 1–33.

Martinson, K.L., Hathaway, M., Jung, H. and Sheaffer, C. (2012). The effect of soaking on protein and mineral loss in orchardgrass and alfalfa hay. *Journal of Equine Veterinary Science* 32: 776–782.

National Research Council (NRC) (1982). *United States-Canadian Tables of Feed Composition: Nutritional Data for United States and Canadian Feeds*, 3rd rev. Washington, DC: National Academies Press.

National Research Council (NRC) (2001). *Nutrient Requirements of Dairy Cattle*, 7th rev. edn. Washington, DC: National Academies Press.

National Research Council (NRC) (2007). *Nutrient Requirements of Horses*, 6th rev. edn. Washington, DC: National Academy Press.

National Research Council (NRC) (2012). *Nutrient Requirements of Swine*, 11th rev. edn. Washington, DC: National Academy Press.

Nelson, A.I., Wijeratne, W.B., Yeh, S.W., Wei, T.M. and Wei, L.S. (1987). Dry extrusion as an aid to mechanical expelling of oil from soybeans. *Journal of the American Oil Chemists Society* 64(9): 1341–1347.

O'Reagain, P.J. and McMeniman, N.P. (2002). Nutrition of sheep under rangeland conditions. In Freer, M. and Dove, H. (eds), *Sheep Nutrition*. Wallingford, UK: CAB International, pp. 263–284.

Revell, D.K., Norman, H.C., Vercoe, P.E., Phillips, N., Toovey, A., Bickell, S., Hulm, E., Hughes, S. and Emms, J. (2013). Australian perennial shrub species add value to the feed base of grazing livestock in low- to medium-rainfall zones. *Animal Production Science* 53(11): 1221–1230.

Smith, O.B. (1991). Fodder trees and shrubs in range and farming systems in tropical humid Africa. *FAO Expert Consultation on Legume Trees and Other Fodder Trees as Protein Sources for Livestock*. Malaysian Agricultural Research and Development Institute, Kuala Lumpur, Malaysia, 14 to 18 October 1991. Available at: www.fao.org/3/T0632E/T0632E04.htm#ch4 (accessed 26 December 2020).

Vandermeulen, S., Ramírez-Restrepo, C.A., Beckers, Y., Claessens, H. and Bindelle, J. (2018). Agroforestry for ruminants: a review of trees and shrubs as fodder in silvopastoral temperate and tropical production systems. *Animal Production Science* 58(5): 767–777.

Westendorf, M.L. and Wohlt, J.E. (2002). Brewing by-products: their use as animal feeds. *Veterinary Clinics Food Animal Practice* 18: 233–252.

Wiley, T. (2009). Tagasaste. *Pastures Australia*. Available at: https://keys.lucidcentral.org/keys/v3/pastures/Html/Tagasaste.htm (accessed 26 December 2020).

7 Feed intake

How animals regulate feed intake

Feed intake is controlled by a complex system involving nerve signals, hormones and hormone-like substances which are made in the digestive tract, brain and fat depots. The control of intake in mammals is described by Dryden (2008) and differences between mammals and birds are discussed by Tachibana and Tsutsui (2016).

In summary, intake control involves the processes described below.

Neurological and hormonal control: Feed intake is controlled by the hypothalamus, a region at the base of the brain. The hypothalamus receives hormonal and neural signals from the digestive tract and other parts of the body which indicate the animal's nutritional status. These signals include messages from stretch receptors in the digestive tract, and hormones from fat deposits and the pancreas.

The mechanisms that control intake motivate, rather than compel. Obviously, the animal would be in trouble if, for example, it had to eat when being attacked by a predator, or if it could not select between feeds on offer or could not choose grazing sites that gave the best return on the energy expended during eating.

Short- and long-term control of intake: Feed intake is controlled over the short term and the long term. Short-term control deals with the start and finish of feeding events. Impulses conducted by the vagus nerve, and hormones like ghrelin, travel to the brain from the digestive tract and these activate 'feeding centres' in the hypothalamus. The animal then eats until signals motivate it to stop eating. These 'satiety' signals include nerve impulses from stretch receptors in the digestive tract, the hormone leptin produced in fat depots, cholecystokinin from the duodenum, and insulin from the pancreas secreted in response to increased blood glucose levels.

Long-term control generally prevents the animal from becoming obese once it has reached its mature size. The main signal involved here is the secretion of leptin from fat depots.

These signals can be over-ridden by the other brain centres, especially the limbic centre. These come into play if the animal is at risk from its environment (e.g. predation, aggression from others, or mating activity) or how the animal perceives the feed it has to eat (i.e. the palatability of the feed).

Energy intake and digestive tract fill are important factors controlling intake: All animals eat to satisfy their energy requirements and will usually stop eating once these have been met. Receptors on the surfaces of intestinal epithelial cells sense glucose, glutamic acid and fatty acids, and sensors in the brain detect amino acids. These signals are especially important in controlling intake in non-ruminant animals such as pigs, poultry and horses.

Ruminants also have these signals, but because their feed is usually more fibrous and thus more difficult and slower to digest (Chapters 3 and 4), digestive tract fill and the osmolarity of the rumen liquor are also important. In the short term, ruminants have a more-or-less constant rumen fill and daily feed intake matches the rate at which previously eaten feed disappears from the rumen. Roughage intake is largely influenced by the rate of passage of undigested feed into the abomasum and small intestine, and by the rate at which the feed is fermented in the rumen – faster passage and fermentation rates allow the rumen to empty faster and thus allow larger DM intakes. Rumen fill is less constant over the long term, as seasonal cold temperatures, and lactation, alter rumen capacity (NRC, 2016).

The relative importance of neuro-hormonal and digestive tract control in ruminants varies with the type of feed being eaten. The behaviour of lot-fed cattle is an example (Fig. 7.1). When we bring cattle into a feedlot from pasture they transition from a fibre-rich feed (grass) to ultimately a concentrate-rich, cereal grain-based feed. As this happens, intake control changes from a situation where

DOI: 10.1079/9781786394453.0007

rumen fill is important to one where the net energy requirement and available energy intake are the controlling factors.

Feed particle size is important for ruminants: Undigested feed has to be reduced to particles smaller than 1.2 mm to have a nearly 100% probability of passing into the omasum (Fig. 7.2). The shape of feed particles also affects their passage – fibres pass more slowly than cuboidal particles. This partly explains why legumes are eaten in greater quantities than grasses. Rumination is important because it is the main way in which feed particles are reduced in size.

We have to strike an optimum feed particle size. While small particles leave the rumen quickly, and this allows higher feed intakes, these small particles are digested less completely because they leave the rumen faster, and provide less protection against rumen disorders. Long pieces of roughage are needed to form the raft which floats above the rumen liquor. The raft promotes rumen movement and rumination (Zebeli *et al.*, 2012), and provides a place for micro-organisms to colonize the feed. Because these particles have to be chewed, this promotes saliva production which helps to maintain rumen pH above 5 and helps to avoid rumen acidosis.

Predicting feed intake

Accurate prediction of the amount of feed that our animals are likely to eat allows us to plan their nutritional management.

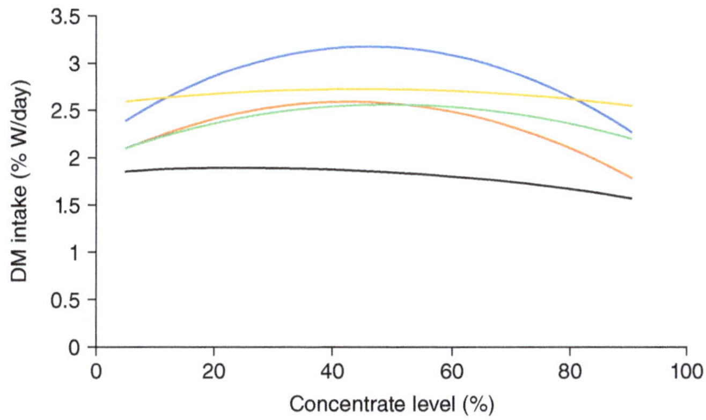

Fig. 7.1. Change in feed intake as the composition of a feedlot ration changes from roughage-rich to concentrate-rich. (Drawn from data in Ribeiro *et al.*, 2001; da Silva *et al.*, 2002; Ítavo *et al.*, 2002; Veloso *et al.*, 2002; Costa *et al.*, 2005; copyright: Gordon McL. Dryden.)

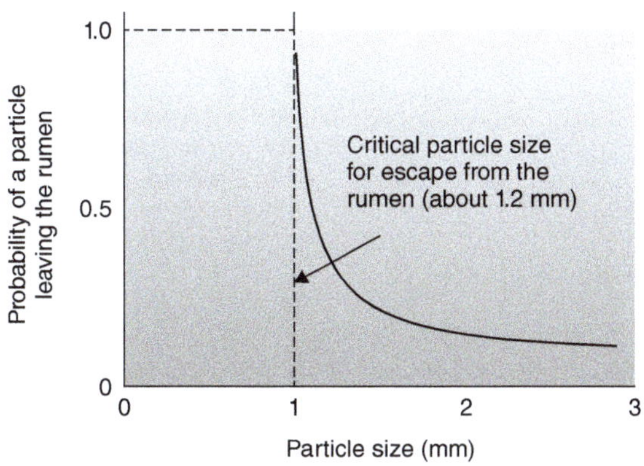

Fig. 7.2. The probability of undigested feed particles escaping from the rumen. (Copyright: Gordon McL. Dryden.)

First, we can use expected intakes to convert daily nutrient requirements into minimum acceptable nutrient concentrations (see Chapter 8). Using this information, we can determine the types of feed ingredients which will meet our animals' requirements.

Second, we can use information on feed intake to predict feed usage, and:

- Plan feed purchases, so that we can take advantage of seasonal availability and price variations.
- Design feed storages, storage capacities and handling facilities – the capacities needed in bins, silos, augers, milling equipment, feed trough capacity, and so on.

Feed intake can be predicted by quite simple relationships based on the animal's live weight and measures of productivity such as milk yields or carcase fatness. Some more complex prediction equations also include environmental factors and measures of feed chemical composition. Nutrient demand also is involved: dairy cows' feed consumption is also influenced by their milk production, and horses' feed intake is influenced by the amount and type of work they do.

Equations to predict intake: Prediction equations are either simple or complex. While the more complex equations are expected to give a more accurate estimate, they do not give an exact figure. For example, the equations for beef cattle in NRC (2000) explain only 12–70% of the between-animal variation in DM intakes, and a series of prediction equations for lactating sows explained only 25% of feed intake variation (O'Grady *et al.*, 1985).

Some feeding standards (e.g. for pigs, poultry and dairy cattle) predict feed intake by dividing the daily energy requirement by the energy content of the feed. This assumes that the metabolizable energy (ME) or NE requirement determines the amount of dry matter (DM) the animal will eat. But we need to be careful; this approach assumes either that an animal's capacity to eat is unlimited (which is not true), or that we are feeding a diet with an NE content which will meet the animal's energy requirement at intakes less than its upper appetite limit.

Should we use a complex or simple equation? This depends on what we want to use the information for: if we want a general idea of the amount of feed we should offer, or of how much storage capacity we need, then a simple equation is easy to use and gives a reasonable estimate.

If we want a more accurate answer, perhaps to calculate a nutrient requirement on a concentration basis rather than as an amount per day, then the more detailed equations which are used in nutrition models (Chapter 10) should give a better answer. These equations can be difficult to use but an Excel spreadsheet or similar will help. Prediction equations are developed from data sets obtained from particular types of animals and feeds. The closer the resemblance between our animals and feeds and the ones used in the data set, the more accurate the prediction will be.

Using prediction equations to understand behaviour: All predictors include live weight (W) or some derivative of it, e.g. standard reference weight (SRW, the live weight of a typical adult of that species and breed), or metabolic size ($W^{0.75}$; described in Chapter 8). This illustrates the connection between the animal's size and its maintenance energy requirement (Chapter 8). Other common prediction variables are the feed's available energy content, the animal's body fat content (as growing animals get bigger, the energy content of their live weight gain increases because they become fatter) and the environmental temperature.

Prediction equations help us to understand the factors which influence intakes. For example, the NRC (2012) equation for predicting the feed intake (FI, g/day) of young growing pigs is:

$$FI = (111 \times W^{0.803}) \times \{1 + [(LCT - T) \times 0.025]\}$$

This shows that intake is first determined by the animal's live weight (W, kg) and increases if the ambient temperature (T, °C) falls below the pig's lower critical temperature (LCT, °C) or decreases if the ambient temperature is above the LCT (see Chapter 19). This behaviour is discussed in more detail below.

Examples of prediction equations: Some examples of simple prediction equations are given in Table 7.1. These are by no means the only examples. For example, Faverdin (1992) lists 25 equations for lactating dairy cattle.

Some cautions:

- The equations in Table 7.1 will not accurately predict individual intakes, although they give a 'ballpark' figure.
- Most of these prediction equations do not differentiate between feeds on the basis of how easily they can be eaten or prehended (which includes grazing and rumination bites and chewing).

Table 7.1. Examples of simple equations to predict the feed intake of domestic animals.

Animal type	Prediction equation[a]	Reference
Poultry		
Broilers[b]	FI = 0.04 × W	Leung *et al.* (2018)
	FI = (AME_n required) / (feed AME_n content)	Poultry Hub (2021)
Laying hens[b]	FI = (AME_n required) / (feed AME_n content)	Hy-Line International (2020)
Pigs		
Growing pigs	DMI = (–0.0003 × W^2) + (0.0499 × W) + 0.1598	Quiniou *et al.* (2000)[c]
Lactating sows	FI = 3 + (0.3 × no. of piglets)	QDPI (1977)
	DEI = 13 + (0.596 × D) – (0.0172 × D^2)	NRC (1987)
Horses		
Weaners, yearlings	DMI = 0.02 × W	Dulphy *et al.* (1997)
Performance horses	DMI = 0.027 × W	Southwood *et al.* (1993)
Brood mares	DMI = 0.02 × W	NRC (2007)
Ruminants (general)		
Growing animals	DMI = 0.027 × W	MAFF (1984)
	FI = 0.03 × W	MAFF (1984)
	DMI = (120/NDF) + (NDFD – 45) × 0.026	Jeranyama and Garcia (2004)
Dairy cattle		
Lactating cows	DMI = (0.025 × W) + (0.1 × MY)	MAFF (1984)
	DMI = 2.726 + (0.015 × W) + (0.372 × FCM)	NRC (2001)[d]
	DMI = (5.4 × W) / [5 × (100 – DMD)]	Conrad (1966)[e]
	DMI = (0.011 × W) / NDF	Mertens (1985)[e]
Sheep		
Wethers	DMI = 0.028 × SRW	CSIRO (2007)[f]
Lactating ewes	DMI = 0.028 × SRW x 1.9 = 0.053 x SRW	CSIRO (2007)[g]
Beef cattle		
Growing steers	DMI = (0.034 × W) + 3.8	NRC (2016)[h]
Lactating cows	DMI = (0.03 × W) + (0.2 x MY) + 5.15	NRC (2016)[h]

[a]In these equations: DMI = dry matter intake (kg/day); FI = air-dry feed intake (kg/day); DEI = digestible energy intake (Mcal/day); W = live weight (kg); SRW = standard reference weight (kg); AME_n = apparent metabolizable energy, N corrected (MJ/kg); D = days into the lactation; MY = milk yield (kg/day); FCM = fat-corrected milk yield (= MY × (0.4 + 0.15 × (milk fat content, %)); DMD = dry matter digestibility (%); NDF = neutral detergent fibre content (decimal); NDFD = NDF digestibility.

[b]Indicative DMI are: 9-week-old male broilers 200 g/day, laying hens 80% lay, 98 g/day; DM intake based on feed providing 12.4 to 13.5 MJ ME/kg DM.

[c]Data reanalysed, this equation applies to growers between 30 and 90 kg live weight in a thermoneutral environment (25°C); the original equation provides for the effect of different ambient temperatures.

[d]Data reanalysed, this equation applies to the second and subsequent months of lactation.

[e]For roughage diets only; Conrad's equation adapted to use DMD rather than indigestible DM.

[f]Assuming that the wether is a mature adult in good but not over-fat body condition; DMI will be reduced if the body condition score is more than 2.5 (on a 5-point scale).

[g]DMI for a ewe at peak lactation (about 1 month after lambing) and in good but not over-fat body condition; DMI falls steadily after peak lactation.

[h]Data reanalysed for cattle eating a diet providing 1.7 Mcal NE_m/kg DM (or 7.1 MJ NE_m/kg DM).

The ways that pasture morphology (e.g. density and grazing height) affects the feed consumption of grazing animals are discussed in Chapter 14, and how the design of feeding equipment can affect intake is discussed in Chapter 17.

- When considering ruminant animals, apart from the relationships of Conrad (1966) and Mertens (1987), the equations in Table 7.1 do not differentiate between intakes of forages and concentrates, or on the basis of the feed's digestibility. We expect that the amount of DM eaten will be controlled by the animal's NE demand if the feed's digestibility is over 70%, while the intakes of feeds with lower digestibilities are more likely to be controlled by digestive tract fill (see Fig. 7.1).

INRA fill unit: The feed data published in Jarrige (1989) include a fill unit (FU), based on the measured

DM intakes of forages by cattle and sheep compared to a reference intake which is the average consumption of some 50 European, temperate (C3) grasses including ryegrasses, cocksfoot, fescues, timothy, brome grass and natural pasture. The reference feed has an organic matter digestibility of 77%.

There are three FU:

- For sheep (SFU): the standard sheep is an adult Texel wether which weighs 60 kg and eats 75 g DM/$W^{0.75}$ per day of the reference forage. Note: this SFU is not the Scandinavian Feed Unit (see Chapter 5).
- For growing cattle (CFU): the standard cow is a 17-month-old Friesian heifer which weighs 400 kg and eats 95 g DM/$W^{0.75}$ per day of the reference forage.
- For lactating cows (LFU): the standard cow is an adult cow which weighs 600 kg, produces 25 L/day of fat-corrected milk (FCM) in the fourth month of lactation, and eats 140 g DM/$W^{0.75}$ per day of the reference forage.

We can measure the animal's voluntary intake capacity using the FU as the unit of measurement. From the DM intakes quoted above, and the fact that for the reference feed FU = 1, we get these intake capacities for the standard animals:

- sheep: 1.62 SFU/day (= $75 \times 60^{0.75}/1000 \times 1$);
- growing cattle: 8.5 CFU/day (= $95 \times 400^{0.75}/1000 \times 1$); and
- lactating cow: 17.0 LFU/day (= $140 \times 600^{0.75}/1000 \times 1$).

The FU are additive for the same FU between different forages, e.g. we can calculate the weighted average of CFU values for several forages to get the total CFU for a mixed feed. Concentrates also have fill units (see INRAE, 2017–2020). These vary according to the composition of the whole feed, including the amount and quality of the roughage.

Example: If we were feeding a mixture (as-fed) of 2 kg of immature ryegrass hay (90% DM, 1.01 FU/kg), 0.5 kg of barley straw (88% DM, 1.58 FU/kg) and 7 kg of dough-stage maize silage (25% DM, 0.31 FU/kg) to a growing steer, the CFU of this mixture (as-fed basis) would be:

$$\text{Total CFU} = (1.01 \times 2) + (1.58 \times 0.5) + (0.31 \times 7) = 4.98$$

or

$$\text{CFU content (as-fed basis)} = 4.98 / (2 + 0.5 + 7) = 0.52 \text{ CFU/kg}$$

Note that the less digestible, more fibrous, barley straw has a higher FU than the highly digestible ryegrass hay, and that the FU for silage is low because these FU are expressed on an as-fed basis.

The intake capacity for a growing heifer is 8.5 CFU/day (see above). This means that the standard animal would be able to eat (8.5/0.52) = 16.3 kg of the hay/straw/silage ration described above.

Using the feed mixture described above, then:

$$\begin{aligned}\text{DM content of the mixture} &= [(\text{amounts of DM from each feed}) / (\text{total as-fed feed})] \times 100 \\ &= \{[(2 \times 0.9) + (0.5 \times 0.88) + (7 \times 0.25)] / (2 + 0.5 + 7)\} \times 100 \\ &= (3.99 / 9.5) \times 100 = 42\%\end{aligned}$$

so

$$\begin{aligned}\text{CFU (DM basis)} &= 0.52 \times (100/42) \\ &= 1.24 \text{ CFU/kg DM.}\end{aligned}$$

The Dutch satiety unit is similar to the INRA fill unit and is described by Blok and Spek (2016).

Practical factors which affect intake

The feed intakes that are suggested by prediction equations are estimates of likely average group intakes. It is rare for animals to exceed these estimates, and much more common for them to eat less (Dryden, 2006). There are several reasons for this, and we should be aware of these reasons so that we can try to avoid them.

Nutrient deficiencies and excesses: Pigs and poultry are sensitive to imbalances in amino acid supply. When we want to maximize feed intake (although we might not want to do that in some cases, e.g. when feeding finishing cattle or pigs, or pregnant sows) we should check that the diet supplies enough essential amino acids. Pigs given diets which are deficient in tryptophan, valine, isoleucine and histidine eat less feed, and interestingly, if the amino acid content of the feed is restricted pigs will eat faster to try to maintain their nutrient intake. Piglets are able to distinguish between diets differing in lysine content and prefer a better-balanced diet over a lysine-deficient one. However, it is not a good idea to simply load the feed with amino acids to try to make sure that there are no deficiencies. Not only is this very expensive, but pigs may eat less feed if they are confronted by excess amino acids, especially excess leucine.

There are similar responses in poultry. Broilers eat less feed if it is deficient in lysine or protein, and both deficiencies and excesses of methionine in relation to cysteine reduce intake. Birds are sensitive to mineral status: intakes are lower if the feed is deficient in available (i.e. non-phytate) P, and chelated Zn sources may improve feed intake over 'inorganic' Zn supplements.

Horses also prefer more nutritious feed, although taste and smell also influence feed choice.

The intake of roughages by ruminants is very much influenced by events in the rumen, as described above. In the short term, where we can assume that rumen fill is approximately constant, the rate that feed leaves the rumen through digestion or by passage of undigested feed to the abomasum equals the rate at which new feed can be eaten to replace it (Fig. 7.3).

Micro-organisms have to colonize feed in the rumen before digestion can begin. The lag time before feed begins to be digested accounts for about 10% of the difference between intakes of different feeds, rate of digestion accounts for another 10%, and passage of undigested feed for about 40%. Diets that are deficient in ruminally available N, P and S are eaten in lower amounts because the population of rumen micro-organisms is reduced, and this affects the rate at which feed is digested. Rumen RAN levels have to be maintained throughout the whole time that feed DM is being digested. This means that slowly digested RAN sources synchronize better with the microbial digestion of fibre. Urea is a good source of RAN but it is very rapidly converted to NH_3 and the uptake of urea-N by bacteria can be very incomplete.

Learning and social behaviour: Animals learn about feeds from their own experience (Chapter 14) through post-ingestive feedback, i.e. what they feel after they have eaten a particular type of feed (Provenza, 1995). They also learn from more experienced members of the herd or flock, often their dam.

When animals or birds are introduced to a new environment, they need time to find their feed and to learn how to use the feeding system. This occurs in all situations: from teaching pasture-fed cattle to adapt to a grain-rich ration fed in a feedlot trough, giving calves milk from a calfeteria for the first time, giving suckling foals a creep feed, moving dairy cattle to a new pasture, or introducing weaned pigs to their new pen and feeding equipment.

To facilitate learning, we should not make feed changes too quickly, and we must ensure that the feed is accessible to each animal.

Introducing new feeds can involve bringing feed to the animal and enticing it to eat, adding a flavour enhancer (e.g. using molasses to mask the taste of urea in a molasses/urea supplement), spreading feed on the ground near the animal (e.g. 'overflow' feeding from poultry pan feeders where feed is allowed to overflow the pan so that day-old chicks can find and easily eat the feed), mixing the new feed with the old in gradually increasing proportions, or simply being patient while animals become accustomed to a novel feed.

Learning is not always successful – e.g. cattle that are suffering from severe protein deficiency because they are grazing a mature, protein-deficient pasture in a drought, may not accept a supplement even though they are suffering and can see other herd members eating the supplement. All we can do here is either to

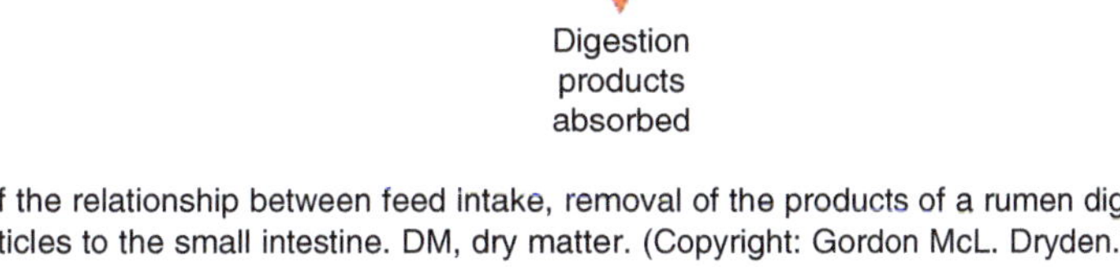

Fig. 7.3. Diagram of the relationship between feed intake, removal of the products of a rumen digestion and flow of undigested feed particles to the small intestine. DM, dry matter. (Copyright: Gordon McL. Dryden.)

separate the problem animal and feed a more acceptable (e.g. a forage-based) feed, or to cull it.

Social pressures within a group (e.g. dominance and leadership) can influence intake. For example, cattle grazing in a very large paddock and given a urea/molasses supplement from a feeder will only stay at the feeder until the leaders are satisfied – less dominant animals will move away with the rest of the herd even though they have not eaten as much as they may want.

Under extensive grazing, pasture intake and the ability to search for good grazing sites can be constrained by the competing demand of caring for young. A cow with a calf at foot cannot travel as fast or as far if she is limited by the need to care for her calf.

Competition for feed: Animals are most often managed in groups because this facilitates resource management, is less expensive than individual housing, and provides for animals' need for contact with others of their type. But group management allows competition for feed between animals. This increases the variability in feed intake and thus the performance of a group of animals. Groups of animals which vary in age, sex or live weight (e.g. in a pen of grower pigs) will exhibit extreme competition for feed. We cannot eliminate competition for feed unless we feed animals individually, and even then they will try to get feed allocated to others.

Animals change their behaviour to try to maintain feed intake. For example, subordinate pigs (Boumans *et al.*, 2018) eat faster for shorter times to maintain their feed intake. Nevertheless, competition can lead to subordinate animals being underfed. Competition for feed can be reduced or eliminated by careful feeder design and by how we manage feeding. We should:

- Check that animals are eating and drinking normally and watch for competition and bullying. Segregate shy feeders or subordinate animals if this is possible.
- Have feed available all the time, if this is practicable.
- Provide feed in several places: this can be by using multiple feeders (e.g. the pan feeders used with growing chicks), dividing the feeding station (e.g. a length of trough) with partitions which are wide enough for only a single animal, or using a 'calfeteria' set up where calves drink from separate teats which draw milk or milk replacer from a common container. This approach is often successful in reducing competition and equalizing intakes.
- Ensure that the feeding system is large enough to give each animal sufficient feeding space. This applies to the design of equipment like feed troughs (bunks) in a feedlot, or chain feeders (a length of open trough served by a conveyer belt) in broiler sheds (Chapter 17). While adequate space helps, it does not necessarily prevent unequal feed intakes as some animals will force others away from the trough even though there is sufficient trough space. Examples are a cow standing lengthwise against (or in) a feed trough, or pigs bullying weaker animals. Recommended feeding spaces are discussed in Chapter 17.
- Automatic electronic feeders reduce the effects of competition and can be used to restrict intakes or to feed special diets if this is needed. These feeders use a transponder attached to the animal (either in an ear tag or on a strap around the neck) to identify each individual and to tailor the amount and type of feed supplied to that individual only. The system can be set up so that access is allowed at certain times, or for a given number of times per day, or to certain feeders. Animals have to be trained to use this equipment, and feeding frequencies and amounts have to be carefully set to avoid animals crowding at the feeder and competing for access (Shrestha *et al.*, 1983).
- Feed animals individually by holding them in separate pens: this ensures correct feed intake for all individuals, but at the cost of a possible breakdown in social cohesion and at a financial cost. Examples are caged laying hens and individually penned breeding sows.

When feeding paddocked sheep or cattle, we can reduce competition by:

- Feeding grain or other supplements by running the feed out in a series of spirals or parallel lines. This reduces 'trailing' behaviour where animals run after the feed bin rather than stopping to eat. Putting supplements in heaps gives subordinate animals a better chance of competing with those that are more dominant.
- Feeding every 3 days, or twice a week. Because we feed out the same total amount of feed as would have been given by daily feeding, the amounts provided at each time are much larger and therefore it is more difficult for an individual to dominate most of the feed. This method is

used during survival feeding when animals are fed strictly limited amounts; it is not recommended for *ad lib* or production feeding.

- Adding salt to supplementary feed: salt limits the intake of dominant animals and this gives subordinate animals easier access to the feed. Methods for doing this are described by Lalman (2018). Cattle will eat an amount of salt equivalent to about 0.1% of their live weight. If we want a 450 kg steer to eat 4.5 kg of a grain supplement each day, then we should be able to achieve this by mixing 450 g salt (i.e. 0.1% of 450 kg) with the 4.5 kg of grain, or feeding a mixture containing 10% salt. We must provide clean, low-salinity water *ad lib* as the cattle will need extra water to excrete the excess Na that they have eaten.

Water availability: One of the earliest signs that animals have inadequate water is that they eat less feed. The water:DM intake ratio is a guide to the amount of water which we would expect a bird or animal to drink when it eats a given amount of feed. Estimates for poultry vary from 1.7 mL to 2.9 mL water/g air-dry feed, with the ratio increasing as the bird ages from 2 to 20 weeks. When converted to DM intakes, these ratios change to 1.9 mL to 3.2 mL water/g DM. Ratios for pigs are about 3.5, 2.6 and 3.5 L/kg DM eaten for weaner, grower/finisher and lactating sows, respectively. Water:DM ratios for ruminants are also close to 3 L/kg.

If the water:DM ratio is used to predict the amount of water needed by an animal, be aware that environmental conditions, as well as the animal's feed intake, influence the water requirement (see Chapter 2).

Weather conditions: An animal's upper and lower critical temperatures (UCT and LCT) map its thermoneutral zone (Chapter 19), which is the range of ambient temperatures in which it can control its core body temperature by means which do not affect its feed intake. Shivering and non-shivering thermogenesis increase heat production, and heat loss is reduced by huddling, seeking shelter, constricting dermal blood vessels and piloerection. Animals sweat, pant, wallow, seek shade, etc. to reduce the body's heat load.

Feed intake falls in hot weather and increases in cold weather. If the ambient temperature is above the animal's UCT, it will reduce its feed intake to try to reduce its heat load, and conversely if the temperature is below the LCT it will eat more feed to try to maintain its core body temperature.

Consequently, feed intake is affected by ambient temperature, humidity and wind speed as all of these affect the heat load. There are also some other factors which influence intake in particular circumstances. Heat loss from birds is increased if the bird loses feathers (i.e. has less insulation), and mud and rain reduce the insulation provided by a cow's coat. Well-conditioned animals are better insulated by their subcutaneous fat.

The ME intake of a laying hen decreases by 1.5% per °C between 12°C and 25°C (SCA, 1983), and the decrease can reach 4% per °C at ambient temperatures over 30°C (NRC, 1994). A grower pig is expected to eat 10–30% less feed at 30°C than at 20°C (NRC, 2012) and must eat more feed if the ambient temperature is below its LCT (which is about 20°C). British or European breed cattle eat about 3% less DM per °C when ambient temperatures are above 25°C.

Weather conditions can affect feed quality, and thus intake, directly. In hot conditions (ambient temperatures higher than about 30°C), freshly cut forage may begin to ferment and become less palatable. Feed which has been affected by rain is also unattractive. This is a major issue for feedlot managers because not only do cattle eat less wet feed, but they may have to be returned to a feed with a higher fibre content if their rumen has to be re-adapted to a concentrate-rich diet after a period of low feed intake.

Diurnal behaviour: Grazing animals show diurnal eating behaviour and feed consumption occurs in several different periods. For example, horses typically have 10 to 15 grazing periods in a day. We need to understand this because we can inadvertently limit feed intake by the way that we manage our animals.

An example: a survey of how farm inputs affected the milk production of dairy cattle in a subtropical region (Rees *et al.*, 1972) showed the expected responses to fertilization, irrigation and use of concentrate supplements, but also indicated that productivity was low on those farms where cows were confined in small 'night-grazing' paddocks. Because daytime temperatures were high, part of the cows' grazing time was in the evening when temperatures were cooler. Feed intake suffered when cows were limited to small grazing areas, and consequently milk yield was reduced as well.

Physical form and accessibility of feed: Animals find it more difficult to consume large pieces of feed. Chopped hay and silage, and pelleted feeds, are more easily prehended. Be careful when feeding pellets to poultry: the pellet must be small enough to be able to be prehended by the bird's beak and swallowed. This is why pelleted feed is passed through crumbling rolls to reduce the particle size before being given to poultry.

A grazing animal's ability to find and prehend its preferred feed is influenced by its ability to access the preferred plant or plant part (Chapter 14). We find this in some pastures where a large, often mature, tussock plant overshadows a smaller plant, or when in the same plant a young leaf is 'protected' by dry mature stems.

We can inadvertently make it difficult for animals to prehend feed if we use badly designed feeding equipment, or use well-designed equipment foolishly. The design and use of feeders is discussed in Chapter 17.

Exercise (work rate) in horses: Energy requirements increase when a horse is active and energy intake tends to increase as well, but there may be more variation due to differences between individual animals than is the result of the training or work regime. Low- and moderate-intensity work does not greatly increase feed intake, although the body condition of working horses may decline. High-intensity work may transiently increase intake but can also depress appetite (Kohnke *et al.*, 1999).

Pregnancy and lactation: Pregnant sows gain live weight easily and they can use this stored energy to contribute to milk production during their lactation. Sows which gain more weight during pregnancy eat less during their lactation than sows which gain less weight in pregnancy (Chapter 8). Managing these gains and losses in live weight is an important part of sow husbandry. Work summarized by O'Grady *et al.* (1985) shows that sows with more previous pregnancies, and those which produce more milk either because they have longer lactations or are nursing more piglets, eat more feed.

The feed intake of heavily pregnant sheep (e.g. ewes carrying twins) may be restricted by the increasing size of the uterus compressing the space available for the rumen (Forbes, 1971). Feed intake can be maintained by a faster rate of passage through the rumen, although this reduces the efficiency of digestion.

The DM intake of lactating cows lags behind their increase in milk production up to peak yield by about 30 days (CSIRO, 2007), as shown in Fig. 7.4. Nevertheless, lactating cows are able to eat 30–50% more feed than dry females because their rumen capacity is larger than a dry cow's. Feeding to get good body condition in cows at parturition helps to overcome the problem of intake lagging behind milk yield.

Feed composition: High fibre contents in poultry feeds can limit their available energy intake, but the response depends on the fibre source (and its

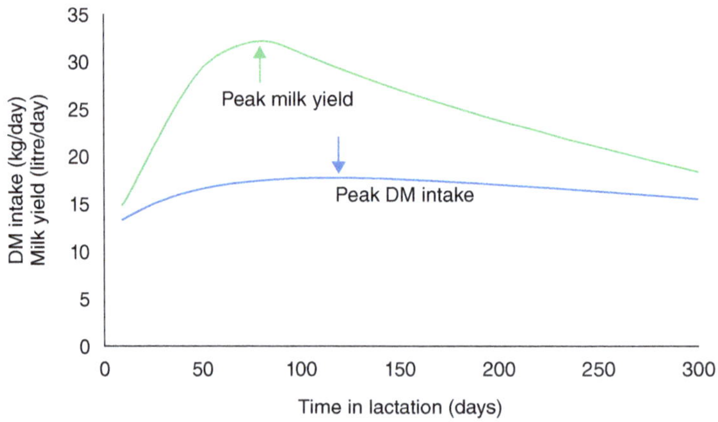

Fig. 7.4. Patterns of milk production and dry (DM) matter intake of lactating dairy cows (milk production follows the Woods curve after the peak, dry matter intakes are calculated from CSIRO, 2007). (Copyright: Gordon McL. Dryden.)

fermentability) and the strain of bird. Modern broiler or dual-purpose meat/layer strains can cope with crude fibre contents of up to about 10% in the feed. However, high feed fibre contents are likely to reduce feed intake. Understanding the birds' responses to dietary fibre is important if we want to use unconventional feeds, such as sugar beet pulp or tropical forage protein sources.

When pigs are given feeds diluted with milled straw or oat hulls, they will increase their intake by as much as 60% to accommodate the indigestible fibre load. Diets with added fat enable sows to eat more ME when ambient temperatures are above their UCT, but this does not apply in more moderate temperatures when they modify their intake to maintain more-or-less constant ME intakes.

Horses, cattle and sheep all tend to eat less fibre-rich feeds, with the response of ruminants being greater than that of horses. The decline in feed intake of sheep and cattle may be due to the increasing difficulty of digesting high-fibre feeds because these are more heavily lignified than the fibre in less fibrous, immature forages, or because high-fibre feeds typically have less ruminally degradable protein or RAN, or to the low palatability of these feeds, or to the resistance of fibrous feeds to chewing. Horses are able to eat more poorly digestible, fibrous feed than ruminants because they do not have a reticulo-rumen to retain long, undigested pieces of feed. Horses grazing the same mature, fibrous pasture as cattle generally maintain better body condition.

Substitution of concentrate for forage: When ruminants fed a roughage diet are also given a concentrate (e.g. grain) supplement, their total DM intake is less than expected because the supplement is substituted for some of the roughage. This effect is more pronounced when the roughage is of high quality, and for grazing animals when there is abundant pasture. Substitution rates are commonly between 0.6 kg and 1.0 kg of concentrate per kg of roughage.

Relationship between intake and performance: residual feed intake and feed:gain ratio

Feed is as much as 70% of the production cost in intensive poultry and pig enterprises, and the production of feed for grazing animals also has a cost. It is important to reduce the amount of feed that we need to use, and one aspect of this is to breed for animals which use feed efficiently. There are two indexes of feed efficiency that we can use.

Feed conversion efficiency (FCE; also called 'feed conversion ratio') is the amount of feed DM eaten compared to the amount of product produced by that animal. The product can be milk, meat, fibre or eggs, so we can have an FCE for milking goats, for example, of 0.95 kg DM/kg of milk (de Oliveira *et al.*, 2014). 'Feed efficiency' is the reciprocal of FCE, i.e. the amount of product for each unit of feed. These measures are useful indicators of how efficiently certain animal types, given particular types of feed, are performing. They are best used as indicators of herd or flock performance.

One of the common expressions of FCE is the feed:gain ratio, i.e. the amount of feed DM eaten compared to the amount of live weight gain produced. This gives an estimation of the nutritional efficiency of different types of animal enterprise. Growing pigs, broilers, beef cattle and sheep fed a concentrate-based diet will have feed:gain ratios of about 3:1 for pigs and poultry, 6:1 to 8:1 for growing lot-fed cattle, and about 5:1 for lot-fed sheep. These between-species differences are partly due to the way that monogastrics and ruminants prehend and digest feeds, and the nature of the digestion end-products used in the animal's metabolism.

Feed:gain ratios differ with the animal's inherent (genetic) growth capability and are influenced by the amount of energy available for growth compared to the animal's maintenance requirement (Chapter 8).

Residual feed intake (RFI; Koch *et al.*, 1963) is the difference between the animal's actual DM intake and the amount of feed DM that an 'average' animal in the flock or herd is expected to eat (Fig. 7.5). RFI can be described as 'high' or 'positive', or 'low' or 'negative'. If an animal eats less than the herd average but still produces the same amount and quality of product, it is more nutritionally efficient than the average. These animals have a low or negative RFI.

There are some important production and behavioural differences between positive and negative RFI animals:

- Although animals with negative RFI eat less feed then positive RFI animals there is usually no difference in growth rate, and the negative RFI animals are more efficient.

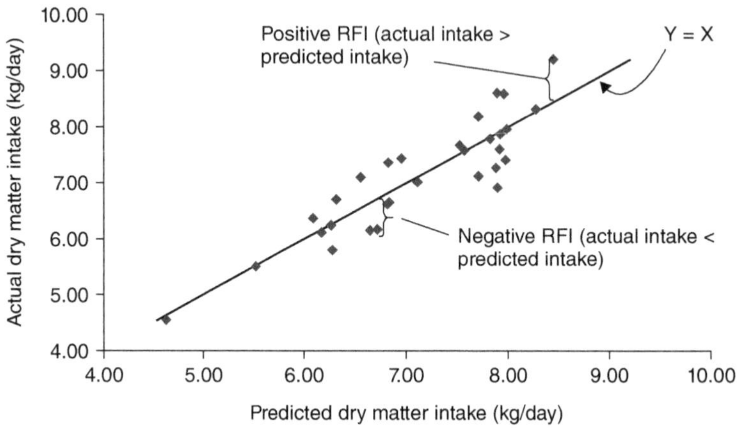

Fig. 7.5. Comparison of actual and predicted dry matter intakes of growing beef cattle. Intakes above the Y = X line have positive residual feed intake (RFI) and indicate that these animals use feed less efficiently; intakes below the line have negative RFI and indicate animals which use feed more efficiently. (From Sainz and Paulino, 2004; reproduced with permission.)

- Lactating cows with negative RFI produce similar amounts of milk as cows with positive RFI.
- Positive RFI pigs and cattle are fatter than those with a negative RFI.
- Negative RFI cattle may have a higher carcase dressing percentage (the 'dressed' carcase is the whole body less the head, hide, hooves and digestive tract).
- Negative RFI cattle, sheep, pigs and poultry eat less and spend less time eating, although they may eat faster.
- Negative RFI cattle kept in pens have similar levels of activity as cattle with positive RFI.
- Negative RFI cattle under feedlot conditions may select more long feed particles than those with positive RFI; this may help to maintain rumen health.
- When grazing under rangeland conditions, negative RFI cows appear to be more heat tolerant, maintain similar body condition scores, and have similar calf weaning weights as positive RFI cows.

The reasons for differences in RFI are not clear, but a great deal of work is currently being done to uncover them. There is evidence that this is a genetically determined characteristic and that negative RFI animals:

- have a somewhat different rumen microbial population;
- have a lower maintenance energy requirement; and
- can produce muscle tissue more efficiently.

Using RFI in practice: RFI is moderately heritable and is worth selecting for, but we need to be able to measure the DM intake of individual animals for at least 6 weeks. This can be done most easily with electronic feeding equipment (Chapter 17). It is best to keep animals in groups so that social factors can influence their feeding behaviour just as they will under normal feeding management.

RFI are mostly measured on growing animals, and we need to measure DM intake and the average daily gain (ADG; growth rate). We then calculate the expected DM intake by regressing DM intake (DMI, kg/day) against metabolic size ($W^{0.75}$, kg) and ADG (kg/day).

While RFI calculations are most commonly based on growth, some workers have included measurements of subcutaneous fat thickness for pigs and lactating cattle, and 'energy-corrected milk yield' for lactating cattle.

References

Blok, M.C. and Spek, J.W. (2016). *CVB Feed Table 2016. Chemical Composition and Nutritional Values of Feedstuffs*. Zoetermeer, The Netherlands: Federatie Nederlandse Diervoederketen.

Boumans, I.J.M.M., de Boer, I.J.M., Hofstede, G.J. and Bokkers, E.A.M. (2018). How social factors and behavioural strategies affect feeding and social interaction patterns in pigs. *Physiology and Behavior* 1: 23–40.

Conrad, H.R. (1966). Symposium on factors influencing the voluntary intake of herbage by ruminants: physiological and physical factors limiting feed intake. *Journal of Animal Science* 25:227–235.

Commonwealth Scientific and Industrial Research Organisation (CSIRO) (2007): *Nutrient Requirements of Domesticated Ruminants*. Collingwood, Vic: CSIRO Publishing.

Costa, M.A.L., Filho, S. de C.V., Paulino, M.F., Valadares, R.F.D., Cecon, P.R., Paulino, P.V.R., de Moraes, E.H.B.K. and Magalhães, K.A. (2005). Productive performance, digestibility and carcass characteristics of zebu steers fed diets with different concentrate levels. *Revista Brasileira de Zootecnia* 34(1): 268–279.

da Silva, F.F., Filho, S. de C.V., ÍtavoL, C.V., Veloso, C.M., Paulino, M.F., Valadares, R.F.D., Cecon, P.R., Silva, P.A. and Galvão, R.M. (2002). Carcass characteristics and biometric of gastrointestinal tract and internal organs of Nellore bulls receiving diets with different concentrate and protein levels. *Revista Brasileira de Zootecnia* 31(4): 1849–1864.

Dryden, G.McL. (2006). Investigating daily changes in food intake by ruminants. In Kebreab, E., Dijkstra, J., Bannink, A., Gerrits, W.J.J. and France, J. (eds) *Nutrient Digestion and Utilization in Farm Animals. Modelling Approaches*. Wallingford, UK: CAB International, pp. 314–327.

Dryden, G.McL. (2008). *Animal Nutrition Science*. Wallingford, UK: CAB International.

Dulphy, J.P., Martin-Rosset, W., Dubroeucq, H., Ballet, J.M., Detour, A. and Jailler, M. (1997). Compared feeding patterns in *ad libitum* intake of dry forages by horses and sheep. *Livestock Production Science* 52: 49–56.

Faverdin, P. (1992). Alimentation des vaches laitières: Comparaison des différentes methods de prédiction des quantités ingérées. *INRA Production Animales* 5(4): 271–282.

Forbes, J.M. (1971). Physiological changes affecting voluntary food intake in ruminants. *Proceedings of the Nutrition Society* 30: 135–142.

Hy-Line International (2020). *Nutritional Levels*. Available at: www.hyline.com/technical-resources (accessed 27 December 2020).

Institut National de Recherche pour l'Agriculture, l'Alimentation et l'Environnement (INRAE) (2017–2020). *INRAE-CIRAD-AFZ Feed Tables*. Available at: www.feedtables.com/ (accessed 27 December 2020).

Ítavo, L.C.V., Filho, S. de C.V., da Silva, F.F., Valadares, R.F.D., Cecon, P.R., Ítavo, C.C.B.F., de Moraes, E.H.B.K. and Paulino, P.V.R. (2002). Concentrate and crude protein levels in growing Nelore bulls diets. Intake and digestibility. *Revista Brasileira de Zootecnia* 31(2): 1033–1041.

Jarrige, R. (ed.) (1989). *Ruminant Nutrition: Recommended Allowances and Feeding Tables*. Paris: John Libbey Eurotext/INRA.

Jeranyama, P. and Garcia, A.D. (2004). *Understanding Relative Feed Value (RFV) and Relative Forage Quality (RFQ)*. Extension Extra. Paper 352. Available at: www.yumpu.com/en/document/read/6339820/understanding-relative-feed-value-rfv-and-relative-forage- (accessed 27 December 2020).

Koch, R.M., Swiger, L.A., Chambers, D. and Gregory, K.E. (1963). Efficiency of feed use in beef cattle. *Journal of Animal Science* 22(2): 486–494.

Kohnke, J., Kelleher, F. and Trevor-Jones, P. (1999). *Feeding Horses in Australia*. Canberra: RIRDC.

Lalman, D. (2018). Supplementing Beef Cows. Oklahoma Cooperative Extension Service. Available at: www.extension.okstate.edu/fact-sheets/supplementing-beef-cows.html (accessed 10 March 2021).

Leung, H., Arrazola, A., Torrey, S. and Kiarie, E. (2018). Utilization of soy hulls, oat hulls, and flax meal fiber in adult broiler breeder hens. *Poultry Science* 97: 1368–1372.

Mertens, D.R. (1987). Predicting intake and digestibility using mathematical models of ruminal function. *Journal of Animal Science* 64(5): 1548–1558.

Ministry of Agriculture Fisheries and Food (MAFF) (1984). *Energy Allowances and Feeding Systems for Ruminants*, 2nd edn. London: HMSO.

National Research Council (NRC) (1987). *Predicting Feed Intake of Food-Producing Animals*. Washington, DC: National Academy Press. Available at: www.nap.edu/catalog/950/predicting-feed-intake-of-food-producing-animals (accessed 27 December 2020).

National Research Council (NRC) (1994). *Nutrient Requirements of Poultry*, 9th rev. edn. Washington, D.C: National Academy Press. Available at: www.nap.edu/catalog/2114/nutrient-requirements-of-poultry-ninth-revised-edition-1994 (accessed 27 December 2020).

National Research Council (NRC) (2000). *Nutrient Requirements of Beef Cattle*, 7th rev. edn. Update. Washington, DC: National Academy Press. Available at: www.nap.edu/catalog/9791/nutrient-requirements-of-beef-cattle-seventh-revised-edition-update-2000 (accessed 27 December 2020).

National Research Council (NRC) (2001). *Nutrient Requirements of Dairy Cattle*, 7th rev. edn. Washington, DC: National Academy Press. Available at: www.nap.edu/catalog/9825/nutrient-requirements-of-dairy-cattle-seventh-revised-edition-2001 (accessed 27 December 2020).

National Research Council (NRC) (2007). *Nutrient Requirements of Horses*, 6th rev. edn. Washington, DC: National Academy Press. Available at: www.nap.edu/catalog/11653/nutrient-requirements-of-horses-sixth-revised-edition (accessed 27 December 2020).

National Research Council (NRC) (2012). *Nutrient Requirements of Swine*, 11th rev. edn. Washington, DC: National Academy Press. Available at: www.nap.edu/catalog/13298/nutrient-requirements-of-swine-eleventh-revised-edition (accessed 27 December 2020).

National Research Council (NRC) (2016). *Nutrient Requirements of Beef Cattle*, 8th rev. edn. Washington, DC: National Academy Press. Available at: www.nap.edu/catalog/19014/nutrient-requirements-of-beef-cattle-eighth-revised-edition (accessed 27 December 2020).

O'Grady, J.F., Lynch, P.B. and Kearney, P.A. (1985). Voluntary feed intake by lactating sows. *Livestock Production Science* 12(4):355–366.

de Oliveira, T.S., Leonel, F. de P., da Silva, C.J., Baffa, D.F., Pereira, J.C. and Zervoudakis, J.T. (2014). Factors affecting feed efficiency in dairy goats. *Revista Brasileira de Zootecnia*, 43(10), 524-529. DOI: doi.org/10.1590/S1516-35982014001000003.

Poultry Hub (2021). *Nutrient requirements of meat chickens (broilers)*. Poultry Hub. Available at: https://www.poultryhub.org/all-about-poultry/nutrition/nutrition-requirements-of-meat-chickens-broilers (also see terms of use at www.poultryhub.org/about/disclaimers/) (accessed 25 March 2021).

Provenza, F.D. (1995). Postingestive feedback as an elementary determinant of food preference and intake in ruminants. *Journal of Range Management* 48(1): 2–17.

Queensland Department of Primary Industries (QDPI) (1977). *Farm Management Handbook*, 5th edn. Brisbane: QDPI, Economic Services Branch.

Quiniou, N., Dubois, S. and Noblet, J. (2000). Voluntary feed intake and feeding behaviour of group-housed growing pigs are affected by ambient temperature and body weight. *Livestock Production Science* 63(3): 245–253.

Rees, M.C., Minson, D.J. and Kerr, J.D. (1972). Relation of dairy productivity of feed supply in the Gympie district of south-eastern Queensland. *Australian Journal of Experimental Agriculture and Animal Husbandry* 12(59): 553–560.

Ribeiro, T.R., Pereira, J.C., de Oliveira, M.V.M., de Queiroz, A.C., Cecon, P.R., Leão, M.I. and de Alvarenga e Melo, R.C. (2001). Influence of nutritional plane on performance of Holstein veal calves. *Revista Brasileira de Zootecnia* 30(6): 2154–2162.

Sainz, R.D. and Paulino, P.V. (2004). *Residual Feed Intake*. UC Davis: Sierra Foothill Research and Extension Center. Available at: www.escholarship.org/uc/item/9w93f7ks (accessed 27 December 2020).

Shrestha, C.M., Spahr, S.L., Puckett, H.B. and Olver, E.F. (1983). Electronic transponder feeder system performance and animal feeding behavior with four feed availability times. *Journal of Dairy Science* 66: 332–340.

Southwood, L.L., Evans, D.L., Bryden, W.L. and Rose, R.J. (1993). Nutrient intake of horses in Thoroughbred and Standardbred stables. *Australian Veterinary Journal* 70: 164–168.

Standing Committee on Agriculture (SCA) (1983). *Feeding Standards for Australian Livestock. Poultry*. Melbourne: CSIRO.

Tachibana, T. and Tsutsui, K. (2016). Neuropeptide control of feeding behavior in birds and its difference with mammals. *Frontiers in Neuroscience* 10: Article 485.

Veloso, C.M., Filho, S. de C.V., Gesualdi Junior, A., da Silva, F.F., Paulino, M.F., Valadares, R.F.D., Cecon, P.R. and Paulino, P.V.R. (2002). Efficiency of metabolizable energy utilization for maintenance and weight gain and metabolizable energy and total digestible nutrients requirements of F1 Limousin x Nellore bulls. *Revista Brasileira de Zootecnia* 31(3): 1294–1301.

Zebeli, Q., Aschenbach, J.R., Tafaj, M., Boguhn, J., Ametaj, B.N. and Drochner, W. (2012). Invited review: Role of physically effective fiber and estimation of dietary fiber adequacy in high-producing dairy cattle. *Journal of Dairy Science* 95(3):1041–1056.

8 Nutrient requirements

The discussion in this chapter describes how animals use nutrients, and their requirements for these nutrients. The prediction equations discussed here do not have to be used in practice by farmers or managers – we can get the information we need from nutrient requirements tables, or better, by using nutritional models (Chapter 10). However, it is useful to understand how this information is generated and presented.

Animals' nutrition should be carefully managed: If we simply give conventional feed to an animal – hay or pasture for ruminants and horses, or a grain-based feed for pigs and poultry – it will often continue to produce the product that we want, whether that is companionship or an economic outcome like fibre, eggs, draught power or meat. Animals can be forgiving of poor nutritional management, but they will only be so:

- for a limited time;
- if the feed fortuitously has enough of each of the wide range of nutrients that the animal needs; and
- usually at the cost of lower productivity and poorer product quality.

Therefore, if we want our animals to be healthy and productive, we must:

- understand the types of nutrients that they need (Chapter 1); and
- know the amount of each nutrient that they need.

It is convenient to divide an animal's nutrient requirements into those for maintenance and those for production.

Nutrient requirements for maintenance

Nutrients are needed to support life processes such as breathing, blood circulation, transport of nutrients and wastes, temperature control, digestion, nerve activity and general muscle activity.

In addition, and very importantly, animal body tissues and cell constituents are continually being destroyed and replaced. This is essential to keep body tissues in a healthy and functioning state. For example, the half-life of liver cells is 4 to 5 days, i.e. half of the liver cells are destroyed and remade in that time. Similarly, enzymes have very short half-lives, e.g. 10 to 30 minutes for ornithine decarboxylase, and 48 hours for acetyl CoA carboxylase. Animals need a wide range of nutrients (including energy and water) to synthesize these molecules and tissues and to deal with the wastes produced when they are destroyed.

The maintenance requirements for nutrients can be defined by the effects of nutrient use on animal physiology and biochemistry: When an animal is not stressed by its environment and is not producing, then:

- The maintenance requirements for energy, amino acids, fatty acids and minerals are the amounts needed each day to keep the animal at a constant live weight and body composition.
- The animal uses water, minerals and vitamins as constituents of enzymes and hormones and to support metabolic processes such as kidney function, secretion of digestive enzymes and bile, and the control of body temperature. The maintenance requirements for these nutrients are the amounts which are needed to maintain proper metabolic function.

The net energy requirement for maintenance is the sum of the energy required for:

- Basal metabolism (the basal metabolic rate, BMR) – the energy used to fuel the life processes described above. The BMR is remarkably constant for eutherian animals and birds. Selected values are:
  Cattle: 0.35 MJ/$W^{0.75}$ per day
  Pigs: 0.32 MJ/$W^{0.75}$ per day
  Poultry: 0.36 MJ/$W^{0.75}$ per day

DOI: 10.1079/9781786394453.0008

$W^{0.75}$ (kg) is the animal's metabolic weight. This is defined in the following text:

- Body temperature regulation – the energy needed to vaporize water from the lungs and to excrete sweat, and energy used in panting, wallowing, huddling, etc. In cold weather, the energy needed to maintain the core body temperature of animals kept outside can raise the maintenance energy requirement to more than twice that of housed animals. Wind and rain reduce the insulation provided by the animal's coat, and thin animals have less subcutaneous fat to provide insulation. Newborn animals have a high maintenance energy requirement because of their large surface area to mass ratio which facilitates the loss of body heat.
- Voluntary movement – the energy used in grazing, eating, playing, etc.

The amount of NE required for maintenance (NE_m, MJ/day) is the sum of these three energy uses:

$$NE_m = BMR + (\text{energy used for temperature control}) + (\text{energy used for voluntary activity})$$

The amount of metabolizable energy (ME) required for maintenance (ME_m, MJ/day) is calculated from the NE_m by allowing for the efficiency of use of ME for this process (conversion efficiencies between ME and NE are described in Chapter 5).

The net protein requirement for maintenance (NP_m, g/day) is the sum of the endogenous losses of N from the body, expressed as the equivalent amount of protein.

The N excreted in urine and faeces is either exogenous or endogenous. Exogenous N comes more-or-less directly from the feed the animal has eaten, e.g. undigested feed protein in the faeces, and that fraction of the urinary urea-N which is derived from the deamination of excess feed amino acids. Endogenous N comes from body tissues and cell constituents which have been turned over during the animal's normal metabolism as described above.

Endogenous N is lost from the body in these forms:

- Endogenous urinary nitrogen (EUN): the main endogenous N constituent of urine is urea, which is the detoxification product of the NH_3 that is produced when amino acids, which had been part of cell proteins, are deaminated (i.e. their amino, $-NH_2$, group is removed). Other important constituents are creatinine which is the excretion product of creatine (an energy storage compound); and purine derivatives which are the excretion products of nucleic acids (see also Chapter 5).
- Metabolic faecal nitrogen (MFN): bacteria from the large intestine and the cell walls of ruminal bacteria, sloughed intestinal cells, mucus, and sometimes plasma protein.
- Detritus (integument) nitrogen – mainly hair and skin cells lost from the body.

Reasonable estimates of endogenous N losses from cattle are (CSIRO, 2007):

$$\text{EUN (g/day)} = 5.92 \times \log_{10}(W) - 6.8$$
$$\text{MFN (g/day)} = 2.43 \times DMI$$
$$\text{Detritus N (g/day)} = 0.018 \times W^{0.75}$$

where: W = live weight (kg)
DMI = dry matter intake (kg/day).

In a manner similar to how we calculate the maintenance energy requirement, the NP_m is:

$$NP_m = [(EUN + MFN + \text{detritus N})] \times 6.25$$

The maintenance protein requirement can also be expressed as the amount of metabolizable protein (MP) needed. See Fig. 5.4 (Chapter 5) for a definition of MP, and for conversion efficiencies (kp) of MP to NP for different physiological processes.

Live weight and metabolic size: The nutrient requirements for maintenance (energy expenditure and endogenous N losses), amino acid requirements, feed intake and other nutritional characteristics vary in proportion to the animal's size – but are often more closely related to metabolic size than live weight.

An animal's live weight is the weight of its whole body, including its digestive tract fill. Because gut fill is variable, and these variations affect the reliability of live weight measurements, live weight is sometimes measured after a period of feed withdrawal. This is called 'shrunk' live weight and is equivalent to the live weight which would be measured after an overnight (16 hours) fast (sometimes called a 'feed curfew') but with access to water. If an actual shrunk live weight cannot be measured, we can take it to be 96% of full live weight.

Metabolic size is the animal's live weight (W, kg) raised to the 0.75 power: $W^{0.75}$ kg (Fig. 8.1). The concept of metabolic size is discussed in detail in Dryden (2008).

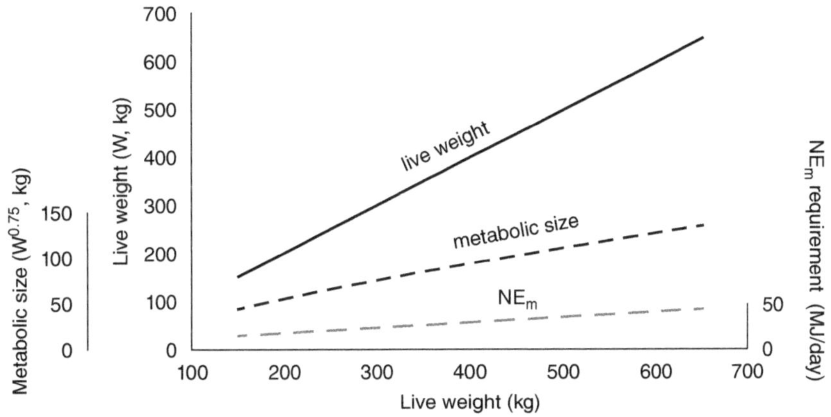

Fig. 8.1. Plots of live weight (W), metabolic size ($W^{0.75}$) and the net energy for maintenance (NE_m) requirement of cattle. NE_m varies in relation to metabolic size rather than live weight. (Copyright: Gordon McL. Dryden.)

Nutrient requirements for production

Domestic animals 'produce' in several different ways. These include:

- producing meat – by growing, i.e. by increasing their body size;
- producing fibre – by growing their pelage (the animal's coat) between periodic harvests (shearing);
- reproducing – this includes the production of eggs, milk and offspring;
- working – including the work of draught animals (e.g. pulling carts, ploughing), and activities such as racing, show-jumping, etc.; and
- companionship – which is achieved by keeping the animal alive and healthy.

We can see from the above list that there are three different types of 'production':

- growth – the increase in the animal's size when new cells are made, or the size of cells increases, or when cells change their chemical composition (e.g. when osteoblasts in developing bone become calcified);
- synthesis of tissues or products which are not part of the animal's body (e.g. foetus, milk and eggs); and
- activity.

The amounts of nutrients the animal needs for these three types of production are its production requirements.

Factorial method for evaluating energy requirements: With this approach we identify each component of a producing animal's energy use and sum them to get the total requirement. For example, a lactating cow's NE requirement is:

$$\text{Total NE} = NE_m + [(\text{milk NE content}) \times (\text{milk yield})] + (\text{NE of developing foetus})$$

We can partition these items further, as in Fig. 8.2. This greater detail allows the animal manager to identify and quantify the effects of the age and breed of cow on the BMR; the effects of ambient temperature, wind speed, humidity and coat condition on the NE required for temperature regulation; and the effects of time in the pregnancy and animal breed on the amount of NE retained in the growing foetus and needed to support foetal growth.

For example: a lactating and pregnant Holstein/Friesian cow weighing 625 kg, producing 35 L/day of 4% fat and 3.5% protein milk in the 120th day of her lactation, 30 days pregnant with an expected calf birth weight of 47 kg, and with no live weight loss or gain. She is grazing a flat paddock, and the ambient temperature is 25°C with no wind or rain (these conditions describe a thermoneutral environment; Chapter 19).

Her total NE requirement can be calculated from these relationships (adapted from NRC, 2001):

A: Energy used for maintenance is calculated from the animal's metabolic weight ($W^{0.75}$, kg), the NE requirement per unit of metabolic weight (a, MJ/kg), and a breed adjustment factor for Jersey and Friesian cattle (F_{breed}). Other adjustments, although not included here, can be made

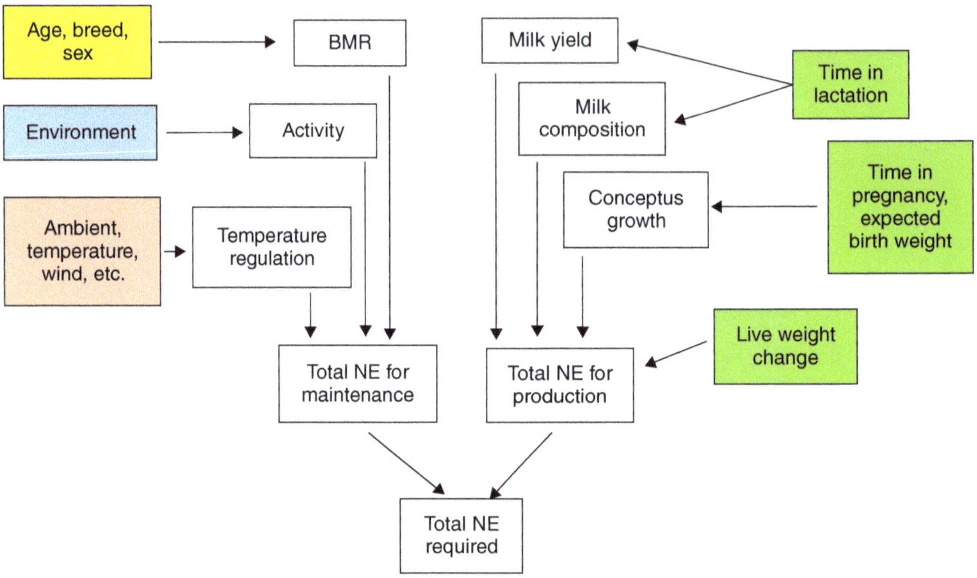

Fig. 8.2. Partitioning of the net energy (NE) requirement of a lactating cow. (Copyright: Gordon McL. Dryden.)

for age, sex and environment characteristics. The calculation is:

$$NE_m = a \times W^{0.75} \times F_{breed}$$
$$= 0.33 \times 625^{0.75} \times 1.12$$
$$= 46.2 \text{ MJ NE/day}$$

B: Energy retained in milk is calculated from the milk yield (MY, kg/day) and composition. We can use this formula developed by Tyrrell and Reid (1965) which uses milk fat (F, %) and protein (P, %) contents to predict the NE content of milk:

$$NE_{milk} = MY \times [(0.376 \times F) + (0.209 \times P) + 0.948]$$
$$= 35 \times [(0.376 \times 4) + (0.209 \times 3.5) + 0.948]$$
$$= 111.4 \text{ MJ NE/day}$$

C: Energy retained in the conceptus (foetus, uterus and placenta) is calculated from the time in the pregnancy (D, days) the expected calf birth weight (CBW, kg), and the efficiency of use of feed energy for foetal growth (k_y):

$$NE_y = \{[(0.0133 \times D) - 0.147] \times (CBW/45)\}/k_y$$
$$= \{[(0.0133 \times 30) - 0.147] \times (47/45)\}/0.218$$
$$= 1.2 \text{ MJ NE/day.}$$

The total NE required by the lactating cow (NE_l, MJ/day) is the sum of the NE required for maintenance plus the NE retained in milk plus the NE retained in the growing conceptus.

$$NE_l = A + B + C$$
$$= 46.2 + 111.4 + 1.2$$
$$= 158.8 \text{ MJ NE/day}$$

Converting NE requirements to ME requirements: The efficiency with which ME is used as a source of NE varies between animal species, feed types and the purpose that the feed energy is used for. These conversion efficiencies are discussed in Chapter 5. To calculate the amount of ME required, we divide the NE requirement for each process (maintenance, growth, milk production, etc.) by the relevant efficiency. However, this calculation can be simplified if we are working with dairy cattle (see Chapter 5 for the reason), and the calculation is:

$$ME_l = NE_l/k_l$$
$$= 158.8/0.62$$
$$= 256.1 \text{ MJ ME/day}$$

Factorial method for evaluating protein or amino acid requirements: As with energy (above), we can identify and quantify each use for any given amino acid. The sum gives us the total amount of the amino acid needed. Lysine is used as the reference amino acid in pig nutrition (the one that all the other essential amino acid requirements are compared to, see below) and we will use it as an example of how a factorial evaluation works.

The lactating sow uses amino acids for maintenance and for milk protein synthesis. The amount of lysine needed by a lactating sow depends on:

- her maintenance requirement;
- the amount of lysine excreted in milk protein; and
- the amount of lysine made available from breaking down (catabolizing) body tissue protein.

It is best to define requirements in terms of available nutrients, and in this example we use standardized ileal digestible lysine (SIDLys). See Chapter 4 for definitions and examples of standardized (or 'true') digestibility.

Calculating the SIDLys requirement is a little more complicated than calculating the NE requirement. We have to measure (or predict) the amounts of lysine which are excreted in milk and obtained from body tissue protein that she has accumulated during pregnancy and metabolizes during the lactation. SIDLys is used with an efficiency of about 67% for milk production and tissue lysine is used with 87% efficiency (NRC, 2012).

Example: a lactating sow weighing 200 kg has a litter of 11 piglets growing at an average of 275 g/day, and she is producing 10.5 kg of milk per day. The sow eats 6.5 kg of feed/day. She has accumulated 20 kg of body weight gain during her pregnancy and loses 15 kg during the 21-day lactation, i.e. 715 g/day. Relationships and data are adapted from NRC (2012) and Tokach *et al.* (2019).

A: SIDLys required for maintenance is the sum of endogenous lysine secreted into the digestive tract (which is calculated from the feed intake, FI, kg/day), plus the lysine in lost skin and hair (which is calculated from the sow's metabolic weight, $W^{0.75}$, kg). k_{lys} (decimal) is the efficiency with which feed SIDLys is used to replace the excreted endogenous lysine.

$$\text{SIDLys for endogenous loss} = [(0.2827 \times FI) + (0.0045 \times W^{0.75})]/k_{lys}$$
$$= [(0.2827 \times 6.5) + (0.0045 \times 200^{0.75})]/0.75$$
$$= 2.77 \text{ g/day}$$

B: SIDLys required for milk protein synthesis is calculated from the lysine content of milk protein and the sow's milk yield. In this example we use an estimate of milk yield (MY, kg/day) and assume milk protein (MilkPr) and protein lysine (MilkPrLys) contents of 4.9% and 7.01%, respectively. k_{lys} is the efficiency with which SIDLys is used for milk protein synthesis.

$$\text{SIDLys for milk} = (MY \times MilkPr \times MilkPrLys)/k_{lys}$$
$$= [(10.5 \times 1000) \times 0.049 \times 0.0701]/0.67$$
$$= 53.83 \text{ g/day}$$

C: Lysine mobilized from catabolized body protein: when the sow loses live weight during her lactation, lysine becomes available from the broken-down body protein. This is the product of the amount of live weight lost (LWC, g/day) and the protein (TissPr, decimal) and lysine (TissPrLys, decimal) contents of this tissue. k_{lys} is the efficiency with which this mobilized tissue lysine is used for milk protein synthesis. We assume that all of the lysine available from body tissue metabolism is directed to milk protein synthesis.

$$\text{Lysine from body tissue} = (LWC \times TissPr \times TissPrLys) \times k_{lys}$$
$$= (715 \times 0.1 \times 0.0674) \times 0.868$$
$$= 4.18 \text{ g/day}$$

Feed SIDLys required by the lactating sow is the difference between the amount of lysine secreted in milk (B) plus the lysine required for maintenance (A), and the amount of tissue lysine available for milk protein synthesis (C).

$$\text{Feed SIDLys} = (A + B - C)$$
$$= 2.77 + 53.83 - 4.18$$
$$= 52.42 \text{ g/day}$$

or, expressed as a concentration in the feed = 0.8% (as-fed).

Ideal protein: Analyses of animal products, e.g. the sow's milk protein or the protein of a bird's lean body tissue, tell us the amounts and ratios of the different amino acids required to make the product. This information allows, in theory, diet formulations which will supply the exact amounts of amino acids needed to meet the animal's maintenance and production requirements. Such an amino acid mixture is called an 'ideal protein'.

Requirements for the other essential amino acids are often expressed in relation to lysine, i.e. using lysine:amino acid ratios. If the diet contains essential amino acids in their correct ratios to lysine, and the lysine content meets the animal's lysine requirement, then we will have provided all the essential amino acids in the required amounts.

The two concepts described above can be combined to give ideal amino acid ratios. This approach is widely used in formulating diets for pigs and poultry.

'Ideal' ratios are based on the amino acid requirements for protein synthesis, although this ignores the other metabolic roles of amino acids. Ideal ratios vary with animal age, sex, product type, level of production, and the use of growth promoters (e.g. ractopamine for grower pigs). To a limited extent, some amino acids can substitute for others, e.g. cystine can provide 50–80% of the requirement for S-amino acids, and tyrosine can provide 50% of the tyrosine + phenylalanine requirement of pigs.

Different authorities have adopted somewhat different 'ideal' proteins (see van Milgen and Dourmad 2015 for examples). Table 8.1 gives the ratios of the essential amino acids to lysine in pig body protein used in the INRAPorc nutrition model (van Milgen *et al.*, 2008); they are similar to the ratios used by NRC (2012).

The information needed to feed animals effectively and safely

When we state an animal's 'requirement' for a given nutrient, we are indicating the amount that it needs for a given function or group of functions, e.g. for maintenance, for growth, for reproduction, or in total. Sometimes, requirements are stated as 'allowances'. These are recommended amounts of nutrient which are sufficient to meet the animal's requirements and which include a small (often 5%) safety margin.

Published 'feeding standards' are lists of recommended nutrient requirements or allowances.

Nutrient requirements can be expressed as daily amounts, or as concentrations in the feed: An animal's daily requirement for nutrients is determined by its type, age, size, physiological status and production level, and it makes sense to specify nutrient requirements in amounts per day.

But when we formulate rations, we have to express nutrient requirements not as daily amounts, but as concentrations in the feed (on either a DM or as-fed basis) so that they match the units used for expressing the nutrient contents in feeds. This is done by dividing the daily nutrient requirement by the amount of feed (DM or as-fed) that we expect the animal to eat, to get the required nutrient concentration (see Chapter 9).

Nutrients, feed constituents and secondary substances: Table 8.2 summarizes the information that is needed for poultry, pigs, horses and ruminants (also see Chapters 1, 2, 5 and 12). This information covers nutrients, feed constituents that are desirable in animals' diets although they are not nutrients, and secondary substances that are present in some feeds and which have adverse effects on nutrient availability, animal health or product quality.

Feeding standards for poultry, pigs, horses, dairy cattle and beef cattle

This section describes feeding standards and discusses some of the factors which affect nutrient requirements. It does not provide detailed data on nutrient requirements – this information is best obtained from current feeding standards or nutritional models.

Information sources: Recommendations for animal nutrient requirements have been developed from research carried out all over the world. Much of this work has been done with the breeds and strains of animals commonly used in temperate regions, and only more recently with tropical animal breeds. We can apply temperate region data generally to all animals of each type, but there are

Table 8.1. Ratios of essential amino acids in pig body protein. (INRAPorc data cited by van Milgen and Dourmad, 2015; reproduced in accordance with CC BY 4.0.)

Amino acid	Amino acid composition of body protein (%)	Amino acid: lysine ratio	Amino acid	Amino acid composition of body protein (%)	Amino acid: lysine ratio
Lys	6.96	100	Ile	3.46	55
Met	1.88	30	Leu	7.17	100
Cys	1.03	30	Phe	3.78	50
Thr	3.7	65	Tyr	2.86	45
Trp	0.95	18	His	2.79	32
Val	4.67	70	Arg	6.26	42

Table 8.2. Feed composition information needed for adequate and safe animal feeding.

Constituent or nutrient	Required information	Comments
Energy	Digestible energy (DE) content Metabolizable energy (ME) content Efficiency of use of dietary ME (k) Net energy (NE) content	 k_m, k_g and k_l and NE_m, NE_g and NE_l are the most important
Protein and amino acids	Total (crude) protein content	Used in ration formulation to indicate the amount of non-essential amino acid in the feed
	Rumen degradability (rate and extent) (dg)	Effective degradability (Edg) is more useful than laboratory measures of dg
	Undegradable dietary protein content (UDP) Ruminally degradable protein content (RDP)	UDP and RDP indicate how well feeds supply ruminally available N and amino acids which bypass degradation in the rumen
	Metabolizable protein (MP) content	
	Total amino acid contents	Amounts of all essential amino acids are important in pig and poultry feeding; lysine and methionine contents are also used in constructing horse and dairy cattle diets
	Available amino acid contents	Availabilities of the limiting essential amino acids (lysine, methionine, tryptophan, etc.) are needed to construct pig and poultry diets
Minerals	Total content of each mineral	In many cases the availability of a mineral depends on the diet composition and age of the animal
	Availabilities or digestibilities of P and Ca	P availability for pigs and poultry is greatly affected by the amount of phytin in the feed; phytin also binds Ca and other minerals
Vitamins	Total contents of each vitamin or vitamin precursor (e.g. carotene for vitamin A)	Needs for specific vitamins, vitamin availability, and the efficiency of conversion of precursors to the active form, vary between animal species
Water	Total amount Salinity	Often a first-limiting nutrient Tolerances vary but must be recognized
Fibre	Total amounts of neutral detergent fibre (NDF) or acid detergent fibre (ADF) in the feed	NDF (total plant cell walls) and ADF (ligno-cellulose) are the usual forms in which the feed fibre content is given
	Amount of physically effective fibre (peNDF)	peNDF is fibre which has a beneficial effect in the digestive tract
Secondary substances	Presence of active form(s) of the substance	Can have serious adverse effects on animal health; tannins at low levels can have beneficial effects on ruminant protein nutrition and may help to control internal parasites

some exceptions: the nutrient requirements of *Bos indicus* cattle and their crosses are slightly different to those of British and European (*Bos taurus*) cattle, and we have to take account of the effects that different environments have on animals, especially the effects of tropical and sub-tropical climates on dairy, pig and poultry nutrition (see Chapter 19).

As well, and importantly, we should avoid using 'old' data. Modern commercial pig and poultry strains have been intensively bred for better performance. They are much more efficient at using feed, and in the case of pigs are much better at depositing lean tissue, and accordingly have somewhat different nutrient requirements to older strains of these animals.

Several authorities have published reliable sets of nutrient requirement recommendations for a wide range of animal types, but not all of these are presented as user-friendly sets of tables or nutritional models. However, the following have easily accessible and usable nutrient requirements recommendations:

- National Research Council (NRC):
  horses: NRC (2007a);
  beef cattle: NRC (2016);
  dairy cattle: NRC (2001);
  sheep and goats: NRC (2007b);
  pigs: NRC (2012); and
  poultry: NRC (1994); an updated revision is being prepared for publication.
  These standards include example nutrient requirement tables and case studies but are best applied by using the nutritional models which are provided as part of each package.
- Institut National de Recherche pour l'Agriculture, l'Alimentation et l'Environnement (INRAE):
  pigs: INRA (2016); and
  ruminants: INRA (2012).
  The nutritional models *INRATION* and *INRAPorc* allow the user to describe animals and feeds, and to formulate rations.
- Commonwealth Scientific and Industrial Research Organisation (CSIRO):
  ruminants: CSIRO (2007); and
  pigs: Pork CRC (2003).
  GRAZFEED, the nutritional model developed from the ruminant standards, is published by Horizon Agriculture (2005–). AUSPIG is a pig husbandry model which addresses all aspects of pig production and management (Chapter 10).

Other regional and national feeding standards are available (see Chapter 5) and commercial poultry breeders provide their own recommendations (see below). Feeding standards which have been developed in individual European countries are gradually coalescing through the sharing of databases from which nutrient recommendations are constructed and are moving towards similar ways of defining feed nutritive value, and energy and protein requirements.

Using feeding standards in practice: Feeding standards are a very useful nutritional tool but they have some limitations. In the first place, nutrient requirement recommendations are estimates. Each standard is derived from a particular data set, and recommendations differ because of this. We can see this in, for example, NE_m coefficients cited for sheep: 0.25 MJ/$W^{0.75}_{kg}$ (NRC, 2007b), 0.27 MJ/$W^{0.75}_{kg}$ (CSIRO, 2007) and 0.22 MJ/$W^{0.75}_{kg}$ (AFRC, 1990); and cattle: 0.31 MJ/$W^{0.75}_{kg}$ (NRC, 2000), 0.38 MJ/$W^{0.75}_{kg}$ (CSIRO, 2007) and 0.36 MJ/$W^{0.75}_{kg}$ (AFRC, 1990).

Secondly, we must appreciate that these recommendations are averages, and are best used to develop feeding programmes for herds or flocks, rather than individuals.

As well, management and environment can influence nutrient requirements. Recommended nutrient requirements will not necessarily work in unusual situations, e.g. when cattle are fed survival rations their NE_m falls by 10% or 20%, and animals recovering from feed restriction initially use feed energy more efficiently. Lactating cows have a higher NE_m than non-lactating animals, and NE_m is also influenced by the distance they have to walk to milking. If we do not control internal parasites the maintenance protein requirement is increased because of blood being lost into the digestive tract. Pigs and birds eat less when the environmental temperature exceeds their upper critical temperature (Chapter 19) and in these circumstances they need diets with higher nutrient levels. Horses are very individual feeders and when this behaviour is combined with the effects of a training or performance programme their feed intakes can be different from those assumed in feeding standards. Birds' feed intake is influenced by the light:dark ratio in barns, and by the effectiveness of temperature control.

And finally, tabulated feeding standards are not universally applicable. They are usually derived from nutritional models and the data have been calculated by assuming an example diet. For example, the NRC (2001) standards for lactating dairy cattle are based on a ration of '15% immature legume silage, 33% normal corn silage, 34% ground high moisture shelled corn, 12% soybean meal', and other ingredients including fish meal (which is a banned ruminant feed in some jurisdictions; see Chapters 6 and 12), and the NRC (2012) pig standards assume 'corn and soybean meal-based diets'. The results strictly apply only to the assumed diet because nutrient availabilities and efficiencies of use vary between different feedstuffs. Nevertheless, we can use published recommendations to get a reasonable idea of an animal's nutrient requirements, particularly if they are fed a ration similar to the one assumed in the modelling exercise. This applies particularly to pigs because the differences in their nutritional efficiencies are relatively small, much less than those seen in ruminant nutrition.

Accordingly, when we choose a feeding standard, we should make sure that:

- Feeding standards suit the user's situation. They must reflect the type of animal and management that we are using, and because they are usually used to check the supply of nutrients from an existing feed or to formulate a ration (Chapter 9), the standards must provide information on the expected feed (or DM) intake, and on the requirements for, at least, those nutrients that will probably limit animal performance.
- Feeding standards are up to date: it is important that we use modern feeding standards which take account of differences between breeds and improvements in animal genotypes. Old standards may not give the performance that we expect from our animals. Poultry and pig genotypes change rapidly, and although horses, cattle and sheep have not been subjected to the same selection pressure, knowledge of nutrition is continually being extended and feeding standards should take account of this.

Feeding standards for poultry: 'Poultry' is a broad classification which includes domestic fowls, turkeys, ducks and geese. Within the domestic fowl class, we have hatchlings, pullets, broilers (birds which will be used for meat), laying hens and breeding hens. Each different species, strain and type of bird has different characteristic feed intakes and nutrient requirements.

Modern layer strains have lower maintenance energy requirements and so produce eggs with greater feed efficiently. But while their total energy requirements are less than those of older strains, their daily requirements for nutrients other than energy are similar, and so we have to formulate diets with higher non-energy nutrient densities when we are dealing with modern genotypes. For example, the diet protein content recommended by Hy-Line International (2020) for layers near peak production increases from 16.3% to 18.1% (as-fed) as the feed intake falls from 100 g/day to 90 g/day.

A large list of nutrients is considered in poultry feeding standards: energy, protein and 12 essential amino acids, linoleic acid (an essential fatty acid), six major minerals, six trace minerals, vitamins A, D, E and K, and nine B vitamins, and vitamin C (ascorbic acid).

Feeding standards for poultry provide, in most cases, recommended nutrient concentrations (usually on an as-fed or 90% DM basis) supported by suggested daily feed intakes. These standards may also give expected daily nutrient requirements, calculated for birds eating different amounts of feed. Sources such as NRC (1994), the Poultry Hub (2021), and companies which breed commercial poultry strains provide nutrient intake and concentration guidelines.

Laying birds eat from 85–120 g of air-dry feed daily, depending on their age and stage in the laying cycle. Birds alter their feed intake to meet their energy requirement, so we do not have to consider their energy requirements when we design rations, provided that diets have at least 10.5–11.5 MJ ME/kg for layers, and 12.5–13.5 MJ ME/kg for broilers. Feed fibre content is a good indication of the available energy content; in general, avoid feeds with more than 3–5% crude fibre.

Growing birds have higher protein and amino acids requirements than layers – from 19–25% protein for broilers (decreasing as the bird gets older) and 15–18.2% for adult layers (decreasing with stage of the laying cycle) (Hy-Line International, 2020). The 12 essential amino acids for poultry are those listed in Chapter 1. Total lysine requirements are between 0.83% and 1.02% for layers and 1.05% and 1.44% for broilers (Poultry Hub, 2021).

The Ca and available P (avP) requirements of laying birds need special attention. They have very high Ca requirements compared to the requirements of other birds because of their need for Ca to make eggshells. Recommended Ca concentrations (Poultry Hub, 2021) for layers increase with duration of the laying cycle from 4.4% to 4.75%, while avP requirements decline from 0.52% to 0.39%. Broilers need from 0.85–1.0% Ca and 0.42–0.5% avP, both declining as the bird ages.

We have to provide for the bird's requirements for the nine B group vitamins (see Table 1.4 in Chapter 1), as well as those for vitamins A, D, E and K. This is because the bird does not have a population of microflora in the proximal digestive tract to provide a source of absorbable B group vitamins. The fat-soluble vitamins (A, D, E and K) have to be provided in the diets of all animals, except for those (such as free-range layers) which are exposed to ultraviolet light and can thus synthesize enough vitamin D to meet their needs. Many of the main ingredients used in poultry diets contain only small amounts of vitamins and so vitamin requirements are always included in poultry feeding standards and in ration formulations.

Feeding standards for pigs: Feeding standards should give separate recommendations for suckling pigs (piglets) and weaners. Suckling pigs get much of their nutrition from the sow but have to be fed a creep feed to prepare them for weaning, while weaners (young pigs about 7.5–30 kg live weight) have been separated from the sow and no longer have access to her milk. Growing pigs include growers (about 30–65 kg live weight) and finishers (up to about 105 kg live weight). These animals use nutrients with different efficiencies, varying according to their breed or strain – some strains deposit lean tissue much more efficiently than others. As well, growers may be given the growth enhancer ractopamine, or immunized against growth hormone. Gilts (young females), boars (entire males) and barrows (castrated boars) have different production capacities and should be fed differently, where this is practicable. Breeding stock – pregnant, transition, and lactating sows, and boars – all have very different nutrient requirements.

Feeding standards may provide estimates of feed or DM intake, but these are not recommendations – pigs' appetites are influenced by their energy requirements. To achieve maximum productivity and feed efficiency, we need to construct a diet in which the cereal grains have been processed to maximize their digestibility, and then to feed it so that each pig can eat as much as it wants. This will allow the pig to maximize its NE intake, and this has to be matched by providing adequate amounts of the other nutrients it needs. Expected air-dry feed intakes of weaners and growers eating a diet containing 13.8–14.2 MJ ME/kg range from 0.27 to 2.7 kg/day (NRC, 2012). Lactating sows eating a similar diet consume about 6.5 kg/day.

ME and digestible energy (DE) are used to express the pig's energy requirement. NRC (2012) use 'effective DE' and 'effective ME'; these have been calculated from measures of NE use and converted to DE and ME (see Fig. 5.1, Chapter 5) using the different conversion factors for weaners, growers and sows which apply to the conventional US corn (maize)/ soybean meal pig diet.

Recommendations for protein and amino acids must deal with each essential amino acid, and the feed's total protein content so as to cover its requirements for non-essential amino acids. Indicative total protein and lysine contents are illustrated in Fig. 8.3). Amino acid requirements vary according to sex (gilts, barrows and entires), live weight, growth rate, and the animal's inherent protein deposition rate (PD). PDs vary from about 115 to 180 g protein/day, and more if they are given ractopamine.

We need detailed information on essential amino acid requirements because the pig, like other monogastric animals and poultry, does not have a microbial buffer in the first part of their digestive tract to even out variations in the dietary amino acid supply. Essential amino acid recommendations may be given as total amounts in the feed, or amino acid apparently digestible in the ileum, or amino acid truly ('standardized') digestible in the ileum (see Chapter 4). They can also be defined in relation to the animal's energy intake – for example, we could

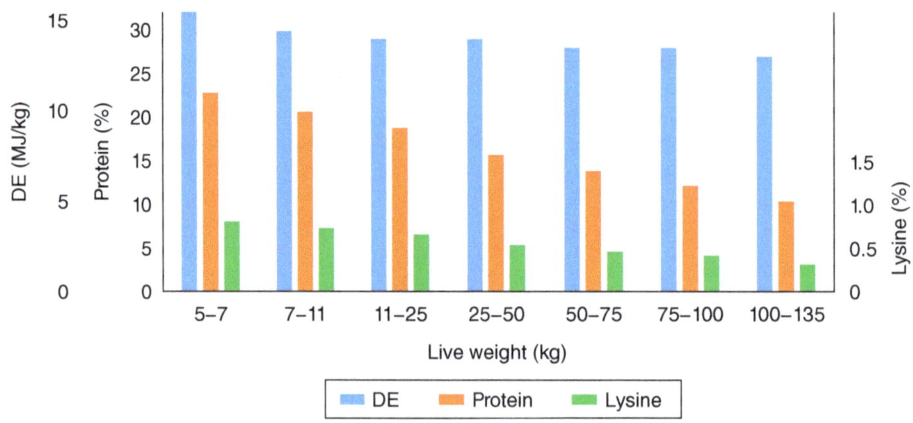

Fig. 8.3. Requirements of growing pigs for digestible energy (DE), protein and lysine. (Drawn from relationships in NRC (2012) and DAFF (2013); copyright: Gordon McL. Dryden.)

specify the lysine requirement of a 60 kg grower pig not as 20.6 g/day, but as 1.44 g/MJ DE. This helps to ensure that the diet will support the synthesis of the amount of lean tissue that the pig is able to generate from its energy intake, and to stop the pig from getting over-fat. Essential amino acid requirements are often expressed in relation to the lysine requirement, so as to reduce wastage of amino acids (see the ideal amino acid ratios in Table 8.1).

Requirements for P can be quoted as 'total' P, 'non-phytate' P, or as 'STTD' P. STTD, or 'standardized total tract digestible' means P that is truly digestible in the whole digestive tract. Recommendations for growers and lactating sows range from 0.45–0.6% Ca and 0.2–0.3% STTD P (NRC, 2012; Tokach *et al.*, 2019). Requirements are affected by growth rate, piglet weaning weight and litter size.

Ca and P requirements can be calculated factorially, while recommendations for other minerals are derived empirically. At the present, both these approaches only estimate mineral requirements, especially those for the trace minerals, so we need to be aware of progress in knowledge about pigs' mineral requirements. Phytase enzyme improves the availability of P and other minerals such as Ca, Zn and Cu (Chapters 5 and 11) and so reduces the amount of supplementary minerals that have to be used.

The fat-soluble vitamins and the B group vitamins are required by pigs. Pigs can synthesize vitamin C and generally do not need supplements of this vitamin. Vitamin D is needed to prevent bone and reproductive disorders in housed pigs, while grazing pigs probably do not need a supplement. Excesses of vitamins A and D can be toxic.

Feeding standards for horses: Equines include domestic horses, donkeys, mules and several wild horse breeds. There is a variety of domestic horses, such as small horses (ponies), large breeds (warmbloods), thoroughbreds and draught breeds. Within each of these classes we have foals, breeding mares, and adults which are used for riding and draught purposes. Riding horses are used for a very wide variety of purposes, ranging from simple pleasure riding, to dressage, jumping, racing (trotting, flat racing and steeplechasing) and endurance events. Each of these work types imposes different demands on the horse and each require very different nutritional treatment.

Estimates of DM intakes are based on live weights and work rates; NRC (2007a) suggests intakes for riding horses equivalent to 2.0–2.5% of the horse's live weight per day. Published feed intake estimates are approximate and it is wise to measure actual feed intakes and to be prepared to adjust the recommended nutrient concentrations to suit each individual horse. Do this as described in Chapter 9.

Horses' energy requirements vary with their temperament and management. Some horses are docile or are confined so that they have little activity, and so their maintenance energy requirement is relatively low. Others are more active or have a more nervous temperament (nervousness is manifested in more activity). These horses consequently have a higher maintenance energy demand. Horses' maintenance DE requirements can vary between 51.5, 55.6 and 60.7 MJ DE/day for horses with 'minimum', 'average' or 'elevated' maintenance requirements, respectively (NRC, 2007a). The work rate of performance or draught horses has an important effect on their energy requirements. For example, the total DE requirement of a 400 kg live weight horse increases from 66.9 MJ DE/day to 111.7 MJ DE/day as the work rate increases from 'light' to 'very heavy' (NRC, 2007a). Physiological state (pregnant or non-pregnant, lactating or non-lactating) also influences the horse's nutrient requirements.

DE is often used to express available energy requirements, although some equine feeding standards use ME. Recommended energy requirements may be derived factorially, from live weight, foetus development, milk production, work rate, etc., or derived empirically from animal responses which have been measured in experiments.

Protein and essential amino acid requirements are both provided in current feeding standards. For example, NRC (2007a) recommends 504 g protein and 21.7 g lysine per day for a resting adult horse weighing 400 kg, equivalent to 6.3% protein and 0.27% lysine (DM basis).

Recommended amounts of major minerals – Ca, P, Mg and K – are usually based on estimated endogenous losses (i.e. excretion of minerals which were once part of the horse's tissues) modified by estimates of how efficiently the mineral in the feed is absorbed from the digestive tract. Absorption rates are modified by animal age, mineral requirement, and if the feed contains substances like oxalic acid or phytate which inhibit absorption.

Recommendations for trace minerals (S, Co, Cu, Fe, I, Mn, Se and Zn), and for the fat-soluble and water-soluble vitamins, are usually empirical recommendations, based on reports of diet concentrations that have appeared to give satisfactory results.

Check that these are up to date because more recent data reflect advances in research techniques.

Feeding standards for ruminants: There are many similarities between the standards for cattle and sheep, and these are discussed in this section.

Typical dairy cattle are Jerseys (mature live weight about 450 kg), Brown Swiss (about 680 kg) and Holstein/Friesians (650–750 kg). Commercial dairy cattle are either growing calves or heifers, cows transitioning between drying-off and calving, or cows in early-, mid- or late-lactation. Transition cows and those in mid or later lactation are assumed to be pregnant, a reasonable assumption for commercial herds.

There are two major species of beef cattle: *Bos taurus* (British or European breeds), and *Bos indicus* or tropical (African and Asian breeds). Within each beef animal class there are suckling calves, weaners, young growing animals (yearlings), heifers (young females which have not had a calf), steers and bullocks (castrated young and older males), breeding cows, and bulls. Growing cattle can also be classed as 'growers' and 'finishers', and these can be fed to grow at different rates. Different beef cattle breeds produce different amounts of milk and have lactations of varying persistency. Most currently available beef cattle feeding standards are designed for commercial *B. taurus* cattle, but they are a useful starting point for all beef cattle types.

Buffaloes, Bali cattle and yaks are used for both milk and meat production. Feeding standards for these species are less well developed than those for standard beef or dairy breeds, but existing cattle feeding standards can be used as a starting point.

Sheep can be divided into four types: wool (e.g. Perendale and Merino); meat (e.g. Dorper and Southdown); dual-purpose (e.g. Corriedale and Texel); and dairy (e.g. Lacaune and Awassi) types. Within these types we have lambs, weaned young stock, hoggets (yearlings), adult ewes (pregnant or lactating or neither), wethers (castrated males) and rams.

When considering ruminant feeding standards, we should note that expected DM intakes vary with animal age and live weight, milk yield and the week of lactation in lactating animals, and foetus development in pregnant females. Feed characteristics, such as the neutral detergent fibre (NDF) and ME contents, also affect intake (Chapter 7). Some feeding standards express nutrient requirements as concentrations in the feed or feed DM, and these can be used to construct a ration (see Chapter 9). But be aware that estimates of DM intake, especially for grazing animals, are not very reliable, and that when nutrient requirements are expressed as concentrations, these values are greatly influenced by the accuracy of feed intake estimates.

Energy requirements can be expressed in a variety of ways (Chapter 5) but ME and NE are often used. Use NE_m recommendations carefully because of the environmental effects on heat loss (wind, rain, low temperatures, etc.) and the NE needed for activity (grazing, walking between pastures and to milking). The NE_m requirement can increase by 250% in adverse environmental conditions.

Ruminant feeding standards must provide recommendations for ruminally degradable protein RDP and UDP which will (i) support synthesis of the amount of microbial crude protein (MCP) which can be produced from the amount of fermentable organic matter provided in the diet (Chapter 5), and (ii) meet the animal's own amino acid requirements.

Some feeding standards give recommended dietary total protein contents, on the basis that:

Total protein = (RDP + UDP)

However, this works in practice only if the feed protein that we intend to use has a similar effective degradability (Edg) to that assumed in the feeding standard recommendations. Suppose that a growing steer needs 730 g RDP and 130 g UDP per day and eats 9 kg DM/day. We can provide the RDP from a diet containing 12% protein if the Edg is 68% or more. At that Edg and protein content, the steer would consume 350 g UDP/day, much more than it needs. However, if the Edg was 85%, then RDP requirement could be covered by a diet with only 9.5% protein, but that diet would provide only 125 g UDP/day. To formulate our ration we should use the actual RDP, UDP and Edg values of the feeds we wish to use, rather than total protein recommendations.

It is increasingly common for feeding standards to give recommended MP intakes:

MP = (digestible MCP) + (digestible UDP)

When considering MP recommendations, we have to be sure that the feed provides enough absorbable amino acids to meet the animal's requirements. Although the amino acid composition of MCP is relatively constant, that of the UDP varies between different feeds.

Very productive dairy cows, wool-type sheep and rapidly growing beef cattle have higher than usual amino acids requirements. Ration formulations for these animals should include data on UDP requirements, and the concentrations of essential amino acids (INRAE, 2017–2020) in the MP passing to the small intestine. Lysine, histidine and methionine, and methionine and cyst(e)ine, are the most likely limiting amino acids for lactating cows and wool sheep breeds.

Feed fibre content is an important consideration for dairy cattle. These animals will produce milk with low fat contents if they are fed diets with low digestible fibre. They need between 25% and 33% NDF with at least 19% NDF from forages (NRC, 2001), corresponding to a dietary roughage content of about 50% (DM basis). Try not to give excessive roughage to high-producing dairy cattle, as diets with more than 44% NDF may restrict feed intake. Concentrate-rich diets fed to beef cattle (commonly, these diets have about 70% cereal grain) should have at least 8% peNDF.

Mineral and vitamin requirements for maintenance, pregnancy, growth and lactation change with live weight and production rate (Fig. 8.4). Requirements can be given as total or absorbable amounts (g/day) and/or total concentrations (%, DM). Most feed libraries provide mineral availabilities, e.g. INRAE (2017–2020) and NRC (2001, 2007b). Note that the availability of minerals varies between different mineral sources. While a factorial approach is used to determine requirements for the major minerals and Cu, most trace mineral and vitamin recommendations are based on empirical studies and so may apply only in general terms to a specific animal type.

Nutrient requirements for pregnancy: The mass, energy, protein and mineral contents of the conceptus (also called the 'gravid uterus') increase with time, and so the nutrient requirements of the dam also increase, particularly in the last trimester. The well-known exponential curve describing foetal weight implies that requirements for pregnancy are important only in the last trimester. This is not correct – do not under-feed pregnant animals at any time because foetal programming occurs throughout pregnancy (Langley-Evans, 2009). For example, kidneys, liver, ovaries and other organs are initiated in early foetal growth, the piglet's immune status can be compromised by under-feeding in early pregnancy resulting in increased post-natal deaths, and a lamb's primary wool follicles are initiated in mid-pregnancy.

Expected birth weights are used to predict the nutrient requirements of pregnant females (CSIRO, 2007; NRC, 2000, 2001, 2007b), so we need accurate estimates of these. Birth weights vary with breed, and the age and body condition of the dam, but useful approximations are 40–50 kg for calves and 3.5–6 kg for lambs.

The efficiencies of use of ME and MP for pregnancy (k_y and kp_y) are much lower than those for maintenance, lactation or live weight gain. This is because nutrients are needed to nourish the uterus and placenta as well as the foetus, whereas we calculate efficiency solely on growth of the foetus.

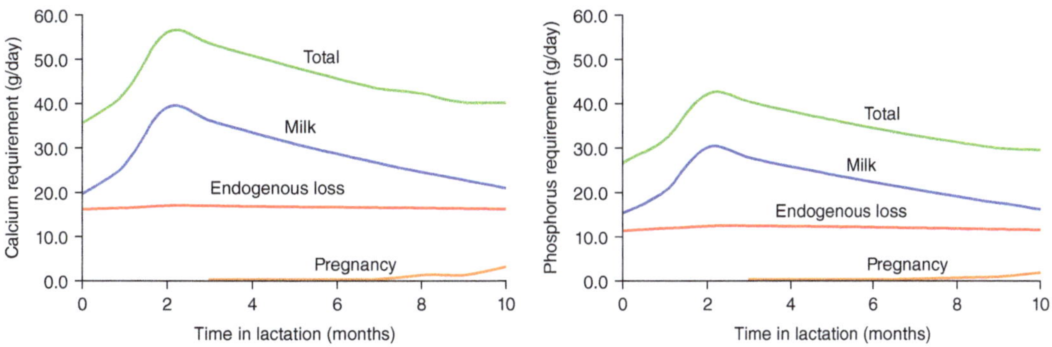

Fig. 8.4. Net calcium and phosphorus requirements of a lactating Friesian cow (650 kg live weight, peak milk yield 30 L/day, DM intake = 0.025 × live weight + 0.1 × milk yield). (Drawn from relationships in CSIRO, 2007; copyright Gordon McL. Dryden.)

Breeding sows pose a problem regarding the efficiency of nutrient use during pregnancy and lactation, and this impacts on how we use nutrient requirement recommendations. Pregnant sows exhibit 'pregnancy anabolism' – they use feed efficiently and accumulate live weight (body tissue) prior to farrowing (Fig. 8.5). However, the more weight gained, the more is lost during the subsequent lactation and the less feed the sow eats during her lactation. This is inefficient use of feed, and weight loss can harm fertility in the next breeding season, so we try to limit live weight gain during the pregnancy.

Feeding lactating cows: The milk yields of Friesian cows fed total or partial mixed rations which have a high concentrate content (e.g. cereal grains and protein meals) can be 35–55 L per day. These are much higher than the yields expected in cows which are managed in a pasture-based system with limited amounts of concentrate supplements and which typically produce 15–25 L per day. The nutrient requirements recommended for highly productive cows will overestimate the requirements of pasture-fed animals.

Beef cattle have lower-yielding (6–15 L/day) and less persistent lactations than dairy cattle and produce milk with typically lower fat contents (2.2–4%) than dairy breeds (see below). Sheep produce 0.5–3.5 L/day with 7–8% fat content, with ewes suckling twins producing more than those with singles.

Milk yield in early lactation can exceed the animal's (especially the dairy cow's) ability to consume feed to support that production (Chapter 7), but the peak milk yield is an important determinant of the whole-lactation yield and its persistency. Consequently, we should have cows and ewes ready for parturition in as good a body condition as possible, as this will allow the mobilization of body tissue as a nutrient source for milk production. However, do not let the pregnant animal get over-fat because this can cause dystocia.

Species, breed, stage of lactation, number of previous lactations and feed composition all affect milk yield and composition, and thus the NE requirement for lactation. Dairy cow milk typically has 3–5% fat, 2.5–3.5% protein and about 4.8% lactose. The fat content, especially, influences the NE content of milk and thus the amount of NE needed to produce it. To simplify nutrient requirement recommendations, we can express a cow's actual milk yield as an amount of 'fat-corrected' (FCM; Gaines, 1928) or 'energy corrected' milk (ECM; Tyrrell and Reid, 1965), which is the amount of 4% fat milk which contains the same amount of NE as the amount contained in the milk actually produced by our cow.

$$\text{FCM yield (L/day)} = (\text{actual milk yield, L/day}) \times [0.4 + 0.15 \times (\text{fat, \%})]$$

$$\text{ECM yield (L/day)} = (\text{actual milk yield, L/day}) \times [0.384 \times (\text{fat, \%}) + 0.222 \times (\text{protein, \%}) + 0.199 \times (\text{lactose, \%}) - 0.108]/3.14$$

Precision feeding

Precision feeding (precision nutrition) is an approach which seeks to minimize nutrient wastage by designing rations which exactly meet the animal's nutrient requirements. If we can do this, then the economics

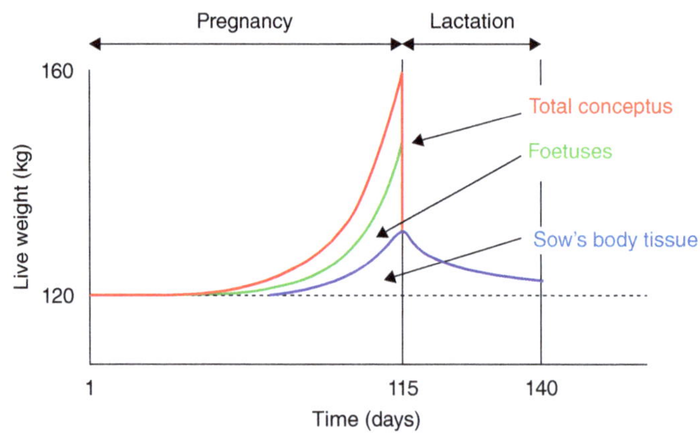

Fig. 8.5. Body weight change during a sow's pregnancy and lactation. (Copyright: Gordon McL. Dryden.)

of animal production are optimized, and adverse effects on the environment (Chapter 19) are minimized. There are several ways to approach precision feeding, these are discussed below.

Do not over- or under-feed animals: Under-feeding restricts animal productivity and eventually leads to welfare issues. Animals need more feed than we may expect – be aware of this, especially when feeding animals which are treated as pets.

If we have to feed less than the animals need in circumstances when feed becomes scarce (e.g. in droughts or after fires or floods; Chapter 16), then consider reducing stock numbers by sale or agistment (leasing grazing in another region where pasture supplies are adequate), or perhaps buying supplementary feed such as cereal grains.

Over-feeding becomes obvious when growing animals become over-fat. It also leads to wasteful feeding behaviour (Chapter 17).

Check the nutrient content of the animals' feed: It is important to be able to recognize the limiting nutrient in an animal's diet (Chapter 1). The amino acids methionine, histidine and lysine can be limiting in dairy cattle feeds. Lysine, together with methionine and other essential amino acids, is often limiting in pig and poultry diets, and glycine and serine may be limiting in poultry feeds. Ruminally available N may limit the productivity of ruminants, particularly when animals are grazing mature (i.e. low-protein) tropical pasture grasses.

Mineral deficiencies, or alternatively mineral excesses, will cause major losses of production and poor animal health. Watch the Ca and P contents of pig diets because the availability of P is reduced in diets where the Ca:P ratio is wider than 1.25:1 (NRC, 2012). Laying birds have a much higher Ca requirement (up to 4.75%; Poultry Hub, 2021) than other animals, and working horses need additional Na (0.3–0.4%, DM; NRC, 2007a). Grazing animals can often be deficient in minerals – many areas have P-deficient soils, and Se, Co and Cu deficiencies also occur in some regions. Get advice before buying mineral supplements for grazing animals because the animals' responses are influenced by their intake of other nutrients, especially energy in regard to P, and S and Mo in regard to Cu.

Ideal amino acid ratios (see above) are used in pig and poultry feeding to improve the efficiency of feed protein use and to reduce environmental pollution caused by animals excreting excess amino acid-N.

Synchronicity of nutrient availability in the rumen is important for the efficient use of RAN and fermentable carbohydrate. Optimizing this requires an understanding of how roughage:concentrate ratios should be managed in animals of different ages (Lascano *et al.*, 2016). Try to manage the behaviour of animals visiting urea supplements, or if this is not practicable then use slow-release urea supplements (Chapter 16).

Nutrient requirement models

Modern feeding standards are based on mathematical models of how the animal uses nutrients, and the factors which determine the amounts of nutrients that they need.

Most authorities provide software based on these models. All of these calculate the animal's nutrient requirements from descriptions input by the user. Some models give estimates of the production levels which can be achieved from feed inputs, others can calculate the animal's nutrient requirements and then formulate a ration from the feeds described in the model feed library or provided by the user.

Nutritional models are discussed in Chapter 10.

References

Agricultural and Food Research Council (AFRC) (1990). AFRC Technical Committee on Responses to Nutrients, Report Number 5, Nutritive Requirements of Ruminant Animals: Energy. *Nutrition Abstracts and Reviews (Series B)* 60(10): 729–804.

Commonwealth Scientific and Industrial Research Organisation (CSIRO) (2007). *Nutrient Requirements of Domesticated Ruminants*. Collingwood, Vic., Australia: CSIRO Publishing.

Department of Agriculture and Fisheries (Queensland) (DAFF) (2013). *Pig production. Nutrient needs*. Available at: www.daf.qld.gov.au/business-priorities/agriculture/animals/pigs/feed-nutrition/nutrients-diets/nutrient-needs (accessed 27 December 2020).

Dryden, G.McL. (2008). *Animal Nutrition Science*. Wallingford, UK: CAB International.

Gaines, W.L. (1928). *The energy basis of measuring milk yield in dairy cows*. Agricultural Experiment Station Bulletin no. 308. Urbana, IL: University of Illinois.

Horizon Agriculture (2005–). *Grazfeed*. Available at: www.hzn.com.au/grazfeed.php (accessed 27 December 2020).

Hy-Line International (2020). *HL Nutritional Levels*. Available at: www.hyline.com/technical-resources (accessed 27 December 2020).

Institut National de Recherche pour l'Agriculture, l'Alimentation et l'Environnement (INRAE) (2017–2020). *INRAE-*

CIRAD-AFZ Feed Tables. Available at: www.feedtables.com/ (accessed 27 December 2020).

Institut Nationale de la Recherche Agronomique (INRA) (2012). *INRATION version* 4.06. Available at: https://inration.software.informer.com/ (accessed 27 December 2020).

Institut Nationale de la Recherche Agronomique (INRA) (2016). *InraPorc version 1.7.1.0*. Available at: https://inraporc.inra.fr/inraporc/history_en.php (accessed 18 March 2021).

Langley-Evans, S.C. (2009). Nutritional programming of disease: unravelling the mechanism. *Journal of Anatomy* 215(1): 36–51.

Lascano, G.J., Koch, L.E. and Heinrichs, A.J. (2016). Precision-feeding dairy heifers a high rumen-degradable protein diet with different proportions of dietary fiber and forage-to-concentrate ratios. *Journal of Dairy Science* 99(9): 7175–7190.

National Research Council (NRC) (1994). *Nutrient Requirements of Poultry*, 9th rev. edn. Washington, DC: National Academies Press. Available at: www.nap.edu/catalog/2114/nutrient-requirements-of-poultry-ninth-revised-edition-1994 (accessed 27 December 2020).

National Research Council (NRC) (2000). *Nutrient Requirements of Beef Cattle*, 7th rev. edn. Update. Washington, DC: National Academies Press. Available at: www.nap.edu/catalog/9791/nutrient-requirements-of-beef-cattle-seventh-revised-edition-update-2000 (accessed 27 December 2020).

National Research Council (NRC) (2001). *Nutrient Requirements of Dairy Cattle*, 7th rev. edn. Washington, DC: National Academies Press. Available at: www.nap.edu/catalog/9825/nutrient-requirements-of-dairy-cattle-seventh-revised-edition-2001 (accessed 27 December 2020).

National Research Council (NRC) (2007a). *Nutrient Requirements of Horses*, 6th rev. edn. Washington, DC: National Academies Press. Available at: www.nap.edu/catalog/11653/nutrient-requirements-of-horses-sixth-revised-edition (accessed 27 December 2020).

National Research Council (NRC) (2007b). *Nutrient Requirements of Small Ruminants – Sheep, Goats, Cervids and New World Camelids*. Washington, DC: National Academies Press. Available at: www.nap.edu/catalog/11654/nutrient-requirements-of-small-ruminants-sheep-goats-cervids-and-new (accessed 27 December 2020).

National Research Council (NRC) (2012). *Nutrient Requirements of Swine*, 11th rev. edn. Washington, DC: National Academies Press. Available at: www.nap.edu/catalog/13298/nutrient-requirements-of-swine-eleventh-revised-edition (accessed 27 December 2020).

National Research Council (NRC) (2016). *Nutrient Requirements of Beef Cattle*, 8th rev. edn. Washington, DC: National Academies Press. Available at: www.nap.edu/catalog/19014/nutrient-requirements-of-beef-cattle-eighth-revised-edition (accessed 27 December 2020).

Pork CRC (2003). *What Is AUSPIG?* Available at: www.porkcrc.com.au/What_is_AusPig.pdf (accessed 27 December 2020).

Poultry Hub (2021). *Poultry Nutrient Requirements*. Available at: https://www.poultryhub.org/all-about-poultry/nutrition (also see terms of use at www.poultryhub.org/about/disclaimers/) (accessed 25 March 2021).

Tokach, M.D., Menegat, M.B., Gourley, K.M. and Goodband, R.D. (2019). Review: Nutrient requirements of the modern high-producing lactating sow, with an emphasis on amino acid requirements. *Animal* 13(12): 2967–2977.

Tyrrell, H.F. and Reid, J.T. (1965). Prediction of the energy value of cow's milk. *Journal of Dairy Science* 48: 1215–1223.

van Milgen, J. and Dourmad, J.-Y. (2015). Concept and application of ideal protein for pigs. *Journal of Animal Science and Biotechnology* 6: 15–25.

van Milgen, J., Valancogne, A., Dubois, S., Dourmad, J.-Y., Sève, B. and Noblet, J. (2008). InraPorc: a model and decision support tool for the nutrition of growing pigs. *Animal Feed Science and Technology* 143: 387–405.

9 Ration formulation

Managing nutrient content and requirement data

Ration formulation is a method of calculating the combination of ingredients which will give a mixture which contains nutrients in specified concentrations. If these concentrations are similar to the animal's nutrient requirements, then we should be able to feed this mixture and get the expected production response. To correctly formulate a ration, we need to have data which is presented in a consistent manner and is appropriate for the type of animal the ration is intended for.

Ration formulation is a useful tool to design animal diets in situations where we can control what, and how much, the animal eats. It is not useful for managing grazing animals because we do not have this control.

Nutrient content and nutrient requirement information is published using either of two bases:

- As-fed basis (also called 'as-received' or 'as-is'), where the relationship between the nutrient or constituent in question and the whole feed including its water is calculated. This basis is used when animals are typically fed feeds based on air-dry ingredients, and which have close to 90% dry matter (DM). Some authorities (e.g. the US pig feeding standards; NRC, 2012) use a standardized as-fed basis where nutrient requirement values are expressed on a '90% DM' basis. Grains, meals and hays have DM contents close to 90%, although the moisture contents of these feeds do vary with ambient temperature and humidity, time in storage, processing, etc.
- Dry matter basis, where the relationship between the nutrient or constituent in question and the feed DM is calculated. Nutrient requirement concentration values for pasture, molasses or silage (which are fed to beef and dairy cattle, sheep, goats and others) all have water contents which are very different from each other, and recommendations for these animals are given on a DM basis.

DM basis values are always larger than as-fed basis values, sometimes substantially so. For example, the protein contents of a high-moisture feed (grass silage, 30% DM) and an air-dry feed (wheat grain, 89% DM) can be given as:

- grass silage: 11.7% protein (DM basis) or 3.5% (as-fed basis); or
- wheat grain: 10% protein (DM basis) or 8.9% (as-fed basis).

Note the different units used here. When a concentration is expressed on an as-fed basis, the units are MJ/kg, g/kg, mg/kg, μg/kg, IU/kg (for some vitamins) and %. If we express the content on a DM basis the units are MJ/kg DM, g/kg DM, mg/kg DM, μg/kg DM, IU/kg DM and % (DM basis).

The difference between DM and as-fed bases is illustrated in Fig. 9.1. Grass silage is chosen for this example because it has a fairly high water content which emphasizes the difference.

If we combine nutrient data from different publications it is essential that they have the same basis of expression.

Sometimes the basis of expression is not given, but the protein or energy contents of a feed with a high water content, e.g. molasses or silage, will indicate which has been used. If the values appear to be low, then the basis of expression is probably 'as-fed'. Mistaking the correct basis does not make much difference for many air-dry feeds, such as cereal grains and their by-products, protein meals and minerals, but assuming the wrong basis of expression will cause substantial errors if we are dealing with moist feeds such as silage, fresh pasture, wet distillers' grains or molasses.

Nutrient content values can be converted between bases: The following method works

DOI: 10.1079/9781786394453.0009

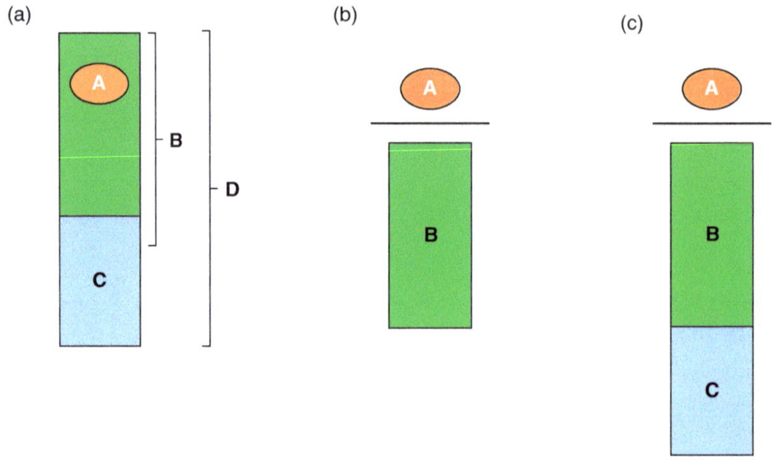

Fig. 9.1. Diagram showing the difference between as-fed and dry matter bases for expressing the nutrient content of feeds; the example feedstuff is grass silage. **(a)** A represents the protein content (200 g), B the total dry matter (1200 g), C is the water content (800 g), and D is the total ingredient (2000 g). **(b)** Protein content on a DM basis = 200/(2000 − 800) × 100 = 16.7% (DM basis). **(c)** Protein content on an as-fed basis = 200/2000 × 100 = 10%. (Copyright: Gordon McL. Dryden.)

for all nutrients and all units of measurement: to convert from as-fed to DM basis: multiply the as-fed basis value by 100/(ingredient) DM%; and to convert from DM to as-fed basis: multiply the DM basis value by (ingredient DM%)/100.

For example: using the data in Fig. 9.1, grass silage has 10% protein (as-fed basis), 16.7% protein (DM basis) and 60% DM.

- Converting from as-fed to DM basis:

  Protein (DM basis) = 10 × 100/60 = 16.7% (DM basis)

- And from DM to as-fed basis:

  Protein (as-fed basis) = 16.7 × 60/100 = 10%

To formulate rations, feed nutrient contents and animal nutrient requirements must be expressed in the same way: Many feeding standards quote nutrient requirements as daily amounts (see Chapter 8). Obviously, feed nutrient contents have to be expressed as concentrations, so this means that the requirement data must also be expressed as concentrations in the feed.

To convert daily amounts to minimum acceptable concentrations, divide the daily amount of nutrient required by the daily amount of feed (total feed or feed DM) that it is expected that the animal will eat.

Example: A yearling horse is to be fed a mixed ration of oat grain, lucerne (alfalfa) hay and wheat bran. The NRC (2007) horse feeding standards give recommended digestible energy (DE) and protein intakes, and information on the nutritive value of our chosen feeds (Table 9.1).

In this example we cannot compare the feed DE or protein contents with the horse's requirements. It makes no sense to compare MJ DE/day with MJ DE/kg DM. However, we can change daily requirements into concentrations if we can make a reasonable estimate of the amount of feed DM that our horse is likely to eat. The NRC (2007) standards suggest that this animal will eat an amount of DM each day equivalent to 2.5% of its body weight. The horse weighs 260 kg, so the expected maximum DM intake is 2.5% × 260 kg = 6.5 kg/day.

The required 62.7 MJ DE must be provided in no more than 6.5 kg DM/day, so the minimum DE content

= 62.8/6.5 = 9.7 MJ/kg DM.

Similarly, the minimum protein content

= [677 / (6.5 × 1000)] × 100 = 10.4% (DM basis).

Table 9.1. Information needed to formulate a mixed feed for a yearling horse. (Data from NRC, 2001, 2007, 2012; reproduced with permission.)

	DE[a]	CP
Requirement[b]:		
Yearling, mature body weight 400 kg	62.8 MJ/day	677 g/day
Feeds:		
Oats[b]	13.9 MJ/kg DM	13.6% (DM)
Grass, cool season, hay, mid-maturity[b]	10.2 MJ/kg DM	19.2% (DM)
Wheat bran[c]	10.1 MJ/kg	15.1%
Grasses, cool season, hay, mid-maturity, 55–60% NDF[d]	11.2 MJ/kg DM	13.5% (DM)

CP, crude protein; DE, digestible energy; DM, dry matter; NDF, neutral detergent fibre.
[a]The units for DE have been changed from Mcal/kg DM to MJ/kg DM.
[b]From NRC (2007)
[c]From NRC (2012)
[d]From NRC (2001)

If there is any doubt that the horse would eat this amount of feed, then to be safe we would have to use a feed mixture which contained more than 9.7 MJ DE/kg DM and more than 10.4% protein.

Nutrient content information must be for the correct animal type: First, values for total DM, protein, mineral and fibre contents are the same for all animal types and we can apply these values across all species. However, animals of different species and ages digest and use feed to differing extents. Avoid using available nutrient values, e.g. DE, metabolizable energy (ME) or net energy (NE), or ruminally degradable protein (RDP) or undegradable dietary protein, or available amino acids, or vitamin contents when they are given in IU, which have been published in pig or poultry feeding standards, for ruminants or horses, or *vice versa*.

Example: In Table 9.1 the wheat bran data has been extracted from pig feeding standards. Pigs digest wheat bran less completely than horses do, and so the DE values included in these feeding standards are lower than those in horse standards (the NRC, 2007, value for wheat bran is 13.5 MJ DE /kg DM). Furthermore, we may decide that the horse feed library does not describe our grass hay very well. 'Mid-maturity' is a fairly loose term, but the NRC (2001) dairy cattle standards have a mid-maturity hay which they describe as having 55–60% neutral detergent fibre (NDF). We decide to use these data, but this brings up a second problem: do horses and cattle digest the sources in grass hay with similar efficiency? The answer is 'no', because of the contribution made by the cow's rumen. So, the DE value published for cattle is not appropriate for our horse.

The units used to describe each nutrient content and requirement must be the same: Values for DE, ME and NE contents are often given as Mcal (megacalories) per pound or per kilogram of feed or feed DM (e.g. NE_m, Mcal/kg) in North America, but in many other places MJ/kg (megajoules per kilogram) is the preferred unit. Similarly, requirements for protein and major minerals are often quoted as %, but also as g/kg. Trace mineral contents are quoted in µg/kg or mg/kg, and vitamin requirements as mg/kg or IU/kg. Conversion factors are given in Chapter 5.

Dealing with variability in the nutritive value of feeds

Published nutrient contents usually differ from those of actual feed samples: There are two reasons for this:

- The nutrient contents of feeds vary with the nature of the raw materials used to produce them and the processing methods used (see Chapter 6).
- The entries in feed tables are averages (means) which were calculated from the selection of data available to the authors when the table was compiled.

Ration formulation risks under-feeding animals: Consequently, using nutrient content data from feed libraries will lead to errors when we formulate rations. There are several ways that we can deal with this (the most effective first):

- Obtain nutrient content analyses for the feed sample in question. While analyses of amino acid, fatty acid, mineral and vitamin contents require a well-equipped lab there are ways in which other useful nutrient content data can be obtained. Near infrared reflectance spectroscopy (NIRS) will rapidly and cheaply predict water, fat and protein contents. NIRS is not within the capacity of most animal managers, but most feed mills routinely make these analyses. Water contents can be rapidly and easily measured with hand-held electronic meters. Use published regression equations (see later in this chapter) to predict energy availability (e.g. ME or AME_n) from NDF, fat and mineral contents; or amino acid contents from the feed protein content.

- The nutrient composition of commercial feeds will be declared on the feed label. In most cases the quoted values will be minimums.
- Use feed libraries that have been prepared for feeds which are produced and used locally, and find feed library entries which match as closely as possible the feed that we wish to use.

Ration formulations may over-state the ration's actual nutrient content: This is because the formulation uses average nutrient content values, and if the data used to calculate the average are normally distributed (form a bell curve), then half of the values encountered in real life will be less than the average.

If it is not possible to analyse the feeds that we intend to use, there are several alternatives to address the under-feeding problem, although all of these have inadequacies:

- Add a safety margin before formulating the ration: this is done by increasing the nutrient requirements by 5 or 10%. This is an arbitrary amount and does not necessarily ensure that the animal gets its correct nutrient concentration in all cases – in fact even a 10% increase might not be enough: note that the lowest protein content reported for maize (corn) grain (INRAE/CIRAD/AFZ, 2017–2020; see below) is 6.7%, only 75% of the average value.
- Reduce the value for each nutrient in each ingredient: this can be done by subtracting an amount from the average (published) value (see below). However, what we might gain in better animal performance we may lose in wasted nutrients, environmental contamination, and increased costs.
- Feed the formulated ration and observe the animals' response: this approach also identifies things like lack of palatability, and undesirable physical characteristics (dustiness, etc.) which can affect intake, and so gives a very complete indication of the ration's overall quality. But this takes some time, and there may be a temporary reduction in animal performance. If we have to alter the nutrient contents, the ingredient composition may have to change, but in most cases we will be able to adjust the nutrient content by simply altering the proportions in the ration of the existing ingredients.

Use the statistical information published for each feed to improve formulation accuracy: Most authorities publish, for each nutrient, the average (mean) content of that nutrient in the feed samples considered in compiling the table, the range (i.e. the minimum and maximum) of contents, and the standard deviation (SD) of the mean. These statistics allow:

- calculation of logical safety margins;
- calculation of a spread of nutrient contents which is likely to encompass the nutrient content of the feed sample that we wish to use; and
- the use of stochastic ration formulation methods.

Example: The protein content of maize grain is given in the INRAE/CIRAD/AFZ (2017–2020) feed tables as 8.9% (DM basis). This is the average value and has an SD of 0.7% and a range between 6.7% and 12.2% (i.e. from 75–137% of the average value). By using the quoted 8.9% protein we are likely to, over time, overestimate the protein content of half of our samples and underestimate the protein content of the other half. As far as animal performance goes, overestimation will have more effect than underestimation because if we think our sample contains more protein than it actually has, this will lead us to formulate a ration which does not meet the animal's protein requirement. To avoid limiting our animals' productivity, we could use the lowest value in the published range, i.e. 6.7%. But this means that we would underestimate the protein content of almost all of our samples, which will lead to producing rations which are more expensive than they need to be because we will include unnecessary protein sources (and these are expensive).

Rather than just using the mean or the range, we can use the SD to calculate a spread of protein contents which include different proportions of the population of samples from which these data were obtained (Table 9.2). Then we decide how conservative we want to be, choose a range of protein contents, and use the lower value of this range. This will reduce the error and the effect on our animals.

Suppose that we want 95% of the maize samples that we encounter to have the same or greater protein content as the value we choose. To do this, we use the protein content which is 2 SD below the average (7.5% in our example) and assume that all of the samples we use have that protein content. This ensures that in 95.4% of cases we would formulate a ration with the minimum required nutrient content.

The method described above is useful for manual and least-cost ration formulations. Another approach, which is quite different to the above, is to use stochastic programming to formulate the ration. This is described later in this chapter.

Using nutrient content and requirement information to check an existing ration

To check the nutrient content of an existing ration or mixture of feed ingredients use the nutrient content and requirement data as discussed in the previous sections.

Example: An adult horse weighs 400 kg and is used for general riding – an hour or two trotting and walking on the flat, and occasionally over low jumps (this is moderate work according to the NRC, 2007). Each day the horse is fed 300 g of soybean meal, 5 kg of pasture hay, 1 kg of oat grain and 50 g of salt (Table 9.3; note – this is an example and not a recommended ration).

There are three things to note about Table 9.3:

- The nutrient contents in this table are given on a DM basis. But this is not mandatory, we can choose whichever basis of expression – as-fed or DM – is most useful or suitable. The data in the NRC, 2007, nutrient content tables are on a DM basis, so they are used as published. However, pig and poultry data are often given on an as-fed basis (as shown in Table 9.1).
- It is useful to know the total amount of feed offered because this should not exceed the animal's expected intake capacity (Chapter 7).
- It makes no sense to add up, or average, the constituent or nutrient content columns – those totals and averages are meaningless.

From the information in Table 9.3 we can calculate the amounts of DE, protein and Na supplied each day using the method shown in Table 9.4. These daily amounts can be converted to nutrient concentrations by dividing by the expected DM intake, as shown in Table 9.5.

Compare the calculated nutrient intakes and contents with feeding standards recommendations: This is a simple process, as shown in Table 9.6. Ensure that the units and basis of expression are consistent between the nutrient requirements and the feed nutrient contents.

From this comparison we see that this ration provides more than enough protein and Na, but is slightly deficient in DE. We could replace some of the soybean meal with oat grain to reduce the protein content (but this would also reduce the DE content) and reduce the added salt content to about 35 g

Table 9.2. Calculating ranges of protein contents which encompass defined proportions of the population of maize grain samples used in the INRAE/CIRAD/AFZ (2017–2020) table. (Copyright: Gordon McL. Dryden.)

No. of SD above and below the mean	Proportion of samples expected to be within this band (mean ± SD)	Range of protein contents (% DM basis)
1	68.2%	8.9 ± (1 × 0.7) = 8.2 to 9.6
2	95.4%	8.9 ± (2 × 0.7) = 7.5 to 10.3
3	99.7%	8.9 ± (3 x 0.7) = 6.8 to 11.0

DM, dry matter; SD, standard deviation.

Table 9.3. Ingredient composition (kg/day, as-fed) and ingredient nutrient contents of a simple horse ration. (Nutrient content data from NRC, 2007; reproduced with permission.)

		Nutrient contents			
Ingredient	Amount (kg, as-fed)	Dry matter (%)	DE[a] (MJ/kg DM)	Protein (% DM basis)	Na (% DM basis)
Grass hay	8	84	8.54	10.8	0.02
Soybean meal	0.3	90	15.6	53.8	0.03
Oat grain	1	90	13.7	13.2	0.03
Salt	0.05	99	0	0	39
Total	9.35	–	–	–	–

DM, dry matter; DE, digestible energy.
[a]The units for DE have been changed from Mcal/kg DM to MJ/kg DM.

Table 9.4. Dry matter and nutrients[a,b] provided by the ration in Table 9.3. (Copyright: Gordon McL. Dryden.)

	Amounts of each nutrient (per day)			
Ingredient	DM (kg)	DE (MJ)	Protein (g)	Na (g)
Grass hay	6.72 (= 8 × 84/100)	57.4 (= 6.72 × 8.54)	725.8 (= (6.72 × 10.8/100) × 1000)	1.34 (= (6.72 × 0.02/100) × 1000)
Soybean meal	0.27	4.21	145.26	0.081
Oat grain	0.9	12.33	118.8	0.27
Salt	0.049	0	0	19.1
Total	7.94	73.49	989.9	20.79

DM, dry matter; DE, digestible energy.
[a]The calculations are shown for grass hay; all the other calculations follow the same method.
[b]The unit for protein is changed from kg to g. This is more convenient for the calculations in Table 9.5.

Table 9.5. Nutrient concentrations in the ration described in Table 9.3. (Copyright: Gordon McL. Dryden.)

Nutrient/constituent	As-fed basis[a]	Dry matter basis[b]
Dry matter (DM, %)[c]	84.9 (= 7.94/9.35 × 100)	100 (= 7.94/7.94 × 100)
Digestible energy (MJ/kg or MJ/kg DM)	7.86 (= 73.49/9.35)	9.26 (= 73.49/7.94) or 9.26 (= (7.86 × 100/84.9)
Protein (%)	10.6 (= (989.9/1000)/9.35 × 100)	12.5 [= (989.9/1000)/7.94 × 100] or 12.5 (= 10.6 × 100/84.9)
Na (%)	0.22 (= (20.79/1000)/9.35 × 100)	0.26 [= (20.79/1000)/7.94 × 100] or 0.26 (= 0.22 × 100/84.9)

[a]To calculate the nutrient concentrations on an as-fed basis (column 2), divide by the total amount of feed (9.35 kg in this example). To calculate on a DM basis (column 3) divide by the total DM amount (7.94 kg in this example).
[b]The alternative calculations in column 3 use the method described previously for converting from an as-fed to a DM basis.
[c]The concentration of DM is always given as a proportion of the whole feed, i.e. on an as-fed basis. The DM content of an ingredient or mixture of ingredients is always 100% on a DM basis.

Table 9.6. Comparison of the nutrient contents calculated in Tables 9.4 and 9.5 and those recommended by NRC (2007; reproduced with permission.)

	Amount per day		Concentration in feed (DM basis)	
Nutrient/constituent	Calculated	NRC (2007)	Calculated	NRC (2007)
Dry matter (DM)	7.9 kg	9 kg[a]	–	–
Digestible energy	73.5 MJ	77.8 MJ	9.26 MJ/kg DM	8.65 MJ/kg DM
Protein	990 g	614 g	12.5%, DM	6.8%, DM
Na	20.8 g	14.2 g	0.26%, DM	0.16%, DM

[a]The NRC (2007) assumes that a horse doing moderate work will eat an amount of DM equivalent to 2.25% of its live weight each day. In this example, 400 × 2.25/100 = 9 kg of DM per day.

(0.035 kg) per day. To fix the DE deficiency we need another ingredient – perhaps maize (corn) grain at 7% of the ration. Another option is to feed 0.5 kg more of the ration each day (we are feeding 1.1 kg DM less than the expected intake limit). This would bring the DE intake up to the NRC (2007) recommended level, but at the cost of substantially overfeeding protein and Na. Among other things, this alternative would increase the cost of feeding.

Ration formulation methods

The methods available for ration formulation include two manual methods – trial and error and the Pearson square. These are both simple, and the Pearson square method is quite rapid, but they cannot handle the complexity of commercial animal rations. In general, it is best to use the more complex, but more accurate, methods that use linear or stochastic programming.

Irrespective of the method used, it is important to decide on the scope of the problem (see below), and to assemble and prepare the nutrient content and requirement data while observing the caveats which are described at the start of this chapter.

Before formulating a ration:

1. Decide on which nutrients to consider in the formulation – there will usually be ten or more. The list will include energy (either TDN, DE, ME, or NE); protein (either total protein, or RDP and UDP or MP depending on animal species); Ca, P, Mg and Na, and trace minerals including Cu, I and Fe; lysine and other essential amino acids (e.g. arginine, histidine, methionine – the list varies according to species and age), essential fatty acids (especially linoleic acid) and vitamins. For ruminants, decide on the maximum level of concentrate ingredients which will be included in the ration.
2. Choose the ingredients: typically, a formulation for a commercial feed starts with a list of 20 or so ingredients for pigs and poultry, or 5 to 10 ingredients for ruminants. Use as large a pool of ingredients as is reasonable, even though it is expected that only some of these will be used in the ration. The larger the feed data base, the more likely it is that the formulation will be successful.

The list of potential ingredients can be very large and somewhat daunting at first sight. But in practice the choice will be influenced by:

- the need to ensure sources of all the required nutrients;
- seasonal availability of feeds, especially cereal grains and forages;
- reliability of supply;
- what is already in store;
- ingredient palatability; and
- the possibility of nutritional disorders caused by lack of fibre or the presence of secondary (toxic) substances in some feeds.

Trial-and-error formulation: This method is a series of guesses and checks:

1. Start with a ration composition that may possibly provide the required nutrient concentrations; or alternatively, the required daily amounts of nutrients.
2. Check the nutrient supply using the method described in Tables 9.4 or 9.5.
3. Change the ingredient composition to make any necessary changes in nutrient supply.
4. Recheck the nutrient contents or daily amounts.
5. Continue this until we are satisfied that we have a suitable ration.

The trial-and-error method is laborious, imprecise, constrained to using only the ingredients that we think will be suitable, and does not guarantee that the final ration is the least expensive. The only advantage that this method has is that the arithmetic is simple.

The Pearson square (also called the 'miller's formula'): This is a simple diagrammatic process used to solve a simultaneous equation of the form:

$$ax + by = R$$
$$x + y = 1$$

where: x and y are the proportions of two different ingredients in the ration
a and b are the contents of the nutrient under consideration, in ingredients x and y

R is the required nutrient concentration.

In the first equation, x and y are the unknowns which are solved for, and a and b are known nutrient contents which are obtained from a suitable feed library. The second equation is the quantity constraint. It ensures that the proportions of the two ingredients sum to 1 (or 100%).

While it is simple to solve this problem if we understand how to solve simultaneous equations, the Pearson square is an easy alternative. To use it:

1. Choose two suitable ingredients to supply the nutrient under consideration. In this example we will formulate a mixture of two ingredients to supply the DE requirement of a growing dairy weaner. The ingredients are maize (corn) grain (16.2 MJ/kg DM) and mature grass hay (8.5 MJ/kg DM). The DE requirement is 12.1 MJ/kg DM.

2. Check that the two ingredient nutrient contents bracket the requirement. In this case the DE contents of hay and grain are respectively lower than, and higher than, the requirement. The Pearson square does not work if the ingredient nutrient contents are both higher than, or both lower than, the requirement.
3. Set out and solve the problem as shown in Fig. 9.2. Work on the diagonals to find the differences between the nutrient contents of the two feeds and the requirement. Always subtract the smaller figure from the larger; this changes with the different ingredients. If the answer is a negative value there is either a mistake in calculation, or the wrong value has been subtracted. If both nutrient contents are either higher or lower than the requirement, the calculations can still give an apparently successful result but the overall solution will be incorrect.
4. To find the answer, read across the figure. The proportion of hay in this example is 53.2%, not 46.8%.

The Pearson square method is very limited in its application to real-life ration formulation tasks. It gives an exact answer for the nutrient under consideration but is constrained to only that single nutrient and the two chosen ingredients and does not guarantee a least-cost mixture as the cost of the ration depends on the prices of the chosen ingredients.

Although the method can be extended to deal with more than one nutrient and additional ingredients can be added to provide these, this extension introduces assumptions and approximations. One approach is to devise a mixture of two or more ingredients and calculate the nutrient content of that mixture, then to consider that mixture as a single ingredient.

With advances in our understanding of how animals use nutrients and the effects of feeds on their health, the list of nutrients and feed characteristics which are now considered when formulating a ration is formidable – 20 to 30 items. This makes ration formulation complex, and simple methods like the Pearson square are simply unable to cope.

Least-cost ration formulation: This method uses linear programming to identify a mixture of ingredients which contains all the nutrients under consideration and guarantees, for the ingredients and nutrients selected, to give a least-cost solution.

Linear programming is too tedious to do by hand or calculator and is only suitable for computer application. However, there are numerous least-cost formulation programs available. The Solver application in Excel has been used (Radhika and Rao, 2010) as the basis of simple Excel-based formulation programs. More usefully, there are free-to-download least-cost formulation programs (e.g. Pesti *et al.*, 2014) and more sophisticated commercial versions which have extensive file-handling capacity. This is an advantage because we can store multiple ingredient data and do not have to input them for each new formulation.

An example – least-cost formulation of a poultry layer ration: In this example there are 14 nutrients and 17 ingredients. The nutrients are protein, lysine, methionine + cystine, arginine, fibre (or

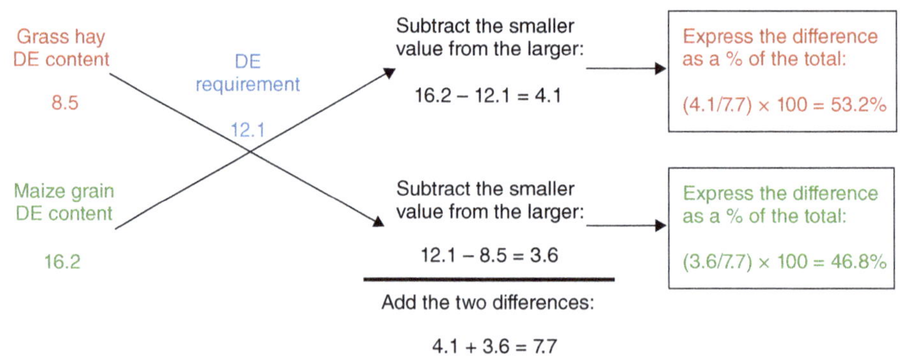

Fig. 9.2. Using the Pearson square. (Copyright: Gordon McL. Dryden.)

alternatively, the proportion of non-concentrate ingredients), Ca, non-phytate P, Na, Mg, vitamin A, vitamin D, vitamin E, vitamin K and linoleic acid. The ingredients in this example are wheat, barley and maize (corn) grains, wheat bran, soybean meal, sunflower meal, canola meal, fish meal, synthetic lysine, salt, dicalcium phosphate, limestone, Mg sulphate, and sources of vitamins A, D, E and K. We would also have to provide mixtures of trace minerals, and of B vitamins; these could be forced into the ration at predetermined levels.

This set of nutrients and ingredients is much larger than the very stripped-down examples that we have seen so far. The number of ingredients and nutrients in this poultry layer example is a much more realistic example of the size of commercial ration formulation problems, although smaller than some real-life commercial ration formulations for pigs or poultry. These might also include the other essential amino acids, other fatty acids, more major minerals, the individual trace minerals and vitamin C.

In this example there are more ingredients than nutrients. We need to set the problem up in this way so that we can successfully formulate a ration.

The equation set in this example has 16 equations. The first 14 equations are the nutrient constraints, the next equation involving the ingredient costs is the cost constraint, and the final equation is the quantity constraint which is included to ensure that the ingredient proportions sum to 1 (or 100%).

$$a_1x_1 + a_2x_2 + a_3x_3 + a_4x_4 \ldots a_{17}x_{17} \geq A$$

$$b_1x_1 + b_2x_2 + b_3x_3 + b_4x_4 \ldots b_{17}x_{17} \geq B$$

.

.

.

.

$$n_1x_1 + n_2x_2 + n_3x_3 + n_4x_4 \ldots n_{17}x_{17} \geq N$$
$$C_1x_1 + C_2x_2 + C_3x_3 + C_4x_4 \ldots C_{17}x_{17} = C$$
$$x_1 + x_2 + x_3 + x_4 \ldots x_{17} = 1$$

Where: $a_1 \ldots n_{17}$ are the contents of the 14 nutrients, *a* to *n*, in each of the 17 ingredients

A, B … N are the required concentrations of the 14 nutrients

$x_1, x_2, x_3, x_4 \ldots x_{17}$ are the proportions of the 17 ingredients in the final ration

$C_1, C_2, C_3, C_4 \ldots C_{17}$ are the costs (e.g. \$ or € or £ or ¥ per tonne) of the 17 ingredients

C is the total cost of the ration.

The purpose of the exercise is to calculate the values for $x_1, x_2, x_3, x_4 \ldots x_{17}$, so that we satisfy all the nutrient requirements and minimize the ration cost (C).

Note that the nutrient constraints are inequalities (≥), where the sum of the terms are not required to equal A (where A is the required nutrient content) but can be greater than A. In some cases, when we set an upper limit for a nutrient or an ingredient, the inequality is ≤ (less than or equal to), and the same reasoning applies.

We have to use this approach because if all the nutrient requirements had to be met exactly the ration formulation problem could not be solved. We can accept this lack of accuracy because animals are able to cope with excesses of most nutrients or ingredients. But be aware that there are some exceptions to this general rule; the problem of nutrient toxicity is discussed in Chapter 1.

The equations above may seem to be abstract and difficult, but we can illustrate how they work by using the example shown in Fig. 9.3. This is a simplified case considering only two ingredients (this is so the constraints can be drawn in a two-dimensional diagram) and two nutrients. The nutrients in Fig. 9.3 are lysine (requirement = 0.69%) and linoleic acid (requirement = 1.0%) and the ingredients are fish meal (containing 0.7% linoleic acid, 4.51% lysine) and maize (corn) grain (2.2% linoleic acid, 0.26% lysine).

It is clear from Fig. 9.3 that the lysine and linoleic acid solutions are very different. This is because the concentrations of these nutrients in the ingredients are also very different. Which solution should we choose? The areas of the quantity line above and to the right of the dotted nutrient constraint lines represent combinations of maize and fish meal which give excess lysine or linoleic acid. The 'lysine' solution will give a ration with a much higher concentration of linoleic acid that is needed, while the 'linoleic acid' solution gives a higher content of lysine than we need. Because both nutrients can be fed in excess without problems, we would choose the solution which gives the lowest cost ration, in this case the 'lysine' solution which has 90% maize grain (the cheapest ingredient) and 10% fish meal.

Useful techniques that can be used with linear programming:

- 'Multi-blending' is formulating two or more rations at the same time. This technique is used

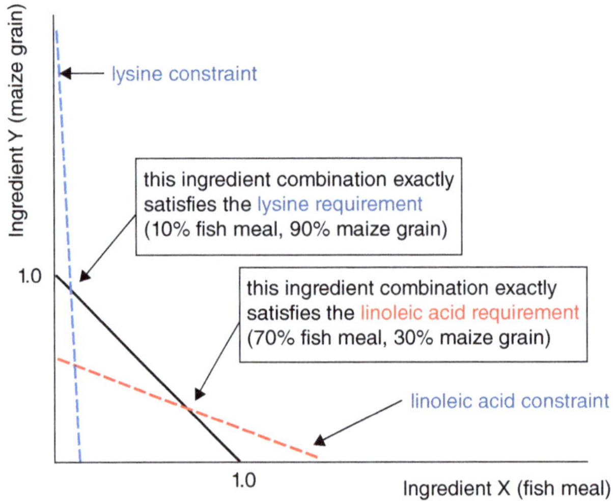

Fig. 9.3. Illustration of nutrient constraints in a least-cost ration formulation problem (dashed lines are the nutrient constraints, the solid line is the quantity constraint). (Copyright: Gordon McL. Dryden.)

by feed mills which produce several different rations. It gives a better result than formulating individual least-cost rations because the program allocates ingredients over both rations so that the overall cost of producing both is minimized. This may not occur if the rations are formulated separately.

- 'Parametric ranging' involves testing the effects of slightly changing the nutrient requirement or ingredient cost specifications. Parametric ranging allows 'what if' questions to be asked, e.g. what happens to the ration composition and cost if the lysine or calcium requirements are reduced? Or what is the effect on the ration composition and cost if the price of wheat grain can be reduced? By asking these questions we might find a cheaper, but still nutritionally adequate, result than if we simply accepted the first 'least-cost' formulation.
- Controlling ingredient use: we can 'force in' or 'force out' an ingredient or limit its inclusion level. This lets us override the least-cost program so that we can use up left-over ingredients and control the use of ingredients which contain poisonous secondary substances (such as gossypol in cottonseed meal), or which may be unpalatable (palm kernel meal), or have adverse effects on product quality (unsaturated fats), or which may be poisonous in excess (such as urea).
- Setting nutrient maximums and ratios: in most cases, we specify the minimum requirements for each nutrient, but there are situations where it is better to put more constraints on nutrient inclusion. For example, nutrient contents can be specified in relation to the amounts of other nutrients. This can help to control mineral availability (e.g. by preventing an excessive Ca:P ratio) or controlling carcase fatness in pigs by ensuring that there is a match between the lysine and ME contents of a ration or using the 'ideal amino acid ratio' approach (Chapter 8). This technique is sometimes called 'nutrient factoring'.
- Sometimes it is advisable to set a maximum content for a nutrient. Some nutrients, e.g. trace minerals (e.g. Cu in sheep diets), and vitamins A and D, are toxic in high concentrations, even though they are essential nutrients.
- Using opportunity costs to determine ingredient buying strategies: least-cost ration formulation programs will give a 'price for inclusion' (or 'opportunity cost' or 'shadow price') for each non-included ingredient. This information is extremely helpful when negotiating purchases because we know exactly what prices we can afford. A second type of shadow price is the new cost of the complete ration if we changed the specification of any nutrient. But always run a check formulation before committing to a new ingredient – the formulation may not be as we expect.

Always check that the formulated ration is suitable for the intended animals:

- Does it have enough fibre to maintain digestive tract health?
- Is it palatable?
- Does it contain excessive amounts of possibly harmful ingredients?
- Are any nutrient ratios unbalanced, e.g. lysine: ME or Ca:P?
- Are there dangerous excesses of any nutrients (e.g. Cu or vitamin D) or ingredients (e.g. urea in ruminant diets)?

And a ration will have to be changed when:

- The animal's nutrient requirements change (e.g. becomes pregnant, is doing a different type of work, or grows larger).
- Ingredients become unavailable.
- The formulated ration turns out to be unsuitable.
- Ingredient prices change.

Stochastic ration formulation is a type of ration formulation which achieves a specified probability of meeting nutrient requirements. It requires data on the average nutrient contents of feeds and the SDs applying to these averages.

Stochastic formulations can be more efficient than linear programmed rations although there is a risk that requiring a high probability of meeting the nutrient requirements will result in a more expensive ration, or that ingredients with a low SD will be selected over others that may have similar nutritional values at lower costs (Tozer, 2000).

Controlling feeding costs

Cost-effective use of animal feed: In most cases the aim in managing domestic animals is to maximize the enterprise's profit. Feed makes up 60% or more of the total costs of an intensive animal enterprise so it is essential that these costs are controlled. To do that, we need to know the components of feed costs and how to minimize these.

The components of feed costs are:

- purchase of ingredients or mixed feed;
- transport of the feed or ingredient to the farm;
- storage;
- processing: milling, mixing, other processes such as pelleting (Chapter 18);
- feeding out (Chapter 17); and
- wastage.

Purchase and transport costs contribute to the landed cost of feeds and nutrients: When considering the cost of ingredients we should calculate the landed cost of the main nutrient that the particular ingredient supplies – e.g. if we are buying protein meal then we calculate the landed cost of total protein or RDP; if we are buying cereal grains we would calculate the landed cost of ME. We then buy the ingredient with the lowest landed cost provided that it is suitable in other criteria such as palatability, freedom from secondary substances, etc.

When buying a pre-prepared mixed feed, we base our choice on the landed cost of the whole feed, not just one of the nutrients in it.

For example: calculating the landed cost of wheat grain:

Cost of wheat in the grower's or trader's silo = \$220/tonne
Transport and handling (100 km journey from the silo to our property) = \$22/tonne

Thus the total cost of a 25-tonne load, landed at our property

= (25 × \$220) + (25 × \$22)
= \$6050
or \$242/tonne or 24.2 c/kg

Because individual feeds should be costed on a 'price per unit of nutrient' basis, we now calculate the landed cost of ME:

ME content = 11.9 MJ/kg
Landed cost of ME = (24.2/11.9) = 2.03 c/MJ

Other feed handling and processing costs: Landed costs account only for the initial purchase price and the cost of transport. We may also have to add processing, storage and feeding-out costs.

The most common type of cereal grain processing is milling through a hammer mill or roller mill (Chapter 18). The costs associated with this include the cost of the electricity needed to power the mill plus equipment maintenance, depreciation and labour costs. These are usually expressed as \$/hour, which we can use to calculate the cost in \$/tonne of processed material by dividing the total hourly cost by the mill's processing rate (tonne/hour). The cost of chopping roughage using a flail chopper or tub grinder is calculated similarly.

Storage costs are a function of the cost of electricity or other fuel used to move ingredients from the delivery vehicle into storage, and the maintenance and depreciation of silos or bins, augers and other equipment. For completeness we could add the costs of feed spoilage.

Feed and ingredient costs can be minimized by careful buying, ration formulation and feed storage: Least-cost ration formulation will generally ensure that the cost of feed is kept to a minimum. Once we have a suitable ration and have decided on which ingredients to buy, the factors which will determine how much of each ingredient we buy at a time are:

- on-farm storage capacity;
- the reliability of supply; and
- stability of the ingredients in storage.

Start by estimating the amount of each ingredient needed from the expected total feed intake (Chapter 7) and the ration composition. If this amount exceeds our storage capacity, then we will generally have to limit the purchase to the amount that can be stored on-site. Other possibilities are to contract for the delivery of additional feed at future dates, or to rent additional storage. When assessing storage capacity, or preparing feeds for animals, it is important to understand the feed's bulk density, i.e. the relationship between mass and volume. Different ingredients, and samples of ingredient, have different bulk densities. The bulk density of any ingredient can change with variations in moisture content and physical form, e.g. whole versus milled grain and mash versus pellets.

If ingredients are not reliably available because of limited supplies (e.g. due to seasonality of supply) or high demand, then we need to compare the costs of storage and possible deterioration during storage, with the cost of a forward contract or of changing to another feed option. Note that most ingredients are available year-round. This applies to cereal grains even though they grow seasonally. Cereal grains are stable in storage and whole grain can be kept for several years provided that it is protected from moisture and vermin.

Often, the unit cost of ingredients or mixed feed is lowest when the material is bought in large quantities, but we do this at the risk of having unused ingredients deteriorate during storage (see below). It is a false economy to buy ingredients in amounts that cannot be used before they deteriorate.

Sources of wastage and ways of dealing with them: There are three ways in which animal enterprises waste feed. These are:

- Loss of feed quality during storage: many ingredients suffer some loss of quality during storage, although whole grain, silage, molasses, protein meals and minerals like salt, limestone and dicalcium phosphate are fairly stable. However, these ingredients lose vitamin activity and some protein during lengthy storage, and fats in milled grain become oxidized. Storage for lengthy periods in substandard facilities risks ingredients becoming wet through exposure to humid air or other water sources (e.g. rain or dew), and consequently becoming good habitats for micro-organisms and insects. Storage facilities need to be weatherproof to limit moisture damage. Vitamins, antibiotics, coccidiostats and rumen modifiers gradually lose potency in storage and it is unwise to use these after their expiry date. Additives do not generally lose all their active principle when they reach this date, and loss of activity generally occurs slowly, but nevertheless, the product's efficacy after the expiry date will be reduced.
- Loss of feed during feeding: feed can be pulled or nosed out of feeders and bins as the animal eats, trodden on, fouled with urine and faeces in animal pens or yards, and dampened and spoiled by rain and very hot weather when fed outside. Feed wastage is usually 3–10% in piggeries and can be considerable (much more than 10%) in roughage feeding systems. Wastage can be reduced as described in Chapter 17.
- Inefficiencies of nutrient use are inherent in how animals use feed and nutrients. Often animals are fed excess amino acids and P so as to make sure that these nutrients are not deficient, but the excesses are excreted and wasted. Although these wastages cannot be easily controlled, feeding excess amino acids and minerals can and should be avoided by using efficient nutritional techniques (Chapters 5 and 8).

References

INRAE/CIRAD/AFZ (2017–2020). *Feed Tables*. Available at: www.feedtables.com/ (accessed 27 December 2020).

National Research Council (NRC) (2001). *Nutrient Requirements of Dairy Cattle*, 7th rev. edn. Update.

Washington, DC: National Academies Press. Available at: www.nap.edu/catalog/9825/nutrient-requirements-of-dairy-cattle-seventh-revised-edition-2001 (accessed 27 December 2020).

National Research Council (NRC) (2007). *Nutrient Requirements of Horses*, 6th rev. edn. Washington, DC: National Academies Press. Available at: www.nap.edu/catalog/11653/nutrient-requirements-of-horses-sixth-revised-edition (accessed 27 December 2020).

National Research Council (NRC) (2012). *Nutrient Requirements of Swine*, 11th rev. edn. Washington, DC: National Academies Press. Available at: www.nap.edu/catalog/13298/nutrient-requirements-of-swine-eleventh-revised-edition (accessed 27 December 2020).

Pesti, G.M., Azain, M.J., Vedenov, D.V. and Bakalli, R.I. (2014). *Windows User-Friendly Feed Formulation for Poultry and Swine*. Research Bulletin 438. University of Georgia Extension. Available at: www.extension.uga.edu/publications/detail.html?number=RB438&title=Windows_User-Friendly_Feed_Formulation_for_Poultry_and_Swine (accessed 27 December 2020).

Radhika, V. and Rao, S.B.N. (2010). Formulation of low-cost balanced ration for livestock using Microsoft Excel. *Wayamba Journal of Animal Science* No. 281076233, pp. 38–41. Available from: www.researchgate.net/publication/277137305_Formulation_of_Low_Cost_Balanced_Ration_for_Livestock_using_Microsoft_Excel (accessed 27 December 2020).

Tozer, R.P. (2000). Least-cost ration formulations for Holstein dairy heifers by using linear and stochastic programming. *Journal of Dairy Science* 83:443–451.

10 Nutritional models

There are many nutritional models, but only a few are used in this chapter to illustrate particular points. Other models which are not mentioned here may be similarly fit for purpose and as capable as those mentioned.

An overview of computer models used in managing farm animals

A computer model is a mathematical description or 'model' or 'simulation' of a process. A nutrient requirements model describes how the animal uses nutrients, and the factors which determine the amounts of nutrients that they need.

Most published feeding standards are based on a nutritional model of this type, and most authorities provide, as part of the feeding standards package, software based on this model which users can use to get specific nutrient requirement data about their own animals in their own environment.

Tactical and strategic models are used in animal management: Models which are used to calculate nutrient requirements are examples of tactical models; they deal with a specific aspect of animal performance.

Strategic models have a much wider canvas. They may contain sub-models which formulate rations, or modules which predict pasture growth and quality and combine this with the generated nutrient requirement data to predict grazing animal performance, and they may predict profit from a combination of production data generated by the model and information on expected market conditions. These models can be used to plan and compare different production strategies.

For examples of tactical and strategic models relating to the dairy industry, see Little *et al.* (2009).

Empirical and mechanistic models differ in the way that they connect an input with a response. Empirical models give a broad overview of the process they describe but do not investigate the physiology or biochemistry of the process, e.g.:

1 kg starch → 0.35 kg fat deposition in a growing pig

A mechanistic model describes the processes which underlie this response, e.g. (very simply):

1 kg starch → 900 g absorbed glucose

800 g glucose available for fat synthesis → 350 g fat

Nutritional models are largely mechanistic, although sub-models of mineral and vitamin nutrition may be empirical. The components of mechanistic models (e.g. nutrient pool sizes and the rates of movement between pools) are determined from experiments with small groups of animals and they are the average responses to nutrient supply and utilization. While these are the expected responses, they may not occur in all situations.

Deterministic and stochastic models: To date, most nutritional models are deterministic, i.e. the outputs from the calculations are determined solely by the values that are given to the various model components. There is little attempt to cater for genetic differences between animals, or variation in feed nutritive values. While 'in practice it is necessary to meet the requirements of as many of the individuals as we can economically' (Heuser, 1941, cited by Fisher, 2015) this is not possible if we use models that are based on average animal responses, because it is likely that we will either under- or overestimate the size of model components when these values are applied to individual animals. The development of stochastic models addresses this problem by giving each step in the mechanistic process a probability. Stochastic modelling is a developing field.

DOI: 10.1079/9781786394453.0010

Nutrient requirements – models or tables?

Published feeding standards demonstrate the limitations of nutrient requirement tables. There are two main reasons for this, discussed below.

Tables do not describe individual animals well enough: Nutrient requirement tables describe animals by breed type, live weight or age and production level. It is not possible to provide data for every increment or combination of these, so published standards aggregate animals into groups (e.g. hens at different stages of lay, growing pigs at nominated live weights, or cows producing milk with specified fat or protein contents) and give only one recommendation for all the animals within each of these groups. This implies that nutrient requirements change in a series of steps as animals move between weeks of the laying cycle, live weights or milk compositions, but this is not the case. Further, the recommendations may be restricted to animals of particular sexes (or mixtures of sex) or genetic quality (e.g. pigs capable of depositing 135 g protein /day, or beef cattle capable of growing at nearly 2 kg/day). If we want recommendations for different animals or production rates, then we would have to alter the recommended values and this would involve making estimates and assumptions. Finally, recommendations for nutrient concentrations are calculated from assumed feed intakes which might be very different from intakes which would be calculated from breed, sex, environment and feed data for individual farms, or measured on different farms.

Tabulated requirement values imply that feed nutrient values are fixed: This is not correct; there is an interaction between the feed type and the way that animals use nutrients, especially energy and protein. For example, the efficiency with which ruminants use metabolizable energy for growth (k_g) varies considerably, depending on the composition of the diet. Some feeding standards tables are based on the requirements of animals fed an example diet, and these will change when the diet composition changes. A tabular value for k_g may be correct if the diet consists of that feed alone, but animals are almost always fed a mixture of feeds, and this will change k_g from the values assumed when the table of requirements was compiled. Nutritional models take this type of variation into account.

Models are much more flexible than tables of requirements. With models we can describe animals and their environment more accurately. We can take into account factors such as breed, actual live weight and age, actual stage of pregnancy or lactation, production levels (e.g. daily egg or milk production, growth rate), type of housing, environmental factors such as ambient temperature and wind speed; and for grazing animals, factors such as rain, mud and pasture topography. From this information we can get a statement of nutrient requirements which is specific for that animal and its environment. In addition, nutrition models can be combined with economic modelling such as least cost ration formulation or market prices for products so that we can investigate the financial outcomes of different feeding and/or marketing scenarios.

Ease of understanding and use: Most feeding standards no longer provide comprehensive tables of nutrient requirements, although they do include some tables of nutrient requirements to provide a modicum of information for those managers who prefer to use tabulated data.

Tables might appear to be simple and straightforward, but they are no easier to use than a model once we have got used to the idea. Nutrient requirement software is easy to install, generally intuitive to use and with easy-to-understand outputs, and comes with a 'how-to-use' manual. We do not have to know how a model is constructed to be able to use it, although it is useful to know something of the reasoning used in their development.

Nutrient requirement models

How nutrient requirements models are constructed: The type of information used in nutritional models is essentially the same for all animal types. All models include equations to describe:

- Feed intake, needed to estimate the amount of ingredients which must be purchased and stored to correctly feed the animal, and to express daily nutrient requirement amounts as concentrations in the feed (Chapter 9). Models provide a predicted feed intake but may allow the user to over-write these estimates with their own measured data.

  Poultry, pig, and some dairy models assume that the bird or animal eats to satisfy its energy requirement and, consequently, that feed intake is determined by this and the energy content of the feed. However, feed intake by ruminants is influenced by rumen fill, digestion and passage into and from the rumen, NE requirements and the NE content of the feed, the animal's physiological state, the environment and other factors. Intake predictions for horses are not as well developed as for other animal types and are based on the animal's live weight and amount and type of activity. See Chapter 7 for more information about factors which influence feed intake.

- Digestion and absorption of nutrients: for pigs and poultry, common measures of nutrient availability are the apparent and standardized (true) total tract digestibilities, or ileal digestibilities, of amino acids, the digestibility or metabolizability of feed energy, and concentrations of non-phytate P (Chapter 5). For ruminants, the models predict the rate of digestion of feed components in the rumen, and rate of passage of undigested feed from the rumen; amounts of MP and/or digestible amino acid reaching the small intestine; measures of energy supply including DE, ME and various forms of NE; and absorbable Ca and P.
- Nutrient demand for maintenance and production: maintenance energy requirements are calculated from the animal's live weight (often its metabolic size which is calculated within the model from the given live weight), breed and sex, physiological status, and the prevailing environmental conditions (temperature, wind speed, etc.); maintenance protein requirements are calculated either from endogenous N losses or from the animal's energy status. Production requirements for energy and protein or amino acids are determined from inputs such as the amount and composition of milk, peak milk yield and time in the lactation; growth rate and the composition (lean, fat and bone) of gain; number of previous parities and days pregnant, etc.
- Nutrient content of feeds: these can be calculated from the feed's chemical composition, but are usually input from an inbuilt feed library, or are provided by the software user.

Example of an animal metabolism component of a deterministic nutrient requirement model: Metabolic models describe the animal's digestive physiology and biochemistry, and consequently how it obtains and uses nutrients. These models consist of statements about pool sizes and the rates and extents at which material is transferred between them.

An example is the calculation of the amount of MP entering the ruminant small intestine and the amount of net protein which is obtained as a result of this. This example is an excerpt from a protein metabolism model developed by CSIRO (2007) and used in the GrazFeed software (Horizon Agriculture 2005–).

The process is illustrated in Fig. 10.1, where the pools are the amounts of protein and fermentable ME eaten, feed protein degraded in the rumen, microbial true protein, endogenous protein entering the stomach, metabolizable protein (digestible protein leaving the abomasum), and net protein

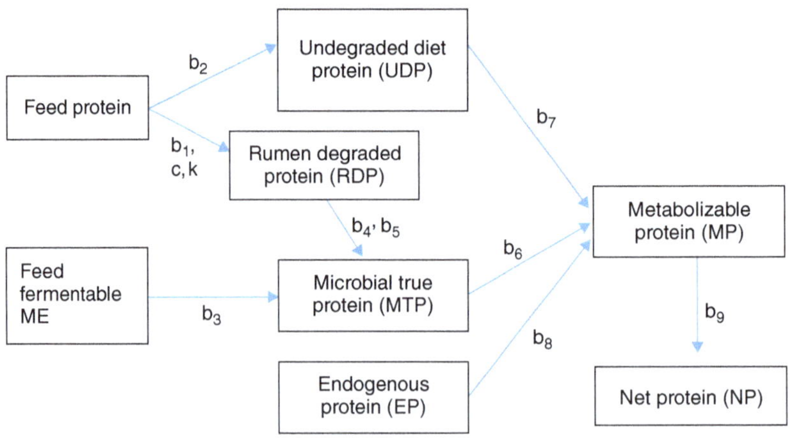

Fig. 10.1. A model of the processes in the rumen which contribute to the production of metabolizable protein and net protein. (Copyright: Gordon McL. Dryden.)

(the protein retained in body tissue or products). The coefficients and rate constants describe how material moves between these pools.

In Fig. 10.1, the symbols represent these coefficients and rate constants (data from CSIRO (2007), reproduced with permission):

b_1 = Edg = A + B (c/(c + k)) = effective degradability of feed protein; this is 50–70% of heat-treated feed protein, 70–80% of tropical grasses protein, 75–95% of temperate grasses protein.

b_2 = (1 – Edg) = effective undegradability of feed protein.

$b_3 = 7 + 6 \times (1 - e^{-0.35L})$ = ratio of microbial protein which is synthesized to the amount of fermentable ME eaten by the animal (g/MJ; fermentable ME is ME from carbohydrates and proteins, but not fats or volatile fatty acids because these are little-used energy sources for rumen micro-organisms). This relationship assumes that only fermentable ME limits microbial protein synthesis, i.e. that nutrients like RAN, S, P and other nutrients are not limiting. L in the formula is the feeding level = amount of ME provided to the animal expressed as a multiple of the ME required for maintenance.

b_4 = proportion of RDP-N and non-protein N captured by rumen micro-organisms; this can reach 80% but can be much less for urea given as a N supplement.

b_5 = proportion of total microbial protein which is true protein; 85%, the rest is nucleic acid N and cell wall N.

b_6, b_7, b_8 = digestibilities of undegradable dietary protein (UDP; bypass protein), microbial true protein and endogenous protein; about 70%, but can vary between 5% and 90%.

b_9 = proportion of absorbed amino acids which are retained in the body; 70% for general tissue protein, 20% for wool protein.

A = amount of quickly degraded (soluble) feed protein.

B = amount of potentially degradable (but insoluble) feed protein.

c = rate at which feed protein is degraded on the rumen.

k = rate at which undigested feed protein leaves the rumen; typically 0.02 to 0.08/hour.

The MP that leaves the abomasum of ruminants is the digestible portion of a combination of microbial protein produced by the growth of bacteria and protozoa in the rumen (microbial true protein, MTP), feed protein which has not been digested by rumen micro-organisms (UDP) and endogenous protein (EP) into the stomach (this consists of rumen epithelial cells, mucus and saliva protein).

The flowchart (Fig. 10.1) shows that the factors determining the amount of MP entering the small intestine (which is what we want to calculate) include MTP and EP. But we cannot measure these easily, and a manager wanting to formulate a ration using the estimates of nutrient requirements based on this model would certainly not have this information. Accordingly, we come back a step and calculate MP from things that we do know, or that there are reasonable published estimates of – the ME contents of the feeds we want to use, the degradability of the protein in these feeds, and estimates of passage rates and digestibilities.

How nutrient requirements are calculated in nutritional models: Nutrient requirements are calculated from inputs such as live weight, genotype (e.g. efficiency of protein deposition in pigs, or egg-laying capacity of poultry) or breed, production level (e.g. growth rate, work by performance horses, milk yield), ambient temperature and feed type.

Example 1 is from NRC (2001) showing the equations used to calculate the amounts of energy and protein needed by a pregnant dairy cow. The most important factors affecting these requirements are the stage of pregnancy (the equation is based on data collected from cows between 190 and 297 days of pregnancy, but NRC, 2001, assumes the requirements to be effectively zero before 190 days) and the expected calf birth weight (relative to a standard birth weight of 45 kg).

$$ME_y = 4.184 \times [0.00318 \times (D - 0.0352) \times (CBW / 45)] / k_y$$

$$MP_y = [(0.69 \times D - 69.2) \times (CBW / 45)] / kp_y$$

where: ME_y = metabolizable energy for pregnancy (MJ/day)

MP_y = metabolizable protein required for pregnancy (g/day)

CBW = calf birthweight (kg)

D = days pregnant (between 190 to 279)

k_y = efficiency of use of ME for pregnancy (= 0.14)

kp_y = efficiency of use of MP for pregnancy (= 0.33)

Example 2 deals with protein deposition in growing pigs. The pig's ME intake determines the amount of energy it has available for protein deposition, and the rate at which it is able to deposit protein in its growing body is related to its live weight. The equations for entire males used by the NRC (2012) to express these concepts in mathematical terms are given below and are illustrated in Fig. 10.2.

$$\text{ME intake (MJ/day)} = 0.004184 \times [10638 \times (1 - e\ (-e\ (-3.803)) \times BW^{0.9072})]$$

$$PD = 151 \times (0.6558 + 0.01274 \times BW - 0.0001039 \times BW^2 + 1.64001 \times 10^{-7} \times BW^3)$$

Where: PD = protein deposition (g/day)

BW = pig body weight (kg)

The equations in these examples may seem difficult, but the calculations are done by the computer. All the dairy cow manager has to do is to provide the expected calf birth weight and the number of days the cow is pregnant, while the feed ME content is either input by the user or calculated within the program from feed library data. The pig farmer has only to provide the pigs' starting live weights, and an estimate of PD if they want to over-ride the default value calculated from the equation.

Using a nutrient requirement model

Describe the animals and their environment: Most of this information is quite simple, things like animal live weight, amount of feed given, ambient temperature, wind speed, and pasture topography (for grazing animals), and so on. Managers know these input values, although some might have to be purposely measured.

It is easy to put data into the model spreadsheet – hover the cursor over the appropriate cell on the screen and enter quantitative values or click to select an option. Just be sure to read the operating manual first so that we know what information is needed, what units to use, and how to access the data input screens.

In some cases, we might have to give detailed information. For example, the NRC (2012) pig feeding standards software asks for an estimate of the expected protein retention rate, and GrazFeed (Horizon Agriculture, 2005–) requires estimates of the expected dry matter digestibilities of pasture components. It is quite likely that we do not know these things; the best option in that situation is to use the default values which are supplied by the software. When we rely on default parameter values, it is a good idea to test a range of possibilities by over-riding the default values (if this is allowed by the program) to get a general view of what happens if the default values are not quite applicable to our situation. Some useful data, e.g. rumen digestion rates and yields of metabolizable protein, are provided in the NRC and INRAE feed nutritive value tables.

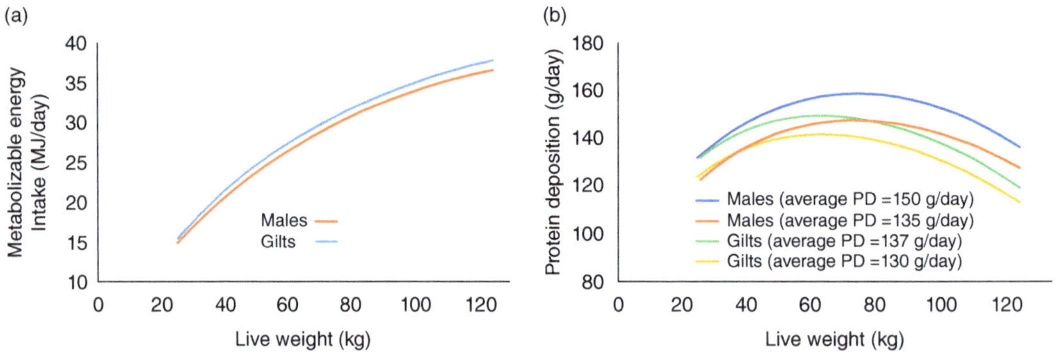

Fig. 10.2. Relationships between live weight and **(a)** metabolizable energy (ME) intake and **(b)** protein deposition for growing pigs. (Calculated from equations in the NRC, 2012, feeding standards for pigs; copyright: Gordon McL. Dryden.)

Model outputs: Running the model to generate the output is as simple as pressing a key on the keyboard. The program uses the equations (which are hidden behind the output screen) to produce the output. Outputs are usually easy to understand, and the model's manual will also describe how to interpret this information.

As well as predicting productivity, some models output information on nutrient use, e.g. a comparison of the nutrients provided by the ration and the animal's requirements, and the partitioning of nutrients like ME, RDP and UDP between different physiological processes. Using this information, we can:

- identify any limiting nutrients;
- adjust the ration composition to improve productivity; and
- investigate 'what if' scenarios – e.g. what will happen if we change the animal's housing by reducing stocking density, or providing shelter from wind and rain or heat, and so on.

The problem of a producing animal's changing nutrient requirements: Any lactating, pregnant or growing animal experiences changes in its nutrient requirements throughout its production cycle. Models predict requirements based on a snapshot of the animal at a given time – whether that is time in lactation or pregnancy, or the live weight of a growing animal or bird. Clearly, requirements determined for that particular case will not apply to other situations. Model compilers address this problem by restricting the model's output to predetermined production intervals. For example, recommendations for growing pigs may be based on 25 kg live weight steps, or monthly periods for lactating dairy cows. This means that we have to reinvestigate the problem for each 25 kg step or month of the production cycle. Nevertheless, we can use a model to get data for an animal of any given live weight, time in pregnancy or stage of lactation.

Strategic (whole enterprise) models

Some models describe the whole management system. These are called strategic models and are used to get a whole-farm view of how to manage animals to get a desired outcome. The benefits of using such a model can be more sustainable use of pasture, better milk or meat production, or minimizing losses of N and P to the environment, etc. These models may have components similar to the INRAE, NRC or CSIRO nutrient requirement models embedded in them, and they may include sub-models which predict the growth and nutritional quality of pasture. Other models include animal breeding and financial sub-models.

An example of a strategic model is the Dutch dairy farm model, DairyWise (Schils *et al.*, 2007; Fig. 10.3), which simulates the 'technical, environmental, and financial processes on a dairy farm'. Like most of this class of model, it has several components: a central program which calculates nutrient requirements, and a sub-model which calculates the farm's pasture grass and silage production. The output can be used to simulate N and P cycling, nitrate leaching, NH_3 emissions, greenhouse gas emissions, energy use, a farm financial budget, and a farm plan which describes material and nutrient flows and their environmental consequences. The latter outputs are very important in places where the intensity of animal production (both housed and on pasture) means that eutrophication of waterways and the accumulation of chemicals on pastures have serious environmental effects.

Some strategic models provide 'expert system' guidance: The outputs from nutritional models can be complex, even though they are provided as tables or figures. However, these outputs can be made more user-friendly by adding a commentary. AUSPIG (Pork CRC, 2003) is an example; it is a strategic pig production model which incorporates a range of sub-models to evaluate feeding and management, and the sale of products (Fig. 10.4). As well, the program includes a module which delivers expert analysis of the model output, such as 'the factor limiting feed intake, the order of limitation and adequacy of essential amino acids and the efficiency of feed energy use' (Pork CRC, 2003).

A grazing animal example is the stocking rate calculator screen in GrazFeed (CSIRO, 2020) where a recommended stocking rate is calculated, the data used in the calculation are shown, and the way that this recommendation can be used is described: 'The value calculated here is the stocking rate that will, in the short term (about 2 weeks), maintain the weight of green herbage at its present level'.

Why do animal managers tend to not use models?

These models are 'decision support tools' – they are designed to provide information which will help

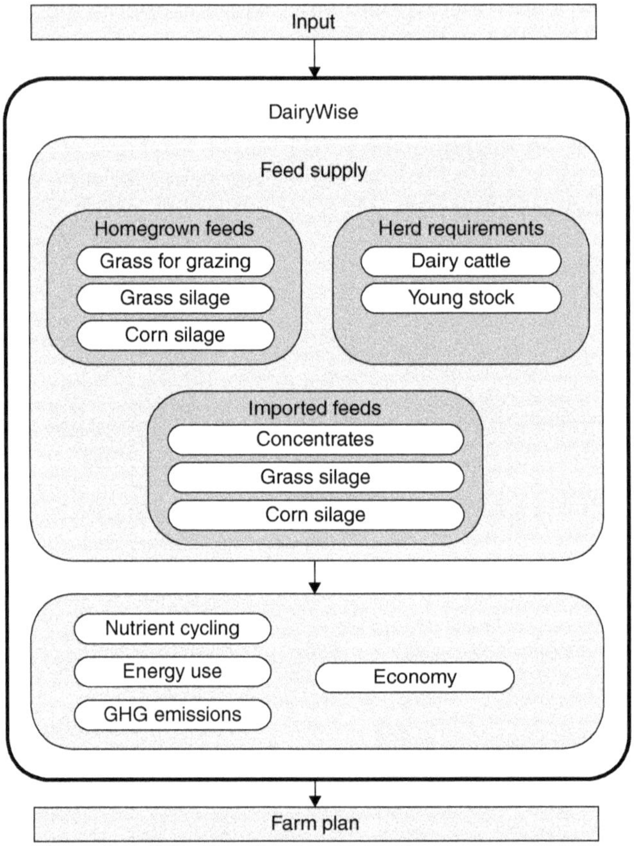

Fig. 10.3. The structure of the DairyWise model. (From Schils *et al.*, 2007; reproduced with permission.)

managers decide on a suitable feeding or management strategy. But apart from the widespread use of linear programming and stochastic programming for ration formulation, the uptake of mathematical models in animal management has not been very rapid. Black (2014) suggests the following reasons:

- In many cases, small changes in farm inputs do not have much effect on farm productivity, so that more detailed assessment of the farming process involves effort and expense for little reward. (However, this does not always apply – Menzies *et al.*, 1992, claimed that AUSPIG improved the profit of a particular pig farm by 500% in the first year it was used.)
- Models do not give real-time outputs. Although true in many cases, this is changing and some animal feeding equipment has inbuilt deterministic models that adjust feed composition and feeding levels in real time.
- Some of the information needed to optimally run the model (e.g. air speeds, humidities, efficiencies of lean tissue growth, days in lactation, categories of pasture quality) is difficult and/or time-consuming to obtain and thus expensive to collect.
- Models focus on 'hard' outcomes, e.g. production levels and product quality, and ignore social issues such as the availability of labour, the need for free time, family interests, and so on.

In addition, animal managers are often not comfortable with mathematics and computing, although this will change as people who are increasingly familiar with using online social platforms, email and the internet, join the rural workforce. However, farmers still have to find the time to input data, run

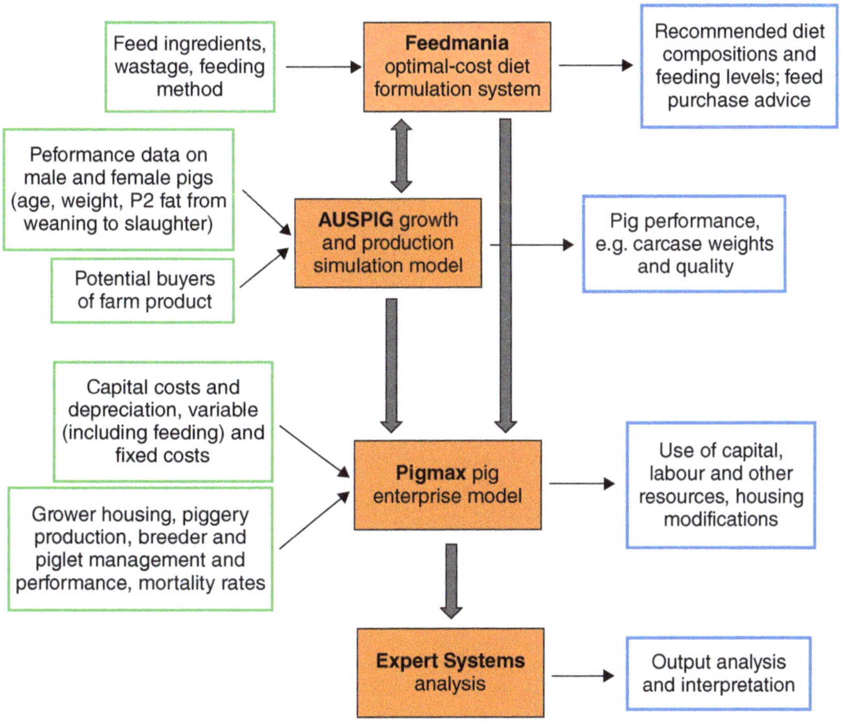

Fig. 10.4. Diagram of the AUSPIG model showing the model components, the required inputs and model outputs. (Copyright: Gordon McL. Dryden.)

the software and assess the result, and then possibly adapt routines or equipment and facilities to introduce new ways of working.

Choosing software

When choosing software, we should look for:

- Parameterization which covers the environment we work in – the program must allow us to define the animal species and breeds, production type and levels, the management system that we wish to work with, and the feed types that we want to use. Note that nutrient use varies between different types of animal and feeds, e.g. the efficiency of utilization of ME for live weight gain varies between feeds, pig strains vary in how efficiently they deposit protein in lean tissue, and there are differences in the nutrient requirements of *Bos taurus* and *Bos indicus* beef cattle. Capacity to define the animal and its environment is especially important if we are using the model to predict the performance of grazing animals because the nutritive value of pasture varies considerably between regions and between seasons, and because these animals are more exposed to the environment than housed animals.
- An easy-to-understand, comprehensive user's manual and good user support.
- A model which does not require an 'expert' level of nutritional knowledge. Some models use data on the nutrient content and digestibility of feeds, or ratios of green:dry material in pasture, as inputs. Default values are usually provided but the model may work better if we can input 'real' values. This requires a thorough understanding of the nutritional environment.
- A good feeds library and ability to add new feeds and modify the inbuilt ones.
- Ability to formulate a least cost, or optimum cost, ration.
- Good file handling capability so that we can store calculations.

The review of 11 dairy models by Little *et al.* (2009) illustrates how tactical and strategic models work, the variety of information that has to be provided by the user to run these models, and the user expertise that may be needed to get the best results from them.

Sources of (tactical and strategic) nutrient requirement models: Several are available, including:

- Ruminants: NRC (2001) dairy feeding standards; NRC (2016) beef feeding standards; CamDairy version 2.4; download from Software Informer (2019); GrazFeed (2007) available from Horizon Agriculture (2005–); and INRATION version 4.06 for beef and dairy cattle, and lactating ewes and does (INRA, 2012).
- Pigs: NRC (2012) pig feeding standards; AUSPIG (Pork CRC, 2003); InraPorc version 1.7.1.0 (INRA, 2016); and Pig Nutrition Optimiser and Pig Growth Model (EFG Software, 2020a).
- Horses: NRC (2007) horse feeding standards.
- Poultry: Broiler Growth Model (EFG Software, 2020b); and Broiler Nutrition Optimiser (EFG Software, 2020b).

New models are always being developed, and it is wise to keep checking updated models as they are developed and published, to assess if they are likely to do the job that we require.

References

Black, J.L. (2014). Brief history and future of animal simulation models for science and application. *Animal Production Science* 54, 1883–1895.

Commonwealth Scientific and Industrial Research Organisation (CSIRO) (2007). *Nutrient Requirements of Domesticated Ruminants*. Collingwood, Vic., Australia: CSIRO Publishing.

Commonwealth Scientific and Industrial Research Organisation (2020). *GrazFeed screen shots*. Available at: www.grazplan.csiro.au/grazfeed/grazfeed-screen-shots/ (accessed 27 December 2020).

EFG Software (2020a). *Pig Programs*. Available at: www.efgsoftware.net/pig-programs (accessed 27 December 2020).

EFG Software (2020b). *Poultry Programs*. Available at: www.efgsoftware.net/poultry-programs (accessed 27 December 2020).

Fisher, C. (2015). An overview of poultry models. In Sakomura, N.K., Gous, R.M., Kyriazakis, I. and Hauschild, L (eds). *Nutritional Modelling for Pigs and Poultry*. Wallingford, UK: CAB International, pp. 1–21.

Heuser, G.F. (1941) Protein in poultry nutrition – a review. *Poultry Science* 20: 362–368.

Horizon Agriculture (2005–). *GrazFeed*. Available at: www.hzn.com.au/grazfeed.php (accessed 27 December 2020).

Institut Nationale de la Recherche Agronomique (INRA) (2012). *INRATION version 4.06*. Available at: https://inration.software.informer.com/ (accessed 27 December 2020).

Institut Nationale de la Recherche Agronomique (INRA) (2016). *InraPorc version 1.7.1.0*. Available at: https://inraporc.inra.fr/inraporc/history_en.php (accessed 18 March 2021).

Little, S., King, R., Lean, I., Rabiee, A. and Breinhild, K. (2009). *A Review of 11 Applied Dairy Nutrition Models Used in Australia*. Summary Report; and Technical Details on How Each Model Works. Melbourne, Australia: Dairy Australia.

Menzies, T., Black, J., Fleming, J. and Dean, M. (1992). An expert system for raising pigs. In *The First Conference on Practical Applications of Prolog*. Available at: www.researchgate.net/publication/2278548_An_Expert_System_for_Raising_Pigs/citations (accessed 27 December 2020).

National Research Council (NRC) (2001). *Nutrient Requirements of Dairy Cattle*, 7th rev. edn. Washington, DC: National Academies Press. Available at: www.nap.edu/catalog/9825/nutrient-requirements-of-dairy-cattle-seventh-revised-edition-2001 (accessed 27 December 2020).

National Research Council (NRC) (2007). *Nutrient Requirements of Horses*, 6th rev. edn. Washington, DC: National Academies Press. Available at: www.nap.edu/catalog/11653/nutrient-requirements-of-horses-sixth-revised-edition (accessed 27 December 2020).

National Research Council (NRC) (2012). *Nutrient Requirements of Swine*, 11th rev. edn. Washington, DC: National Academies Press. Available at: www.nap.edu/catalog/13298/nutrient-requirements-of-swine-eleventh-revised-edition (accessed 27 December 2020).

National Research Council (NRC) (2016). *Nutrient Requirements of Beef Cattle*, 8th rev. edn. Washington, DC: National Academy Press. Available at: www.nap.edu/catalog/19014/nutrient-requirements-of-beef-cattle-eighth-revised-edition (accessed 27 December 2020).

Pork CRC (2003). *What Is AUSPIG*? Available at: https://camdairy.software.informer.com/2.4/ (accessed 27 December 2020).

Software Informer (2019). *CamDairy 2.4* . Available at: www.camdairy.software.informer.com/2.4/ (accessed 27 December 2020).

Schils, R.L.M., de Haan, M.H.A., Hemmer, J.G.A., van den Pol-van Dasselaar, A. *et al.* (2007). DairyWise, a whole-farm dairy model. *Journal of Dairy Science* 90(11): 5334–5346.

11 Feed additives

This discussion, including that of the use of antibiotics and growth promoters in animal feeds, does not take account of laws which might apply in different countries or whether the registration of a particular product is confined to particular types of animal, because these vary between jurisdictions. Neither does it take account of 'off-label' uses, e.g. by veterinary prescription, which may be permitted in different jurisdictions. Antibiotics or other additives may be used to treat diseases and these uses are not discussed in this chapter.

We can augment our animals' feeds to get better productive performance and improve their digestive tract health. For monogastric animals, these techniques focus on using ionophores and probiotics to maintain or improve gut health and feed enzymes to improve digestibility or mineral availability. For ruminants, the focus is on protecting nutrients from degradation in the rumen or protecting the animal from the adverse effects of excessive starch fermentation in the rumen.

Metabolic modifiers

Several substances which promote more efficient growth and/or nutrient use are used in meat and milk production. These include somatotropin which is a hormone that directs nutrient use into lean tissue growth, hormones such as oestrogens (in steers) and androgens (in heifers) which improve feed conversion efficiency and growth, and immuno-castration which inhibits the action of gonadotrophin-releasing factor, which in turn reduces the synthesis of testosterone and other hormones. However, these are given by injection or implant and so are not relevant to this discussion of feed additives.

β-Adrenergic receptor agonists: Ractopamine and zilpaterol direct feed energy use away from fat deposition in favour of lean tissue growth, particularly in ruminant animals (Dunshea *et al.*, 2005) where they improve growth and feed conversion efficiency, and increase muscle size (Lean *et al.*, 2014).

Ractopamine is used in pig feeds to improve carcass lean content, although we get less tender meat with less intramuscular fat (de Almeida *et al.*, 2012). It is essential that the pig is given enough amino acids in its feed to enable the effect of ractopamine to be expressed. Ractopamine changes the amino acid composition of muscle protein and the NRC (2012) recommends increasing the available lysine content in growing pig diets by 25%.

Conjugated linoleic acid: This is used in growing pig diets to reduce fat deposition. It may help to avoid problems of soft fat in pigs which are fed feeds which contain amounts of unsaturated fatty acids, such as we find in cereal grains, rice bran, peanut and soybean meals, and other products.

Antibiotics, coccidiostats and anthelmintics

Ionophore and non-ionophore antibiotics have been used to improve animal productivity: It has been common practice since the 1960s to add subtherapeutic levels of antibiotics to the feed or water of intensively-managed poultry, pigs and cattle. This helps to improve animal performance and health by limiting the growth of pathogens, improving the health of the intestinal epithelia, and possibly by reducing competition between the animal and digestive tract microbes for nutrients. Antibiotics promote improved growth and feed conversion efficiency and help to maintain better animal health. There can be benefits in both intensively and extensively managed animals.

Antibiotics will change the composition of the volatile fatty acid pool produced in the rumen and promote propionic acid production over

DOI: 10.1079/9781786394453.0011

acetic acid. This is associated with an improvement in the efficiency of energy use by the host animal, but also a decline in milk fat content because acetic acid is a precursor of milk fat. Antibiotics will also reduce the amount of CH_4 produced in the rumen.

Many jurisdictions have banned or controlled the use of antibiotics in animal feeds: The use of antibiotics, especially the non-ionophore ones, as feed additives has been controversial in animal industries for some time (UK Parliament, 1989). The main concern is that using antibiotic doses which do not kill most of the target microbial population is likely to promote resistance to the antibiotic in these organisms. There are more and more instances where we find this resistance developing, and cross-resistance which has developed in other microorganisms. This reduces the effectiveness of those antibiotics when they are used in animal and human medicine to treat diseases. As well, drug residues occur in animal products, e.g. poultry meat (Patel *et al.*, 2018), unless withholding periods are observed.

Feed antibiotics have now been completely banned in the European Union and several other countries, and the use of individual antibiotics is limited in others to use by veterinary prescription.

The growth in demand for 'organic' food products has meant that antibiotic use has been subjected to further scrutiny and criticism. As a general rule, we cannot offer products from animals that have been given antibiotics in their feed for sale through the 'organic' food products marketing chain.

Antibiotic use in feeds has not been restricted without consequences. There has been an increased incidence of bacterial diarrhoea, weight loss and mortality in pigs (weaners and adults), and of clostridial necrotic enteritis in broilers, after the ban on antibiotic use came into effect in the European Union (Casewell *et al.*, 2003).

We need something to take the place of antibiotics, but without the accompanying risks to general human and animal health. Possible ways are:

- Probiotics can replace sub-clinical levels of antibiotics in weaner pig feed without adverse effects on growth, but we cannot be certain of getting this result.
- Clay minerals may give a similar response in some situations, e.g. in pig and poultry feeds where they may act against *Clostridium* spp. and *Escherichia coli* bacteria.
- Maintain good management – housing, feeding, weaning protocols, hygiene, stock density, handling, transport – so that animals are robust enough to withstand diseases.

If we intend to use antibiotics, then we should use only those which are not used in human or animal medicine to treat specific diseases; ionophores are an example. Using dedicated equipment (bins, augers, feeders) for medicated and non-medicated feeds will reduce the likelihood of cross-contamination. In all cases, we must check that a proposed use is currently legal.

Ionophore antibiotics can improve animal production: The range of ionophore antibiotics used in animal feeds includes monensin, lasalocid, salinomycin, narasin and several others.

Ionophores improve ruminant animal production by altering the bacterial population of the rumen. Gram-positive bacteria are more sensitive than Gram-negative bacteria to these antibiotics. The remaining microbial population uses propionic acid, rather than acetic acid, as a 'H sink' to mop up the H produced as they ferment feed constituents, especially carbohydrates (see Chapter 3). These changes in the bacterial population can:

- Improve feed conversion efficiency: savings in feed costs of 5 to 10% are frequently quoted by the lot-feeding industry, because cattle eat less feed when monensin is in the ration. The recommended inclusion rate for monensin is 25 mg active monensin/kg feed dry matter (DM).
- Reduce the degradation of protein in the rumen and thus increase the proportion of undegradable dietary protein in the diet – this may increase the amount of essential amino acid reaching the small intestine, depending on the amino acid profile of the undegraded protein.
- Increase the proportion of propionic acid in the rumen VFA mix and reduce acetate and CH_4 production – these changes increase the amount of glucose precursor absorbed by the animal (propionic acid is a glucogenic VFA) and reduce greenhouse gas production.
- Prevent rumen pH falling excessively: ionophores kill the rumen bacteria which produce lactic acid and this helps to avoid the adverse effects of a low rumen pH (Chapter 13).

Ionophores are used in pig and poultry feeds. Monensin, narasin, lasalocid, salinomycin and semduramicin are, or have been, used to control coccidiosis in poultry, a disease which causes diarrhoea and can be fatal. Coccidiostats are used primarily for broilers, breeding hens and replacement pullets. With pigs, monensin and narasin have been, or presently are, used to control diarrhoea and coccidiosis, especially in weaner pigs. Narasin is also registered for improving feed conversion efficiency and growth rates in growing pigs.

Ionophores must be used carefully:

- Always read the label and use the product according to the label directions. Ionophore use varies, e.g. not all ionophores are registered for use in sheep.
- Use the correct dose. Ionophore dose rates vary with animal type; they can be poisonous if they are fed at two or three times the recommended dose, and ineffective if too little is used. DPIR, NT (2016) has a list of toxic levels of monensin for different animal species.
- Horses and sheep are especially susceptible to ionophore poisoning. Very low levels of monensin, 1 mg/kg live weight, will poison horses; 4 mg/kg live weight will kill sheep.
- Pigs are less susceptible to monensin toxicity than horses or sheep. However, if pig feeds also contain tiamulin (a non-ionophore antibiotic) this will exacerbate the toxic effect of monensin, and there have been cases where feeds that contained both of these antibiotics caused severe poisoning.
- Observe the required withholding periods before selling products from animals which have been fed ionophores. Information about withholding periods is readily available.

Several non-ionophore antibiotics are or have been used in animal feeds: Two important examples are:

- Virginiamycin used with cattle, sheep and horses to reduce the risk of acidosis and laminitis. It can also be given to poultry and pigs to improve growth rates and feed conversion efficiencies, but these uses are not legal in some jurisdictions.
- Tylosin effectively reduces the risk of liver abscesses in lot fed cattle. The registration of this and other macrolide antibiotics for growth promotion has been revoked or subjected to tight control in many countries, including the European Union, New Zealand, Canada, Australia and the United States.

Pro(eu)biotics and prebiotics

Probiotics (also called 'eubiotics' or 'direct-fed microbials') are preparations of bacteria and/or yeasts which are intended to improve animal health and performance. They are administered by being mixed with the feed.

Probiotics are defined by the Food and Agricultural Organization of the United Nations and the World Health Organization as: 'live micro-organisms, that when administered orally at adequate concentrations, provide a beneficial effect beyond that of their nutritional value'. The organisms used in probiotics should be able to survive passage through the glandular stomach (i.e. resist enzymes and low pH), have antimicrobial properties, adhere to mucus and epithelial cells in the intestines, and be able to withstand the conditions that they are subjected to during probiotic production and through the marketing chain.

Typical probiotic organisms are the bacteria *Lactobacillus* spp., *Enterococcus faecium*, *Pediococcus acidilactici*, *Bifidobacterium animalis*, *Bacillus subtilis* and other *Bacillus* spp., the yeast *Saccharomyces cerevisae*, and the fungus *Aspergillus oryzae*. Additional probiotics studied in ruminants have included *Bacillus* and *Faecalibacterium* spp.

Probiotics improve animal health and performance (Yan and Polk, 2011) by:

- Preventing pathogenic micro-organisms from colonizing the intestinal walls; probiotic organisms do this by competing for adhesion sites.
- Stimulating the animal's immune system by acting on the epithelial cells which produce immunoglobulins and stimulating responses from the host's intestinal epithelial cells.
- Inhibiting or inactivating bacterial toxins by affecting gene expression, and by secreting enzymes which destroy bacterial toxins, e.g. *Lactobacillus* can interfere with the genes responsible for toxin production by *Salmonella* and *E. coli*.
- Reducing the pH of the large intestine – some of the common probiotic organisms are *Lactobacillus* spp., which produce lactic acid and other end-products. Lactic acid reduces the pH and this produces conditions which are unsuitable for some pathogens. In addition, the presence and activity of lactobacilli encourage the proliferation of *Veillonella* and other bacteria which use lactic acid as an energy source.

- Competing with other bacteria for nutrients.
- Improving the digestibility of feed constituents.

Effectiveness of probiotics in poultry: Probiotics have been shown, in some cases, to improve the tenderness, texture and juiciness of chicken meat, leg strength in broilers, to increase egg weight and eggshell thickness, and decrease cholesterol in egg yolk. Probiotics can be mixed with the feed given to hatched birds or given to the embryo before it hatches (called '*in ovo*' administration) by injecting the probiotic into the egg's air sac at day 12 of incubation.

Probiotics for pigs: Giving pigs probiotics may improve the digestion of DM, protein and energy, increase feed intake, improve feed use efficiency, and increase growth rate (Liaoa and Nyachotib, 2017). Pig meat quality can be improved, with lower drip loss and better redness. Probiotics may reduce NH_3 and H_2S emissions from pig manure.

Probiotics for horses: Giving probiotics to performance horses may reduce the amount of blood lactate after exercise, but this effect probably depends on the bacterial and other species in the probiotic (Schoster *et al.*, 2014). Results to date suggest that probiotics are not always helpful for horses, and they can have adverse effects in foals.

Probiotics for ruminants: *Lactobacillus acidophilus* and *Propionibacterium freudenreichii* are often used in dairy cow probiotics, as well as yeasts, especially *Saccharomyces cerevisiae*. These probiotics may (but not always) reduce rumen lactate concentrations, increase rumen pH and fibre digestion, and promote better milk production. In addition, there have been some reports of improved feed utilization efficiency and live weight gain. Probiotics can change the chemistry of rumen fatty acids to increase the proportions of desirable fatty acids in milk and meat. Lactate-utilizing bacteria (e.g. *Megasphaera elsdenii* and *Selenomonas ruminantium*) may reduce rumen lactate concentration and help to protect grain-fed cattle against rumen acidosis.

Probiotics are usually fed mixed in a concentrate mixture, such as a dairy concentrate supplement, or a beef feedlot ration. They can also be fed to grazing animals; dairy cattle grazing a pasture which had been sprayed with probiotic (mainly *Lactobacillus* spp.) produced more, higher protein content, milk (Olchowy *et al.*, 2019).

Prebiotics: These are polysaccharides which are fed with probiotics and provide the probiotic microbes with sources of feed which are not able to be digested by the animal's gastric or intestinal enzymes (see Chapter 3) and which specifically help the probiotic organisms to grow. Prebiotics include fructo-oligosaccharides and inulin (these are both β1-2-linked chains of fructose molecules), mannan-oligosaccharides (α1-6- and α1-2-linked chains of mannose), xylo-oligosaccharides (chains of β1-4-linked xylose molecules), and yeasts and yeast cell walls (which are rich in mannan-oligosaccharides), and yeast metabolites.

A mixture of probiotic and prebiotic is sometimes called a 'synbiotic'.

Is it worth using probiotics, or not? Although probiotics have been used for more than 20 years, and although mainly positive responses have been listed in the above discussion, there is still a lack of consistent evidence about how reliably probiotics give positive responses, especially in ruminants and horses. Part of the problem is that the animal's basal diet and management affect how well the probiotics work.

If we are going to use a probiotic then:

- As a general rule, choose a probiotic which is guaranteed to contain live organisms. Although there are some reasons for expecting positive results from dead organisms (mainly because of the presence of their end-products in the preparation), we should expect better results from probiotics which contain living organisms, present either as metabolizing cells or as spores. It is sometimes difficult to determine if the culture is active, especially if we have doubts about how it has been stored.
- Be aware that the composition and activity of some commercial probiotics can be variable. Look for the organisms named in the preceding discussion.
- Do not expect uniformly positive results.

Feed enzymes

Enzymes are often added to pig and poultry feeds to improve protein digestibility and P availability, and to counteract the effect of β-glycans on the digestibility of cereal grains.

Using added enzymes to digest non-starch polysaccharides (NSPs) in cereal grains: Some cereal grains, e.g. barley and oats, have substantial amounts of NSPs – polysaccharides made of glucose, xylose and other monosaccharide molecules linked by β bonds. These cannot be digested by the animal's intrinsic α-amylases (from the salivary glands and pancreas) and they affect the availability of nutrients in cereal grain-rich diets (see Chapter 12).

There is a large number of commercially available enzyme products which can be added to feed to degrade these substances: mannanases, glucanases, cellulases, xylanases, other carbohydrases (a general term for enzymes that digest carbohydrates) and proteases (enzymes that digest protein).

Added carbohydrase enzymes can increase pig growth rates by up to 20–60 g/day and poultry growth by 4–9%, and it can be beneficial to use them (Torres-Pitarch *et al.*, 2017). However, several factors impact on the result that we get:

- The type of grain used in the ration: e.g. mannanase is effective with maize (corn) based diets and may also be effective with other grains, while xylanase plus β-glucanase are effective with diets based on wheat, maize, barley, or rye. Enzymes are substrate-specific and must match the types of β-glycans which predominate in the cereal grain we are using. Generally, we can expect better results from using a complex of enzymes, rather than a single enzyme.
- The enzyme's activity: look for enzymes which are heat stable, because these are most likely to resist the heating effects of pelleting and extrusion (Chapter 18) if the feed is processed in this way.
- Enzymes may improve the digestibility of β-glycans in the diet but this effect might not be carried over into improvements in growth rate or feed efficiency.
- Enzymes are more likely to improve the digestibility of low-quality, high-fibre feeds.

Should we use carbohydrase enzymes? The answer depends on the relative cost of the feed and the added enzyme, and the price we get for the animal product. A review of recent research (Torres-Pitarch *et al.*, 2019) indicated that including enzymes in pig diets gave a positive response in 25% of cases, but there were some negative responses and in many cases there was no response at all. A similar situation applies to poultry, even though about 70% of commercial poultry feeds have added enzymes.

Proteases: These are also available for adding to pig and poultry diets. These help to digest proteins which are not readily digested by the pig's or bird's intrinsic protein-digesting enzymes (Chapter 3). These enzymes are relatively new and have not been widely used, but it seems that adding proteases to pig diets may improve protein digestion and growth rate but may not affect feed efficiency.

Adding phytase to break down phytic acid: Phytic acid is the main P-containing substance in cereal grains and other seeds (see Chapters 5 and 12), and pigs and poultry are unable to break this down. So, when these animals are fed grain-rich diets they either become P deficient or have to be given extra P as a feed supplement. Neither of these options is acceptable. Adding extra P increases the cost of the feed, and if animals excrete excess P this P-enriched effluent can pollute waterways. Letting an animal become P deficient is foolish because the animal is less productive, and we contravene animal welfare standards because P deficiency depresses feed intake and can cause lameness and other bone disorders.

As well as its effects on P availability, phytase can improve the availability of energy, protein and some minerals (Chapter 8).

Phytase activity is measured in phytase activity units (FTU). Phytases are usually included in pig feeds to give about 500 FTU/kg, with similar or higher levels in poultry feeds.

Should we use phytase in pig and poultry feeds? Yes, the evidence is clear that phytase makes the P in seeds and grains more available, reduces the need to include extra sources of P, and can improve the availability of other nutrients.

Protected nutrient sources

Some nutrients are degraded in the rumen as a result of digestion and metabolism by rumen micro-organisms. The destruction of essential amino acids and the saturation of unsaturated dietary fatty acids are two important adverse effects; as well, there are potential advantages from protecting starch from rumen degradation.

We can treat feed ingredients to make their protein, starch and fat unavailable to rumen microbes.

Protected amino acid sources: The aim is to deliver essential amino acids into the small intestine where they can be absorbed. Crystalline (or 'synthetic') amino acids can be protected by coating the amino acid particle with a long-chain fatty acid layer, or a pH-sensitive polymer (Rossi *et al.*, 2003). Another option is to make the amino acid resistant to degradation by attaching an acetyl group to one of its amino groups (review by Menchu, 2019). However, it is important that the coating can be broken down in the small intestine so that the amino acid can be absorbed.

For dairy cattle, methionine and lysine are usually the most limiting amino acids, with histidine and phenylalanine the next limiting. Feeding protected lysine and methionine to lactating dairy cattle is likely to slightly increase milk protein content but may not have much effect on milk yield (Lean *et al.*, 2018).

Wool and other fibres (e.g. cashmere and angora) are rich in keratin, a protein which contains a great deal of cystine. When the animal's diet is deficient in cystine, or methionine (a cystine precursor), sheep and goats may respond positively to supplements of rumen-protected methionine or cystine. Wool growth increases of more than 30% have been reported (e.g. Dryden *et al.*, 1969), and in some cases there is greater live weight growth.

Other responses to rumen-protected amino acids include improved immunoglobulin G (IgG) lambs, higher lamb birth weights, and better antioxidant status in adult sheep.

Some feed proteins have natural protection against rumen degradation: These include corn gluten meal and dried brewers' grains, which combine high protein contents and high (more than 50%) levels of rumen protection (NRC, 2000). Other feeds that have high protection rates, but lower total protein contents, include mature brome and timothy hays, dried lucerne (alfalfa) meal, cereal straws, maize (corn) and sorghum grains, and dried beet pulp.

The susceptibility to ruminal degradation of the amino acids in the UDP of different feeds varies. But there is a tendency over all the feeds which have been tested, for essential amino acids (Chapter 1) to be less susceptible than non-essential ones. The most resistant is phenylalanine, with methionine and tyrosine also tending to resist rumen degradation. Unfortunately, because it can be a first-limiting amino acid, lysine is one of the essential amino acids most susceptible to degradation in the rumen (but see below).

Heating is a commonly used method of protecting feed protein from rumen degradation: Heat denatures proteins and can make them less easily degraded by bacteria. A wide variety of processing conditions has been tested, e.g. heating at 125°C for 3 minutes, heating at 150°C for 1 hour, cooking a wet (30–50% water) mixture until the water content had decreased to 12%, steaming at 100°C for 4 minutes, then holding at 100°C for 16 minutes, autoclaving at 127°C for 30 minutes.

Conventional expeller extraction of oilseeds (a process which involves heating the meal; Chapter 6) and other processing methods that include heat treatment, such as pelleting and extrusion (Chapter 18), also make feed protein less degradable in the rumen.

While heating is commonly used (especially as a side-effect of oil extraction), and reduces the degradability of feed protein, there is no control over the extent of protection, and some amino acids, especially lysine, are likely to bind to carbohydrates and become unavailable.

Formaldehyde treatment is an alternative method of protecting feed protein from digestion by rumen micro-organisms (Gulati *et al.*, 2005). Added formaldehyde (usually 0.3–0.6% formaldehyde relative to the protein content) makes the feed protein resistant to attack by rumen micro-organisms. The increase in UDP can give better animal production. Feeding formaldehyde-protected protein meals to lactating dairy cows can give small (about 10%) increases in milk yield and may also increase milk protein content. Animals which have a high amino acid demand, or which are fed low-protein diets, or which are recovering from a period of under-feeding, respond to formaldehyde-protected feeds.

Over-protection, by using excessive amounts of formaldehyde, will protect feed protein from ruminal degradation but will also prevent it from being digested in the small intestine, and will make amino acids, especially lysine, unavailable.

Formaldehyde can be added to pig and poultry feeds to control *Salmonella* and moulds (Ricke *et al.*, 2019).

Regulations about using formaldehyde-treated feeds vary between jurisdictions. For example, it cannot be used as a feed additive in the European Union, is not used in Japan, South Korea or New Zealand, but can be used in the USA. Formaldehyde is carcinogenic and thus it presents a danger to people who work with this material. Treated feeds are considered to be safe provided that all the unreacted formaldehyde has been removed.

Other methods to reduce the rumen degradation of feed protein:

- Tannins will partially protect (the response is dose-dependent) oilseed meal protein and silage protein from degradation in the rumen. This technology has not been widely adopted in practical animal feeding.
- Added xylose has been used to produce non-enzymatic browning – chemical binding of amino acids and sugars – which reduces the degradability of protein in the rumen. Again, this technology has not been widely adopted.

Should we feed protected amino acid and protein supplements to ruminant animals? The responses which have been recorded to feeding protected amino acids are quite variable, and it is difficult to predict when animals will respond positively to protected amino acid supplements. In general, we should not expect positive responses if the diet provides enough of these amino acids in the feed's undegradable protein.

Positive results have been reported more often from feeding ingredients which have natural or artificial protein protection, than from feeding protected amino acids. These responses are more likely to occur high-producing dairy cows, rapidly growing cattle, and sheep which require high levels of cystine for wool growth.

Protected starch: When starch is fermented in the rumen, we risk a rapid fall in rumen pH and the diseases which can follow from that (Chapter 13).

Some starch has natural protection against rumen digestion. Maize and sorghum starches have slow rates and low extents of degradation, whereas wheat, barley and rye starches have rapid rates and high extents of degradation in the rumen.

There are some chemical treatments which protect at least some of the starch from fermentation in the rumen (Humer and Zebeli, 2017). Formaldehyde treatment of milled grain protects starch because it reacts with the protein matrix that surrounds starch granules in the endosperm cells. Tannic acid added at 1 to 5% of the grain DM will reduce the rate at which bacteria attack starch granules.

Protected fats: There are some good reasons for adding protected fat to ruminant animals' (mainly dairy cows') diets. When the protected fats arrive in the small intestine they are digested, and the freed fatty acids are absorbed and used as energy sources or contribute to milk fat and the inter- and intramuscular fat in meat. The result is to increase milk production and growth, and to (slightly) reduce the proportions of saturated and *trans* fatty acids (Chapter 1) in animal products.

If we want to add fat to ruminant diets, we should bear in mind these things:

- Rumen bacteria digest dietary fats by breaking the ester bond between the fatty acids and the glycerol backbone. They use the glycerol, but not the free fatty acids, as an energy source. However, rumen bacteria do use the released fatty acids as H sinks. Rumen bacteria generate a great deal of H (Chapter 3) which has to be dealt with in some way. Bacteria use much of this H to synthesize VFA but some is transferred to unsaturated fatty acids in the feed in processes that generate saturated and *trans* fatty acids. The resulting altered fatty acids are incorporated into milk and meat.
- Fatty acids, especially long-chain polyunsaturated fatty acids, are toxic to bacteria, especially those that digest plant fibre. A practical upper limit to the unprotected fat content of a ruminant's diet is 7%, otherwise rumen function is adversely affected. Note that we rarely reach these levels when typical ruminant feeds are fed – forages and cereal grains have only about 3% fat.

For both of these reasons, we want to prevent bacteria from metabolizing, or being exposed to, excessive amounts of dietary unsaturated fatty acids. There are several ways to protect unsaturated fatty acids being hydrogenated to saturated fatty acids (Gadeyne *et al.*, 2017). We can:

- React free fatty acids with Ca to form a Ca soap, or with amino acids to form a fatty acid amide. In both cases, we get some, although incomplete, protection of the fatty acids against rumen hydrogenation.
- Encapsulate fat droplets in a resistant protein coating. The coating can be made by reacting

protein with formaldehyde or with reducing sugars (e.g. lactose) to form a structure which is resistant to microbial digestion and protects the fat that it covers. Formaldehyde is the most commonly used chemical, and it causes amino acid chains within the protein to cross-link. Reaction with reducing sugars (the Maillard reaction) also forms a resistant structure but this method gives less protection than the formaldehyde method.
- Form a protein/lipid gel. This contains cross-linked proteins which give quite high (about 30%) protection of the lipid.

All these methods have advantages and disadvantages. They all protect a varying proportion of the protected fatty acid (from 1% to 45%; formaldehyde treatment is the most effective), all are fairly expensive to perform, and all except Ca soaps involve the use or possible production of potentially toxic substances.

Chemical buffers, clay minerals, acidifiers and alkalizing agents

These are substances which are added to feeds to protect ruminant animals from the adverse effects of excess starch fermentation in the rumen (see Chapter 13), and they may potentially replicate the effects of antibiotics in feeds.

Clay minerals: These include kaolinite, zeolite, montmorillonite and bentonite, and are used in ruminant (especially feedlot) feeds and in pig and poultry feeds, to improve animal performance and health. They have also been used to promote binding of feed ingredients during the manufacture of pelleted feeds (Chapter 18).

Clay minerals in ruminant feeds control rumen pH by trapping H^+ ions within the clay lattice. They can also trap heavy metals and mycotoxins. While this should work in theory, and there have been some promising results, especially with North American products, in practice we find that the source of these clay minerals affects the response we get. Clay minerals are usually added at 1–2% (sometimes up to 4%) of the feed, or approximately 0.5 kg per day for adult cattle. These are quite large amounts and can dilute the feed's nutrient content. Larger amounts can have adverse effects on milk production and rumen health.

Pigs may also respond well to clay minerals at 0.5 to 3% of their diet (Subramaniam and Kim, 2015). Increases between 1.5 and 9% have been reported for live weight gain, feed intake and feed conversion efficiency, and clay minerals can reduce the incidence of diarrhoea. However, the recorded responses to clay supplementation have been inconsistent and some workers have obtained no response.

In poultry feeds, clay minerals may improve egg production (size and shell strength) and reduce the incidence of wet droppings.

Alkalizing agents: These are used to control the drop in rumen pH which happens when starch and other easily fermented constituents are digested and metabolized by rumen micro-organisms, with the production of VFAs and possibly lactic acid (Staples and Lough, 1989).

Calcium oxide and Mg oxide have a direct chemical effect on rumen pH. They react with H to form Ca and Mg hydroxides, which reduces the H concentration in the rumen liquor and thus increases the pH. As well, these alkalis may reduce propionate production with an accompanying increase in milk fat content. Ca and Mg oxides are added to cattle diets at 0.5–1.5% in the feed DM.

Na bicarbonate sets up a carbonic acid/bicarbonate buffering system like the one produced by bicarbonate ions in saliva. Bicarbonate reacts with H to give carbonic acid; this reduces the H concentration and prevents the rumen pH from falling. Dairy cattle which are fed rations containing Na bicarbonate have a higher acetate:propionate ratio in their rumen liquor and produce milk with a higher fat content. Na bicarbonate is included at about 1.5% in cattle diets.

Acidifiers: When organic acids such as formic, propionic, butyric, fumaric, citric and lactic acids are added to pig and poultry diets (at levels of about 1 to 2%) they reduce the pH of the feed. This inhibits the growth of pathogenic micro-organisms in the feed and, after it has been eaten, in the digestive tract. The result is (sometimes slightly) improved productivity.

Inorganic acids can also be used, and hydrochloric and phosphoric acids (but not sulphuric acid) at about 0.5% of the diet give similar improvements as those from organic acids. When using these acids, be very careful to not exceed the recommended dose and to mix the acid evenly through the feed.

Cautions about the use of additives in animal feeds

To use additives in our animals' feed we must:

- Check that the use is legally permitted: in some jurisdictions the use of antibiotics and hormones is banned.
- Use the substance exactly as it says on the label.
- Find out if any withholding periods (withdrawal periods or export slaughter intervals) are required before meat, milk or eggs from the treated animal can be sold. These periods might be imposed because of the requirements of importing countries. Withholding periods must be observed.

We risk affecting the animals' health, and exceeding maximum residue limits in animal products, if we misuse additives. This puts our animals, our enterprise, and the country's export trade in jeopardy.

Clay minerals, ionophores and other antibiotics, alkalis and chemical buffers can be helpful, but we should not use them to cover deficiencies in good animal management.

References

de Almeida, V.V., Nuñez, A.J.C. and Miyada, V.S. (2012). Ractopamine as a metabolic modifier feed additive for finishing pigs: a review. *Brazilian Archives of Biology and Technology* 55(3). Available at: www.scielo.br/scielo.php?pid=s1516-89132012000300016&script=sci_arttext (accessed 30 December 2020).

Casewell, M, Friis, C., Marco, E., McMullin, P. and Phillips, I. (2003). The European ban on growth-promoting antibiotics and emerging consequences for human and animal health. *Journal of Antimicrobial Chemotherapy* 52(2): 159–161.

Department of Primary Industry and Resources, Northern Territory (DPIR, NT) (2016). *Ionophore Poisoning. Fact sheet.* Available at: www.dpir.nt.gov.au/__data/assets/word_doc/0007/496726/fs-ionophore-poisoning.docx (accessed 30 December 2020).

Dunshea, F.R., D'Souza, D.N., Pethick, D.W., Harper, G.S. and Warner, R.D. (2005). Effects of dietary factors and other metabolic modifiers on quality and nutritional value of meat. *Meat Science* 71(1): 8–38.

Dryden, G.M., Wickham, G.A. and Cockrem, F. (1969) Intravenous infusion of cysteine and wool growth of Romney sheep. *New Zealand Journal of Agricultural Research* 12(3): 580–587.

Gadeyne, F., De Neve, N., Vlaeminck, B. and Fievez, V. (2017). State of the art in rumen lipid protection technologies and emerging interfacial protein cross-linking methods. *European Journal of Lipid Science and Technology* 119(5), 1600345.

Gulati, S.K., Garg, M.R. and Scott, T.W. (2005). Rumen protected protein and fat produced from oilseeds and/or meals by formaldehyde treatment; their role in ruminant production and product quality: a review. *Australian Journal of Experimental Agriculture* 45(10): 1189–1203.

Humer, E. and Zebeli, Q. (2017). Grains in ruminant feeding and potentials to enhance their nutritive and health value by chemical processing. *Animal Feed Science and Technology* 226: 133–151.

Lean, I.J., Thompson, J.M. and Dunshea, F.R. (2014). A meta-analysis of zilpaterol and ractopamine effects on feedlot performance, carcass traits and shear strength of meat in cattle. *PLoS One* 9(12): e115904. www.doi.org/10.1371/journal.pone.0115904.

Lean, I.J., de Ondarza, M.B., Sniffen, C.J., Santos, J.E.P. and Griswold, K.E. (2018). Meta-analysis to predict the effects of metabolizable amino acids on dairy cattle performance. *Journal of Dairy Science* 101(1): 340–364.

Liaoa, S.F. and Nyachotib, M. (2017). Using probiotics to improve swine gut health and nutrient utilization. *Animal Nutrition* 3(4): 331–343.

Menchu, S. (2019). *Ruminal Protection and Intestinal Availability of Rumen-Protected Methionine and Lysine in Lactating Dairy Cows.* All Graduate Theses and Dissertations. 7451. Available at: www.digitalcommons.usu.edu/etd/7451 (accessed 30 December 2020).

National Research Council (NRC) (2000). *Nutrient Requirements of Beef Cattle,* 7th rev. edn. Update. Washington, DC: National Academies Press. Available at: www.nap.edu/catalog/9791/nutrient-requirements-of-beef-cattle-seventh-revised-edition-update-2000 (accessed 27 December 2020).

National Research Council (NRC) (2012). *Nutrient Requirements of Swine,* 11th rev. edn. Washington, DC: National Academies Press. Available at: www.nap.edu/catalog/13298/nutrient-requirements-of-swine-eleventh-revised-edition (accessed 27 December 2020).

Olchowy, T.W.J., Soust, M. and Alawneh, J. (2019). The effect of a commercial probiotic product on the milk quality of dairy cows. *Journal of Dairy Science* 102(3): 2188–2195.

Patel, T., Marmulak, T., Gehring, R., Pitesky, M., Clapham, M.O. and Tell, L.A. (2018). Drug residues in poultry meat: A literature review of commonly used veterinary antibacterials and anthelmintics used in poultry. *Journal of Veterinary Pharmacology and Therapeutics* 41(6): 761–789.

Ricke, S.C., Richardson, K. and Dittoe, D.K. (2019). Formaldehydes in feed and their potential interaction with the poultry gastrointestinal tract microbial community–a review. *Frontiers in Veterinary Science* 6: 188. DOI: 10.3389/fvets.2019.00188.

Rossi, F., Moschini, M., Masoero, F., Cavanna, G. and Piva, G. (2003). Rumen degradation and intestinal digestibility of rumen protected amino acids: Comparison between in situ and in vitro data. *Animal Feed Science and Technology* 108(1–4): 223–229.

Schoster, A., Weese, J.S. and Guardabassi, L. (2014). Probiotic use in horses – what is the evidence for their clinical efficacy? *Journal of Veterinary Internal Medicine* 28(6): 1640–1652.

Staples, C.R. and Lough, D.S. (1989). Efficacy of supplemental dietary neutralizing agents for lactating dairy cows. A Review. *Animal Feed Science and Technology* 23(4): 277–303.

Subramaniam, M.D. and Kim, I.H. (2015). Clays as dietary supplements for swine: A review. *Journal of Animal Science and Biotechnology* 6(1): 38. DOI: 10.1186/s40104-015-0037-9.

Torres-Pitarch, A., Manzanilla, E.G., Gardiner, G.E., O'Doherty, J.V. and Lawlor, P.G. (2017). Effect of feed enzymes on digestibility and growth in weaned pigs: A systematic review and meta-analysis. *Animal Feed Science and Technology* 233: 145–159.

Torres-Pitarch, A., Manzanilla, E.G., Gardiner, G.E., O'Doherty, J.V. and Lawlor, P.G. (2019). Systematic review and meta-analysis of the effect of feed enzymes on growth and nutrient digestibility in grow-finisher pigs: Effect of enzyme type and cereal source. *Animal Feed Science and Technology* 251: 153–165.

UK Parliament (1989). *Select Committee on Science and Technology*, 7th report. Available at: www.publications.parliament.uk/pa/ld199798/ldselect/ldsctech/081vii/st0706.htm#n27 (accessed 30 December 2020).

Yan, F. and Polk, D.B. (2011). Probiotics and immune health. *Current Opinion in Gastroenterology*, 27(6): 496–501.

12 Disorders caused by feed-borne pathogens and poisons, and nutrient deficiencies

Mycotoxins

General comment about moulds: Moulds damage the appearance of feeds (see below), especially grains, and are often toxic to livestock. There are several thousand different mycotoxins (mould poisons) and there are some which are frequently found in animal feeds and which have important effects on animal health (Hocking, 2003).

A worldwide survey of unprocessed cereal grains (Lee and Ryu, 2017) indicates the extent of this problem: aflatoxins were detected in 55% of tested samples, ochratoxin A in 29%, fumonisins in 61%, deoxynivalenol in 58% and zearalenone in 46%, with the extent of contamination varying considerably in different parts of the world. The effect of mould contamination can be limited by identifying and removing affected grains from sale. However, if the feed is processed, e.g. a mixture of milled grains and other ingredients, we may not be able to detect mould contamination.

The six most serious mould poisons are described below.

Aflatoxins (produced by *Aspergillus* spp. moulds): There are four of these: B1, B2, G1 and G2. Aflatoxin B1 has the most serious effects (Arapcheska *et al.*, 2015). Aflatoxins are found in contaminated maize and peanuts, as well as other cereal grains. *Aspergillus* colonize growing crops and are present in higher amounts in crops that have been drought-affected, subjected to temperature stress or to insect attack. The infection can be transferred to stored feeds if they are damp and warm. Aflatoxins cause haemorrhage, liver damage, genetic defects in embryos, and tumours. Affected animals show reduced milk, egg and meat production, and severely affected animals are likely to die. Be very careful when feeding lactating dairy cows because about 5% of the ingested aflatoxin is converted to a toxic metabolite (aflatoxin M1) which has been found in milk and manufactured dairy products (Serraino *et al.*, 2019).

Ochratoxins (*Aspergillus* and *Penicillium* spp.): There are three ochratoxins, the A form (OTA) is the most toxic (Denli and Perez, 2010). OTA has been found in all types of cereal grains, both tropical and temperate. OTA damages animals' kidneys (especially in pigs) and livers and causes birth defects. In general, OTA reduces productivity, including growth rate, efficiency of feed use, and egg production and shell quality. Ruminants are less susceptible than monogastric animals and poultry. Ochratoxins can accumulate in animal products – dairy and meat, and so can affect humans.

Deoxynivalenol (DON or vomitoxin; produced by *Fusarium* spp.): This mould contaminates cereal grains (e.g. wheat, barley, sorghum and maize; Pestka, 2007). Its effects are most severe in pigs, while poultry, horses and ruminants are much less susceptible. Large doses to pigs cause severe vomiting, acute diarrhoea, lack of muscle coordination, and sudden death. DON also appears to make animals more susceptible to disease by impairing the functioning of the immune system. The most common effect in pigs is that they refuse contaminated feed, or if DON is ingested, they reduce feed intake and thus are less productive.

Fumonisins (produced by *Fusarium* spp.): These three mycotoxins (FB1, FB2 and FB3) are found in grains and forages (especially maize (corn) silage) throughout the world (EFSA CONTAM Panel, 2018). Fumonisins cause mild to fatal toxicity in the liver, kidney and heart in horses, pigs, cattle, sheep, chickens, and cause blind staggers in horses and lung oedema in pigs. In practice, the risk of adverse health outcomes from exposure to fumonisins

DOI: 10.1079/9781786394453.0012

is very low for ruminants, low for poultry and horses, but potentially concerning for pigs.

Zearalenone (ZEN; produced by *Fusarium* spp.): Is an oestrogenic substance which can cause a range of reproductive effects in animals, especially pigs and sheep (EFSA CONTAM Panel, 2017). It is related to the resorcylic acid lactone compound used in some countries as a growth promoter in beef cattle. ZEN is found in mouldy cereal grains and their by-products (especially bran and millrun), and in cereal straws and silages (especially maize silage). It also occurs in many pastures. ZEN concentrations are usually low in recently harvested grain, but they increase if infected grain is stored with moisture greater than 30–40%. ZEN has been found in mouldy hay, high-moisture maize grain and pelleted feed rations. Cattle and poultry are resistant to the effects of ZEN, but sheep and pigs are susceptible. Ovulation rates and lambing percentages are reduced in affected ewes, and prepubertal gilts have heavier uteruses and swollen vulvas, mature sows have longer oestrous cycles and may have fewer live piglets, and boars may have reduced sperm production. If animals are fed high levels of ZEN, some of this appears in the milk of sheep, cows and pigs. If poultry are given feed with high levels of ZEN some may appear in egg yolks but there are minimal levels in chicken meat.

Ergot: Is an alkaloid mycotoxin produced by the mould *Claviceps purpurea* (Coufal-Majewski *et al.*, 2016). It has a long history of causing disease in humans. Ergot alkaloids are absorbed from the digestive tract and cause blood vessels to contract and this can stop the flow of blood to the animal's extremities – ears, hooves, tail. The symptoms of ergot poisoning in animals include rough coat, inability to tolerate heat, unusual nervousness when forced to move, loss of ear and tail tips, and in severe cases the legs and hooves are affected with swelling of the hoof above the coronet and sometimes the hooves being lost. Pregnant mares affected by ergot may have difficulty foaling, or have small, weak or stillborn foals.

Recognizing feed contaminated with mould: The signs of mould growth are dampness, unusual colours (black, orange, yellow or white growths on the feed), an 'off' or musty smell, and sometimes the partial loss of the non-fibre part of the feed. Feed that has these characteristics should not be used, and we should be careful not to touch it with bare hands. Mould development can also encourage mite and insect infestation.

● To prevent the growth of moulds we should keep stored feed dry and cool – it is important that the moisture content of grains and protein meals is less than 13.5%. Grain is sometimes harvested at higher moisture content than 12% or 13%, either by accident or if it is intended for processing as high-moisture grain. Even when grain is harvested at the correct moisture content, it is usually stored in silos or bins where it may absorb moisture from the air (Chapter 17).

It is always wise to test the moisture content of grain before it is put into storage, if this is possible, and to make other arrangements if it is too damp. Moist grain can be artificially dried (at a cost), or possibly mixed with dry grain to give an average moisture content which is safe to store. Both approaches are too expensive and impractical for small-scale animal managers, so prevention is much better than cure.

Phytoestrogens

Phytoestrogens are plant substances made in the cells of some pasture legumes, and which cause reproductive problems in grazing animals, especially sheep. The condition was first identified in sheep grazing red and subterranean clovers and was called clover disease.

Phytoestrogens are similar to the endogenous oestrogen synthesized by the animal. Phytoestrogens bind to oestrogen receptors in cells and prevent normal oestrogen metabolism, either by interfering with the expression of genes which are involved in reproduction or by directly affecting the action of the endogenous hormone.

There are several types of phytoestrogens (Reed, 2016); those which are relevant to this discussion are the isoflavones (genistein, daidzein, glycitein, formononetin and biochanin A are the main compounds in this group) and coumestans (coumestrol). The phytoestrogens which are of most practical importance for grazing animals are the isoflavones in subterranean and red clovers (*Trifolium subterraneum* and *T. pratense*) and coumestans in lucerne (alfalfa; *Medicago sativa*). Phytoestrogens also occur in soybeans (*Glycine max*), peas (*Pisum sativum*), lima beans (*Phaseolus lunatus*) and pinto beans (*P. vulgaris*).

Disease caused by phytoestrogens: The ingested phytoestrogens markedly impair reproduction. Different phytoestrogens have different effects on the animal's physiology, but they have adverse effects on many mammalian species (e.g. horses, cattle, sheep and pigs), and in practice, particularly in sheep and cattle (Reed, 2016).

Sheep affected by isoflavones have:

- Reduced conception rates (reductions of 10 to 80% have been reported) because ovulation rates are reduced.
- Fewer live births from those which get pregnant because of increased embryonic losses. Progesterone production is reduced during pregnancy and this results in the foetus being aborted.
- Lambs which may be born weak and die soon after birth.

And affected sheep may suffer from:

- dystocia (lambing difficulties) which is implicated in poor mothering, birth of weak lambs and neonatal lamb deaths;
- uterine prolapse;
- swollen external genitalia; and
- secretion of a milky fluid from the mammary glands of castrated males and non-pregnant females.

The latter two effects are temporary and if the animal is removed from the feed then the symptoms disappear after about a month. However, if ewes are fed oestrogenic feed for a long time, the effects become permanent because of changes in their reproductive tract which makes them unable to store sperm and thus for their ova to become fertilized.

Avoiding phytoestrogen disease: To protect animals against this disease, do not graze breeding ewes on pastures which contain red or subterranean clovers, and do not feed raw soybeans or raw linseed to breeding females. Avoid clover cultivars which are known to be oestrogenic; older cultivars are more likely than newer ones to have significant levels of phytoestrogens because plant breeders now identify unsuitable new varieties, and they are not released onto the market.

Oestrogens are present in higher amounts in fresh, green forage. Mature, dry clover forage and hay made from this are less likely to have potent levels of oestrogens. Oestrogens levels are substantially increased if the plant is N deficient or water-stressed.

Mycoestrogens: Some moulds which grow on cereal grains, or on dead and decaying matter in pastures or are present on hay or silage made from the grains, produce zearalenone (ZEN; discussed above under 'Mycotoxins').

Bacterial, viral and prion diseases transmitted by feed

Several diseases can be contracted by eating contaminated feed. In some cases, the feed has simply been exposed to, and carries, the disease organism, in the same way as clothing and equipment can carry disease; an example is Newcastle disease of poultry. However, the diseases listed here are those where the infectious agent (usually a bacterium or a virus) is carried in the feed itself because the feed either contains inadequately processed animal carcase meal products made from infected animals, or has been a growth substrate for disease organisms.

Salmonellosis: Feed which has been contaminated by faeces, particularly those of rodents and birds, may be infected with *Salmonella* bacteria which grow and multiply, especially if the feed is stored in warm, damp conditions (Dar *et al.*, 2017). These bacteria invade the epithelial cells lining the digestive tract, causing enteritis (inflammation of the digestive tract and diarrhoea). Enteritis with septicaemia occurs in newborn calves, lambs, foals, fowl, and piglets when *Salmonella* infects the blood's macrophages.

Animals which are affected by salmonellosis have a fever, foul-smelling diarrhoea with mucus and sometimes blood, abdominal pain, and can become dehydrated. Affected pigs may have difficulty defecating, and pregnant females may abort. The onset and seriousness of salmonellosis is often related to the animal experiencing stress – e.g. inadequate feeding, being put into a new social group, being transported for long periods, etc.

We cannot visually identify feed that is loaded with *Salmonella*, but dampness and heat indicate conditions which allow the growth of this organism.

Botulism: This is a usually fatal disease caused by toxins produced by *Clostridium botulinum*. Animals usually encounter this organism when they eat something which is contaminated by the bacterium. This can be a feed ingredient, e.g. poultry litter (which has been sometimes fed to cattle; see Chapter 6), or an animal can ingest the bacterium if they eat decaying carcases. The disease is described in the 'Bone Chewing' section below.

Bovine spongiform encephalopathy (BSE, 'mad cow' disease): BSE is a neurological disease of cattle where affected animals progressively become nervous or aggressive, very sensitive to touch or sounds, have difficulty standing, and lack coordination. The disease is fatal and there is no treatment (US Food & Drug Administration, 2018). The disease has been found in cattle in the United Kingdom, several European countries, Israel, Japan, Canada and the USA.

The disease agent is a protein molecule, called a 'prion'. Prions make newly formed protein molecules change their shape and thus become non-functional. When this happens in the brain, we get lesions where cells have disappeared and leave open spaces, hence 'spongiform' in the name of the disease.

The disease has two consequences: first, it is fatal and would be a major hazard to a country's cattle industries, and second, there is a possibility that people who eat infected beef may contract the fatal brain disease, variant Creutzfeldt–Jakob disease (vCJD).

Inadequately processed meat and bone meal made from sheep infected with scrapie is possibly the source of prions which infected UK beef cattle in the late 1980s. Many jurisdictions have banned the feeding of carcase meals and milk products to ruminants because of the possibility that they might be a vector for the transmission of BSE (Chapter 6). Some jurisdictions have banned all animal protein meals from being fed to ruminants, including fish meals and poultry product meals. Fish and poultry meals do not carry prions, but the reasoning is that it is difficult to distinguish between protein meals made from mammal carcases and those from other animals except by DNA testing.

Diseases of pigs:

- African swine fever (ASF) causes fever, vomiting and diarrhoea, abortion, and death within 6 to 13 days; it can be fatal in 100% of cases. ASF virus is transmitted to pigs which feed on infected meat. The virus can remain infectious for 3–6 months in uncooked pork products but is destroyed by heat.
- Aujeszky's disease is highly contagious. It causes neurological symptoms in young animals, respiratory illness in older pigs and reproductive losses in sows. Mortality rates in very young piglets can be high, although older animals typically recover. The disease can be transmitted to other species if they come into contact with infected pigs. Eating infected pig tissues can transmit the virus.
- Classical swine fever causes fever, cyanosis of the skin especially of ears, limbs, tail and snout, constipation followed by diarrhoea, breathing difficulties, ataxia and death. It is transmitted when pigs eat inadequately processed food wastes.
- Swine vesicular disease (SVD) causes lameness and affected animals are reluctant to move. Vesicles appear in infected pigs above the coronet and between the claws. The whole hoof can sometimes be lost. SVD occurs in pigs which have eaten meat scraps and swill derived from infected pigs. The virus remains active in tissues of dead animals.

Foot and mouth disease (FMD): This is a serious, highly contagious disease affecting cloven-hoofed animals, including ruminants (e.g. sheep, cattle, goats, deer), pigs and camelids (e.g. camels, llamas and alpacas).

FMD is usually passed on through aerosols or contact with infected clothing, etc., but it can also be transmitted by contact with infected feed (DEFRA, 2002). These feeds include milk, and meat meals where the pH has remained above 6.0.

Reducing the risk of contracting feed-borne diseases: We can avoid, or at least reduce the risk of, transmitting feed-borne diseases by vaccinating at-risk animals. This is easy to do (with care), and although it is expensive it is much less than the cost of losing an animal.

Do not feed materials which might harbour disease organisms. Importantly, this includes animal carcase meals and swill (Chapter 6). Recognizing infected or contaminated feed can be difficult, but we should be very wary if the feed:

- is discoloured – has white, black, yellow or orange patches which are in contrast to the expected feed colour;
- has an 'off' odour – musty or mouldy or sharp;
- feels warm and moist – this indicates good conditions for bacterial and mould growth; or
- will be fed to ruminants and seems to include meat meals.

Secondary substances in animal feeds

Secondary substances (also called 'anti-nutritive' or 'anti-quality' or 'non-nutritive' substances or 'plant poisons') are chemicals which plants produce to protect themselves against insects, predation by grazing animals and microbial diseases. These are very useful to the plant, but they can have very adverse effects on animals.

Secondary substances are tannins, alkaloids, organic acids, etc. (D'Mello, 1992) which can:

- be poisonous or otherwise affect animal metabolism;
- reduce the availability of nutrients in the feed;
- change the taste of the feed;
- affect the storage lives of animal products; or
- affect the taste and appearance of animal products.

Table 12.1 lists the secondary substances in animal feeds which cause problems when these feeds are fed to domestic animals. Where individual feeds are listed, they also contain the secondary substances listed under 'general'.

Protease inhibitors (trypsin and chymotrypsin inhibitors): These secondary substances are proteins which inhibit the action of a variety of proteases (enzymes which digest proteins; Clemente *et al.*, 2015). The seed protease inhibitors protect the germinating seed against insect and microbial proteases. Unfortunately for our animals, they are also active against trypsin and chymotrypsin which are important protein-digesting enzymes secreted from the pancreas.

Proteins are damaged by heat, and so these inhibitors are not active in oilseed meals which have been heat treated during their manufacture. However, raw, ground legume seeds still have active protease inhibitors.

Protease inhibitors prevent protein digestion in the small intestine by pigs and horses, and pre-ruminant calves, lambs and kids. Affected animals are less productive. As well as limiting the amount of amino acids absorbed from the small intestine, this stimulates the synthesis of more proteases which increases the animal's requirement for dietary protein.

Phytate (phytin or phytic acid): Is a P storage compound found widely in seeds and up to 75% of the seed P can be in this form (Chapter 5; Li *et al.*, 2016). Phytic acid also binds Ca, Mg, Zn, Pb, Mn, Mg, Co and Fe. While phytate-P is mostly unavailable to pigs, different poultry species (e.g. turkeys compared to meat chickens) and birds of different ages are able to digest different proportions of phytate-P. Ruminants are more able to get P from phytate than monogastric animals because the substance is partly digested by rumen micro-organisms. Nevertheless, the non-phytate-P contents of cereal grains are a general measure of their available P. Pigs, poultry and horses that are given a diet rich in cereal grains must be given a mineral P supplement, or the enzyme phytase has to be added to the diet to release P from phytate (see Chapter 11).

Phytin also affects the activities of intrinsic digestive enzymes and reduces the availability of carbohydrates and amino acids.

Tannins: There are hydrolysable tannins where tannin monomers are bound to a carbohydrate molecule (e.g. glucose), and condensed tannins where several monomers are bonded together. Both occur in feeds (although condensed tannins are the most common) and both affect the feed's nutritive value (Mangan, 1988). The effects of plant tannins are very variable because the chemistry of tannins, and their concentrations in feeds, are also variable.

Tannins can have a variety of effects in ruminants. Some effects are adverse – tannins can make feeds taste astringent and this can reduce feed intake in some cases, and condensed tannins bind to plant cell protein and make it unable to be digested in the rumen. If condensed tannins are released freely into the rumen liquor they can bind to and inactivate the microbial enzymes which digest cellulose.

However, tannins in feeds for ruminants do not have uniformly adverse effects. Although they make the major plant protein, rubisco, less available to degradation by rumen bacteria this increases the undegradable dietary protein content of these feeds, which is often a useful outcome because the tannin–rubisco complex disassociates in the abomasum and the protein can be digested in the small intestine. As well, tannins can work as an anthelmintic – they have been reported to kill internal parasites in sheep, goats and deer. Tannins can also bind to plant cell protein and stop them forming a protein foam which contributes to bloat (Chapter 13).

When feeds which contain tannins are fed to non-ruminants, they have generally adverse effects: reduced digestibility of dry matter (DM) and energy because tannins bind to and inactivate digestive enzymes, formation of tannin–protein complexes which cannot be digested, inhibition of the animal's own proteases, and production of

Table 12.1. Secondary substances in animal feeds. (From Dryden, 2008; reproduced with permission.)

Feed	Secondary substance	Effect on animals
Grain legumes (pulses)		
General	Protease inhibitors	Increased endogenous N excretion and reduced protein digestibility in non-ruminants, including pre-ruminant calves, lambs and kids
Oilseeds		
General	Phytic acid	A molecule which contains P in an unavailable form; phytic acid also binds Ca, Mg, Zn and several other trace minerals and prevents their absorption from the intestine (see below and Chapter 5)
	Unsaturated fatty acids	Some are essential (Chapter 1), but too much can produce unappealing pork fat
Soybean (raw soybean meal)	Protease inhibitors	(See grain legumes)
	Haemagglutanins	Possibly bind to mucosal cell membranes and reduce nutrient absorption, coagulate red blood cells
	Phytic acid	(See general)
	Oestrogens	Too little for any effect
	Saponins	Haemolytic but too little for any effect
	Goitrogens	Cause thyroid gland enlargement (goitre) by preventing the binding of I in the thyroid gland, and thus the synthesis of thyroxine
	Anti-vitamins	Increase requirements for vitamins A, D, E, B12 and pyridoxine. Variable effects from reduced growth and fertility to nervous disorders and death
Peanut (peanut meal)	Goitrogens	(See soybeans)
Lupin (sweet) (seed)	Quinolizidine alkaloids	Blurred vision, nausea
	Protease inhibitors	(See soybeans)
	Tannins	(See soybeans)
	Saponins	(See soybeans)
	Phytic acid	(See soybeans)
Rapeseed (canola meal)	Goitrogens	(See soybeans)
	Erucic acid	Can cause fat deposits in heart tissue, young pigs are the main animal type at risk
	Sinapine	Causes a fishy taint in eggs
	Tannins	Bind to proteins and render them indigestible
Cottonseed (white cottonseed, cottonseed meal)	Gossypol	Temporary male infertility; toxic in non-ruminants, less so with ruminants because gossypol binds to ruminal protein before it can be absorbed. May cause green yolk colouration in eggs
	Phytic acid	(See cereal grains)
	Cyclopropanoid fatty acids	Colours egg white (pink); can reduce fertility in hens
Linseed (linseed meal)	Cyanogens	Produce HCN on fermentation (note that linamarin may be hydrolysed by bacterial fermentation and by seed enzymes)
	Phytic acid	(See soybeans)

Continued

Table 12.1. Continued.

Feed	Secondary substance	Effect on animals
Sunflower (sunflower meal)	Chlorogenic acid	Feeding high levels of sunflower meal can stain eggshells
Grass and legume forage		
Legume forage	Tannins	Bind to soluble proteins and make them unavailable in the rumen
Sorghum forage	Cyanogenic glucosides	Very poisonous for all animals; symptoms include laboured breathing, frothing at the mouth, staggering, and rapid death
	Nitrite	Binds to haemoglobin and prevents oxygen transport to cells
Temperate grasses	Nitrite	(See sorghum forage)
Tropical grasses	Oxalate	Binds to Ca and makes this mineral unavailable to non-ruminants
	Nitrite	(See sorghum forage)
Cereal grains		
General	Phytic acid	(See soybeans)
	Unsaturated fatty acids	(See oilseeds)
	Non-starch polysaccharides	
Pearl millet grain	Phytic acid	(See soybeans)
	Goitrogens	(See peanuts)
Sorghum grain	Tannins	(See soybeans)
Triticale grain	5-alkyl-resorcinol	Reduced feed intake, growth depression
Fodder trees		
General	Tannins	(See oilseeds)
Leucaena spp. (leaf)	Mimosine	Mimosine causes hair loss especially in horses and sheep, mouth ulcers, and poor growth; its rumen metabolites 2,3- and 3,4-DHP cause goitre – cattle, sheep, goats, pigs and horses are affected
Insects		
Insect meals	Contaminants in insect feed, including chitin	Variable effects depending on the type and level of these in the feed, and the uptake of these into the insect pupae and larvae. Housefly larvae meal can carry active disease organisms

poisonous substances if the tannin macromolecule is hydrolysed. As a result of this, pigs and poultry which are fed tannin-containing feeds such as sorghum grain and some plant protein meals show reduced growth and performance (Jansman, 1993).

Gossypol: Is a polyphenol which the plant produces in its seeds as a protection against insect attack. It causes a variety of symptoms in poultry, pigs and young ruminants – it damages liver, kidney, and heart tissue, and depresses feed intake and growth, and causes infertility in males because of damage to the sperm and the germinal cells in the testes (Garland, 2015).

Gossypol is present in raw cottonseed (i.e. 'white' or 'fuzzy' cottonseed) and in the protein meal made from this. Heating cottonseed will bind cottonseed protein to gossypol, but this does not inactivate all of the gossypol and reduces the availability of seed protein, especially the essential amino acid lysine. Animals fed cottonseed meal respond well to supplementary ferrous salts. These bind to gossypol and inactivate it. Lower-gossypol cotton cultivars are being developed.

Non-starch polysaccharides (NSPs): These are large cellulose-like molecules which cannot be digested by intrinsic animal digestive enzymes, e.g. amylase.

They are, therefore, particularly troublesome in pig and poultry diets. The main NSPs in cereal grains are β-glucans (which are chains of glucose molecules joined by β1-3 and β1-4 glycosidic bonds) and arabinoxylans (also long-chain molecules which are made of arabinose and xylose molecules). These substances are found in barley, rye and oats, wheat and triticale (which is a wheat/rye hybrid).

These large molecules have two main effects on monogastric animals. The indigestible NSPs reduce the amount of digestible organic matter in the feed. This is especially important when the feed contains 60% or 70% (sometimes more) cereal grains, as is the case for most commercial pig and poultry diets. Also, some β-glycans make the intestinal contents viscous and this stops feed particles from contacting the intestinal epithelial cells and the digestive enzymes which are located in the membranes of these cells and stops nutrients from being absorbed from the small intestine.

We can reduce the effects of NSPs in pig and poultry diets by adding β-glucanase and xylanase enzymes to the feed. These enzymes break down the NSPs and improve animal performance (Chapter 11).

Mimosine: This is a non-protein amino acid which is found in all parts of the leucaena tree. It can cause major ill-effects in all animals, but especially sheep, cattle, goats, pigs, poultry and horses (CSIROpedia, undated). Ruminants (especially sheep) and horses lose hair, and pregnant sows may resorb embryos or give birth to piglets with deformed limbs.

Mimosine is metabolized into two products by rumen bacteria: 2,3- and 3,4-di-hydroxy-pyridone (DHP). 3,4-DHP is also produced by plant enzymes when leucaena leaf is macerated. The two forms of DHP are goitrogenic, that is, they interfere with thyroxine synthesis by preventing the incorporation of iodine. Affected animals develop a large, swollen thyroid gland. This form of goitre does not respond to I supplements.

Rumen inoculation with the bacterium *Synergistes jonesii* is the best way of reducing the effects of mimosine in ruminants; this bacterium degrades mimosine and 2,3- and 3,4-DHP, and inoculation has contributed to reducing the adverse effects of leucaena feeding (Annison and Bryden, 1998). It is not necessary to inoculate all the herd as the bacterium will spread from treated cattle to other animals grazing in the same herd. While cattle treated with *S. jonesii* become resistant to the effects of mimosine and much more productive, there are some caveats: *S. jonesii* preparations lose their effectiveness if they are exposed to air or stored for long periods without exposure to mimosine or DHP. In addition, some treated cattle still absorb DHP and are thus exposed to the risk of goitre.

Mimosine toxicity in sows can be reduced by feeding 1% ferrous sulphate in the diet, as the Fe forms a chelate with mimosine, which is then excreted.

Cyanide poisoning: The cyanogenic glucosides linamarin and lotaustralin in linseed meal, and dhurrin in some sorghum (*Sorghum almum*), Sudan grass (*S. sudanense*) and Johnson grass (*S. halepense*) forages and in raw cassava root, release the highly poisonous hydrocyanic acid (HCN) when they are metabolized by rumen bacteria (in the case of forages) or seed enzymes (in the case of linseed) (Business Queensland, 2018).

The cyanide potential is highest in sorghum forage crops which are recovering from stresses such as drought, insect attack or cold weather, and may be increased by N fertilizers. Haymaking does not alter the cyanide potential. The only safe way of avoiding cyanide poisoning is to not feed suspect forage (either fresh or dry). Giving a S supplement, e.g. feeding *ad lib* a salt block containing 10% S, will help to detoxify cyanide by converting it in the rumen to thiocyanate, but this is not a certain way of preventing cyanide poisoning. Sorghum grain does not contain cyanogenic glucosides.

Linseed is used to make linseed meal, and its cyanide potential is reduced by heating the seed. This inactivates the enzymes which produce HCN from linamarin. Linseed is heated when the oil is extracted by the expeller extraction process. Less heat is applied in solvent extraction.

Nitrate/nitrite poisoning: Plants absorb N from the soil as nitrate (NO_3) and this is translocated to the leaves. Normally, given good conditions for photosynthesis, this NO_3-N is then converted to amino acids and protein. If conditions do not favour photosynthesis, e.g. cold, overcast weather or water stress, then the nitrate accumulates in the stem and leaves.

Nitrate has a caustic effect on the digestive tract and will cause diarrhoea and colic. However, in ruminants, NO_3 is usually converted to nitrite (NO_2) by rumen micro-organisms, and usually then to NH_3 which is used to synthesize amino acids. If the amount of NO_2 exceeds that which can be converted to NH_3, NO_2 accumulates and is absorbed into the animal's blood where it combines with haemoglobin to form methaemoglobin, which cannot transport oxygen. Sheep, cattle, horses and pigs can be affected, in that general order of increasing susceptibility. Young animals are more at risk.

Many plants can accumulate NO_3 under appropriate conditions (EFSA CONTAM Panel, 2009). These include brassica and soybean forages, cereal forages (maize, sorghum, millet, wheat, oats and barley), lucerne (alfalfa), subterranean clover, and some ryegrass varieties. High soil N contents will also contribute to high plant NO_3 contents, and run-off water from heavily fertilized paddocks can also contain poisonous concentrations of NO_3. In addition, bacteria growing on damp forage may reduce NO_3 and produce a poisonous amount of NO_2.

Animals suffering from NO_2 poisoning show symptoms within a few hours of eating the at-risk forage. They have increased heart rate, rapid, laboured breathing, general weakness, vomiting, and may die. Chronic poisoning causes reduced feed intake, lower production (e.g. milk and live weight gain), and abortion (EFSA CONTAM Panel, 2009).

We can reduce the risk of NO_2 poisoning by recognizing the risk factors and giving hungry animals a non-poisonous feed before they are allowed to graze an at-risk pasture.

Oxalate (oxalic acid): Found in the leaves of some pasture plants, oxalate binds Ca in an insoluble and unavailable form. In practice, the Ca-binding effects of oxalate are largely observed in horses because these animals absorb Ca in their small intestines but cannot degrade oxalate until it reaches their large intestine. Rumen micro-organisms destroy oxalate, and this protects ruminants from the effects of oxalate poisoning, although a sudden, large intake by hungry animals will overwhelm this capacity (Rahman *et al.*, 2012).

Grasses which can have deleterious amounts of oxalate include kikuyu (*Pennisetum clandestinum*), buffel grass (*Cenchrus ciliaris*), setaria (*Setaria sphacelata*), green panic (*Megathyrsus maximus* var. *pubiglumis*), para grass (*Urochloa mutica*) and pangola grass (*Digitaria eriantha*). Oxalic acid contents are highest in young leaves and after a period of wet weather. The level increases during the night and decreases during the day, so if we have to graze suspect pastures it is best to do this in the late afternoon. About a third of the Ca in lucerne (alfalfa, *Medicago sativa*) is bound as the oxalate (Ward *et al.*, 1979) but the high Ca content of this plant makes it a useful source of Ca.

Horses grazing the tropical grasses listed above are at risk of osteodystrophia fibrosa (ODF or 'big-head'). The common name for this condition describes one of the most easily seen symptoms – the horse develops swellings along the nose as Ca is withdrawn from bones. There are three stages to the disease: at first, horses have a mild, shifting lameness, sometimes creaking joints, and may arch their back. In the second stage, fractures and sprains can occur and the facial bones become enlarged ('big-head'). The horse may have difficulty breathing, infected sinuses and may develop a cough especially when stressed. In the third stage, the horse loses body condition, becomes anaemic and may die. ODF is reversible in the early stages by feeding a Ca supplement such as limestone or legume hay, or by removing the horse from the at-risk pasture. A supplement of 350 g of limestone plus 650 g of dicalcium phosphate mixed with 1.5 kg of molasses will provide enough Ca for one horse for one week.

Feed taints in eggs, milk and meat: Some feeds have constituents which cause feed taints in animal products.

One of the most widely reported taints is a fishy taint in eggs caused by sinapine in rapeseed meal (including the 00 canola variety which has been bred to have very low levels of erucic acid and goitrogens). Bird genotype and intestinal micro-organisms, as well as the feed's sinapine content, are implicated and the problem is greatest for birds which lay brown-shelled eggs. Fish oil, which contains long-chain unsaturated fatty acids, will confer a fishy taint on chicken meat, probably due to the fatty acids being oxidized when the meat is cooked.

Meat and milk from pasture-fed animals have different tastes to those from animals fed concentrate-rich diets, and a large number of chemical compounds are involved (Frank, 2016). Off-flavours in sheep meat are caused by *Brassica* spp. (turnip, swede, kale and rape) forages and lucerne (alfalfa). Milk tastes differently if it is from cows fed a concentrate-rich diet rather than pasture or silage. The roughage-fed cow's milk has a 'feed' flavour which can taste 'off', especially if we are expecting a blander taste. Propanol and ethanol are found in small amounts in silage and can give a taint to milk. Lactones in chicory (*Cichorium intybus*) forage produce a bitter taste in milk, although cows have to be fed a large amount for several days for this to happen. Feeding rapeseed meal to dairy cows can produce a fishy taint in milk and the reason appears to be the same as for the similar taint in eggs.

Feed processing can reduce secondary substances in oilseed meals and grain legumes: When oilseeds are processed, either the ground seed is heated and pressed to extract the oil, or alternatively is immersed in a solvent such as hexane which dissolves the oil. The 'pre-press solvent extraction' process uses both methods (Chapter 6). Thus, the resulting protein meal obtained after the seed oil is extracted has been subjected to at least two processes – milling ('grinding') and heating.

Raw seed is prepared for oil extraction by being passed through a roller mill or hammer mill. This breaks the seedcoat and reduces the particle size. There is little chemical change because although grinding can increase the temperature of the meal a little, there is no effect other than on particle size. So raw oilseed meals have similar nutritional properties as the original seed, including the same amount of active secondary substance.

Heating is used as part of the oil extraction process in pre-press and expeller extraction processes. Heat makes it easier to physically separate the oil from the rest of the seed. This heat will completely or partially destroy (depending on the substance and the temperature and duration of heating) protease inhibitors, lectins, hemagglutinins, the plant enzymes which produce the active form of some poisonous secondary substances (e.g. releasing HCN from linamarin), and phytin. However, there are many secondary substances which are not inactivated by heat.

How to reduce the impact of secondary substances on susceptible animals: Pigs, poultry, horses, and pre-ruminant calves, lambs and kids (i.e. which have not developed a functioning rumen), are the most susceptible to secondary substances. We can limit the adverse effects of secondary substances by not feeding raw oilseeds and their meals, and raw grain legumes, to susceptible animals. In particular, be careful when feeding 'full-fat' soybean meal to make sure that the meal has been heat treated. White ('fuzzy') cottonseed is an exception to the general rule; it can be fed to non-breeding cows and steers *ad lib* because these animals are not as greatly affected by gossypol as entire (breeding) males, and because cattle will self-limit the amount of white cottonseed that they eat.

- In some cases, we can reduce the effects of secondary substances if we are careful about the amounts of feed we use. This applies in particular to oilseed meals (cottonseed, rapeseed meals); grain legumes (bitter lupins, raw cowpeas, raw navy beans); some cereal grains (oats, triticale); and some forages (sorghum, temperate grass and forage cereal species). Recommended inclusion levels for some common feeds in pig diets are given in Table 12.2.

Table 12.2. Suggested maximum inclusion levels of ingredients in pig diets. (From Dryden, 2008; reproduced with permission.)

Feedstuff	Main secondary substance(s)	Suggested maximum inclusion level
Cottonseed meal	Gossypol	3–5% for sows; 10–15% for growers
Linseed meal	Linamarin	5%
Rapeseed (canola) meal	Erucic acid, goitrogens	0–3% for breeding stock; 5% for young pigs; 10–15% for growers/ finishers (except for '00' cultivars)
Soybean meal	Protease inhibitors (see Table 12.1)	No limit for heat-treated meal; nil for raw soybeans
Cowpea[a]	Protease inhibitors	15% for adults; nil in creep feeds and diets of weaners
Mung bean[a]	Protease inhibitors	10% for processed beans; 5% for raw beans
Navy bean[a]	Protease inhibitors, lectins	25% for heat-treated meal; nil for raw beans
Triticale grain	5-alkyl-resorcinol	40–50% for mature pigs; nil for young pigs
Rye grain	Tannins, phytin	20% for adult pigs; nil for young pigs

[a]Unless otherwise indicated, the suggested inclusion limits for grain legumes are for the raw seed

- We should manage grazing carefully by not letting hungry stock graze pastures that contain plants which can cause nitrate/nitrite or cyanide poisoning, or which have high oxalate contents. If there is no alternative but to use these forages, try to manage grazing so that animals have access at times of the day when the secondary substance is likely to be at its lowest level. It may be possible to use supplements which can mitigate the effect of the secondary substance, e.g. S to counter cyanide poisoning, or dicalcium phosphate to provide available Ca in feeds containing Ca oxalate.

Parakeratosis and zinc deficiency

Parakeratosis is a disease of pigs, cattle and poultry which occurs when they are fed a diet which is Zn deficient or where the availability of Zn is impaired. A deficiency of essential fatty acids (linolenic and linoleic acids) has also been suggested as a contributing factor to parakeratosis.

Zn is an essential mineral; it is a co-factor for several enzymes and is involved in protein synthesis. A deficiency reduces appetite, and causes growth depression (Fig. 12.1), slow wound healing, hair loss, impaired immune status, and impaired reproduction and testicular development.

Ca reduces the availability of dietary Zn by binding Zn in an insoluble Zn/Ca/phytin complex which cannot be absorbed. Zn will also bind directly to phytin forming a stable, insoluble and unabsorbable complex.

Parakeratosis in pigs: The recommended level of Zn for growing pigs varies from 50 mg/kg (NRC, 2012) to 110 mg/kg (Blum, 1989). Zn deficiency can be simply a result of feeding ingredients that have low Zn contents (e.g. maize and sorghum grains and some grasses) or because Zn availability is compromised by phytin or excess Ca. If the Ca content of a growing pig diet is above about 1.2% (compared to their normal requirement of 0.55–0.72%), this will precipitate parakeratosis.

Parakeratosis starts with the development of reddened plaques which become thick, black scabs. This is first seen on the fore and hind limbs, but then progressively covers the rest of the body. There are cracks in the skin between the scabs and these are often infected.

Affected animals eat less feed and drink less water, and generally have the Zn deficiency symptoms that are described above. Pigs recover from Zn deficiency very quickly – within 3 weeks – when they are given a Zn supplement.

Parakeratosis in cattle: This is rare but has been reported in cattle which were grazing Zn-deficient pastures in several countries: Guyana, Venezuela, Finland, Norway, USA and South Africa. Cattle with parakeratosis have bald spots where hair has been lost, with the skin between the legs being the worst affected. Zn-deficient cattle have reduced appetite and impaired growth.

Zinc deficiency in poultry: Birds that suffer from Zn deficiency have the same responses as pigs and cattle – reduced appetite and performance (Leeson, 2015). They typically grow frizzled (curled rachis and barbs) and rough feathers and develop a severe

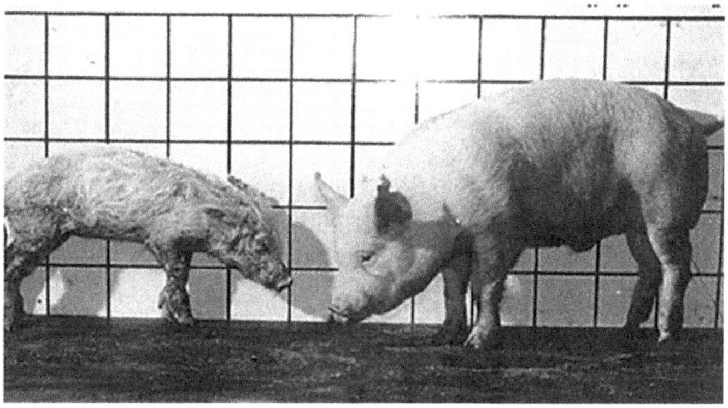

Fig. 12.1. Effects of zinc deficiency in pigs: growth depression and parakeratosis. (Photo by J.H. Conrad and M.W. Beeson, Purdue University; reproduced with permission.)

dermatitis on their feet. Hens may lay fewer eggs. Severely affected birds will die. Embryos from Zn-deficient birds may die before hatching and have severe skeletal deformities. If chicks hatch from these eggs they are weak and are unable to stand, eat or drink, and have laboured breathing. Any disturbance is likely to cause them to die. Chicks that hatch normally but are fed a Zn-deficient feed develop short legs with thickened hock joints.

How we can avoid a zinc deficiency: While chemical analysis might suggest that a diet has enough Zn, we should check the diet Ca and phytin contents. Diets which are based on cereal grains and soybean meal pose a particular risk because these ingredients contain high phytin levels (between 0.75% and 2.25 % dry matter basis) and, in the case of cereal grains, have very low (sorghum), to low (barley and maize (corn)) or moderate (wheat) Zn contents.

To deal with this problem we can:

- add phytase to the ration (Chapter 11); or
- add extra Zn from sources such as Zn oxide or carbonate, or a Zn chelate such as Zn methionine.

Bone chewing

Osteophagia: Animals chew bones presumably to try to correct P deficiencies. Bone chewing is mostly seen in beef cattle grazing pastures growing on P-deficient soils but has been reported in dairy cattle, buffaloes, goats and sheep, and in deer during periods of P stress such as lactation and antler growth.

It is likely that P-deficient cattle recognize bones as a P source, and that the stimulus to this is the smell of the bones (Dixon *et al.*, 2018). This behaviour, and the response to the availability of bones, is confined to P-deficient animals because if a P supplement is given the chewing behaviour stops.

Nevertheless, bone chewing is not a very effective way of correcting a P deficiency. A 400 kg live weight beef cow growing at 0.5 kg/day needs 10 g Ca and 4 g P per day. To get this much mineral the animal would have to eat about 50 g of dry bone, or a cube of bone about 5 cm on each side. But bone-chewing animals eat only a fraction of this amount.

Botulism: Caused by infection by *Clostridium botulinum* bacteria, is a major adverse side effect of osteophagia (PIRD, 2018). Carcasses can carry large *C. botulinum* loads, especially if there is still soft tissue associated with the bones. When the animal eats the bones and/or soft tissue it ingests the bacteria, which release the botulinum toxin. The symptoms include a sudden occurrence in a herd of weakness and paralysis, and animals which are unable to eat or drink. Death of infected animals occurs between 12 hours and 3 weeks after infection.

Cattle which are pastured on P-deficient country and which are likely to have access to animal carcases should be vaccinated against botulism.

Photosensitization

Photosensitization is caused by the excitation by ultraviolet light of molecules which are present in the blood. When these molecules pass through capillaries in the skin in those parts of the animal which are not protected by hair or pigmented skin, such as ears, muzzle, udder and feet, the excitation of these molecules causes damage to cell constituents including the cell's DNA.

Animals which are affected by photosensitization have swollen and sun-damaged, blistered and peeling skin, and hair loss. Cattle, sheep, goats and horses are the most commonly affected animals. The condition can also occur in poultry.

There are two forms of photosensitization (Hussain *et al.*, 2018):

- Primary photosensitization occurs when animals eat plants which contain substances which are excited by ultraviolet light. When these substances are absorbed into the blood and pass through blood vessels in unprotected skin, they cause the symptoms described above.
- Secondary (hepatogenic) photosensitization is when animals eat plants that contain substances which damage liver function or eat pasture that has been contaminated with fungi which do the same thing. Chlorophyll, present in all green plants, is attacked by micro-organisms in the ruminant digestive tract, and this yields phylloerythrin, a degradation product of chlorophyll. Phylloerythrin is absorbed into the blood and is usually excreted via the liver, but if the liver is damaged, excretion is impaired. Phylloerythrin accumulates in the blood and is excited by ultraviolet light, causing the effects described above.

Secondary photosensitization is the most common form in domestic animals. Plants like lantana (*Lantana camara*), some *Brachiaria* spp. and *Megathyrsus* spp. grasses, red clover (*Trifolium pratense*), lucerne (alfalfa; *Medicago sativa*), *Brassica* spp. and green couch grass (*Cynodon dactylon*) contain substances which can cause liver damage, with resulting secondary photosensitization. The disease facial eczema is a type of photosensitization caused when the liver is damaged by the mycotoxin sporidesmin, produced by the mould *Pithomyces chartarum* which can infest ryegrass pastures.

References

Annison, E.F. and Bryden, W.L. (1998). Perspectives on ruminant nutrition and metabolism. I. Metabolism in the rumen. *Nutrition Research Reviews* 11: 173–198.

Arapcheska, M., Jovanovska, V., Jankuloski, Z., Hajruali-Musliu, Z. and Uzunov, R. (2015). Impact of aflatoxins on animal and human health. *International Journal of Innovative Science, Engineering and Technology*, 2(2): 2015. Available at: www.researchgate.net/publication/283856306_IMPACT_OF_AFLATOXINS_ON_ANIMAL_AND_HUMAN_HEALTH (accessed 30 December 2020).

Blum, J.C.A. (1989). INRA – Elevage des Monogastriques. *L'alimentation des animaux monogastriques: porc, lapin, volailles*, 2nd edn. Paris, FRA: INRA.

Business Queensland (2018). *Cyanide and nitrate poisoning from sorghum crops*. Available at: www.business.qld.gov.au/industries/farms-fishing-forestry/agriculture/land-management/health-pests-weeds-diseases/livestock/cyanide-nitrate-sorghum (accessed 30 December 2020).

Clemente, A., Arques, M.C., Dalmais, M., Le Signor, C., Chinoy, C., Olias, R., *et al.* (2015) Eliminating anti-nutritional plant food proteins: the case of seed protease inhibitors in pea. *PLoS One* 10(8): e0134634. DOI: 10.1371/journal.pone.0134634.

Coufal-Majewski, S., Stanford, K., McAllister, T., Blakley, B., McKinnon, J., Chaves, A.V. and Wang, Y. (2016). Impacts of cereal ergot in food animal production. *Frontiers in Veterinary Science* 3: 15.

CSIROpedia (undated). *Leucaena toxicity solution*. Available at: www.csiropedia.csiro.au/leucaena-toxicity-solution/ (accessed 30 December 2020).

Dar, M.A., Ahmad, S.M., Bhat, S.A., Ahmed, R., Urwat, U., Mumtaz, P.T., Bhat, S.A., Dar, T.A., Shah, R.A. and Ganai, N.A. (2017). *Salmonella typhimurium* in poultry: a review. *World's Poultry Science Journal* 73(2): 345–354.

Denli, M. and Perez, J.F. (2010). Ochratoxins in feed, a risk for animal and human health: control strategies. *Toxins (Basel)* 2(5): 1065–1077.

Department for Environment, Food and Rural Affairs (DEFRA) (2002). *Origin of the UK Foot and Mouth Disease Epidemic in* 2001. Available at: http://adlib.everysite.co.uk/resources/000/095/936/fmdorigins1.pdf (accessed 30 December 2020).

Dixon, R.M., Fletcher, M.T., Goodwin, K.L., Reid, D.J., McNeill, D.M., Yong, K.W.L. and Petherick, J.C. (2018). Learned behaviours lead to bone ingestion by phosphorus-deficient cattle. *Animal Production Science* 59(5): 921–932.

D'Mello, J.P.F. (1992). Chemical constraints to the use of tropical legumes in animal nutrition. *Animal Feed Science and Technology* 38(2–3): 237–261.

Dryden, G.McL. (2008). *Animal Nutrition Science*. Wallingford, UK: CAB International.

EFSA CONTAM Panel (2009). Nitrite as undesirable substances in animal feed – scientific opinion of the panel on contaminants in the food chain. *EFSA Journal* 1017: 1–47. Available at: www.efsa.onlinelibrary.wiley.com/doi/10.2903/j.efsa.2009.1017 (accessed 30 December 2020).

EFSA CONTAM Panel (2017). Risks for animal health related to the presence of zearalenone and its modified forms in feed. *EFSA Journal* 15(7): e04851. Available at: www.efsa.onlinelibrary.wiley.com/doi/full/10.2903/j.efsa.2017.4851 (accessed 30 December 2020).

EFSA CONTAM Panel (2018). Risks for animal health related to the presence of fumonisins, their modified forms and hidden forms in feed. *EFSA Journal*, 16(5): 5242, 1–144. Available at: https://www.efsa.europa.eu/en/efsajournal/pub/5242 (accessed 30 December 2020).

Frank, D. (2016). Impact of brassica and lucerne finishing feeds and intramuscular fat on lamb eating quality and flavor. A cross-cultural study using Chinese and non-Chinese Australian consumers. *Journal of Agricultural and Food Chemistry* 64 (36), 6856–6868.

Garland, T. (2015). *Overview of gossypol poisoning. MSD Veterinary Manual*. Kenilworth, NJ: Merck Sharp & Dohme Corp. Available at: www.msdvetmanual.com/toxicology/gossypol-poisoning/overview-of-gossypol-poisoning (accessed 30 December 2020).

Hocking, A.D. (2003). Microbiological facts and fictions in grain storage. In Wright, E.J., Webb, M.C. and Highley, E. (eds), *Stored Grain in Australia 2003. Proceedings of the Australian Postharvest Technical Conference, Canberra, 25–27 June 2003*. CSIRO Stored Grain Research Laboratory, Canberra. Available at: www.storedgrain.com.au/wp-content/uploads/2013/06/10.pdf (accessed 30 December 2020).

Hussain, S.M., Herling, V.R., Rodrigues, P.H.M., Naz, I., Khan, H. and Khan, M.T. (2018). Mini review on photosensitization by plants in grazing herbivores. *Tropical Animal Health and Production* 50(5): 925–935.

Jansman, A.J.M. (1993). Tannins in feedstuffs for simple stomached animals. *Nutrition Research Reviews* 6: 209–236.

Lee, H.J. and Ryu, D. (2017). Worldwide occurrence of mycotoxins in cereals and cereal-derived food products: public health perspectives of their co-occurrence. *Journal of Agricultural and Food Chemistry* 65: 7034–7051.

Leeson, S. (2015). Mineral deficiencies in poultry. Zinc deficiency. *MSD Veterinary Manual*. Kenilworth, NJ: Merck Sharp & Dohme Corp. Available at: www.merckvetmanual.com/poultry/nutrition-and-management-poultry/mineral-deficiencies-in-poultry (accessed 30 December 2020).

Li, X., Zhang, D., Yang, T.Y. and Bryden, W.L. (2016). Phosphorus bioavailability: a key aspect for conserving this critical animal feed resource with reference to broiler nutrition. *Agriculture,* 6: 25. Available at: www.mdpi.com/2077-0472/6/2/25/pdf (accessed 30 December 2020).

Mangan, J.L. (1988). Nutritional effects of tannins in animal feeds. *Nutrition Research Reviews* 1: 209–231.

National Research Council (NRC) (2012). *Nutrient Requirements of Swine*, 11th rev. edn. National Academies Press. Washington, DC. Available at: www.nap.edu/catalog/13298/nutrient-requirements-of-swine-eleventh-revised-edition (accessed 30 December 2020).

Pestka, J.J. (2007). Deoxynivalenol: Toxicity, mechanisms and animal health risks. *Animal Feed Science and Technology* 137(3–4): 283–298.

Primary Industries and Regional Development Western Australia (PIRD) (2018). *Botulism in cattle*. Available at: www.agric.wa.gov.au/livestock-biosecurity/botulism-cattle (accessed 30 December 2020).

Rahman, M.M., Abdullah, R.B. and Wan Khadijah, W.E. (2012). A review of oxalate poisoning in domestic animals: tolerance and performance aspects. *Journal of Animal Physiology and Animal Nutrition* 97: 605–614.

Reed, K.F.M. (2016). Fertility of herbivores consuming phytoestrogen-containing *Medicago* and *Trifolium* species. *Agriculture-Basel* 6: 35; DOI: 10.3390/agriculture6030035.

Serraino, A., Bonilauri, P., Kerekes, K., Farkas, Z., Giacometti, F., Canever, A., Zambrini, A.V. and Ambrus, Á. (2019). Occurrence of aflatoxin M1 in raw milk marketed in Italy: exposure assessment and risk characterization. *Frontiers in Microbiology* 10: 2516.

US Food & Drug Administration (2018). *Bovine Spongiform Encephalopathy (BSE) Questions and Answers*. Available at: www.fda.gov/vaccines-blood-biologics/safety-availability-biologics/bovine-spongiform-encephalopathy-bse-questions-and-answers (accessed 30 December 2020).

Ward, G., Harbers, L.H. and Blaha, J.J. (1979). Calcium-containing crystals in alfalfa: their fate in cattle. *Journal of Dairy Science* 62(5): 715–722.

13 Feed-related diseases

Some of the disorders discussed in this chapter can be caused by disease organisms as well as by feeds and feeding methods. These descriptions do not include any discussion of other possible origins of these diseases or describe ways in which these diseases should be treated in sick animals. If we suspect that an animal is ill, then the most sensible thing to do is to call a veterinarian. As a general rule, good animal management includes carefully watching animals for signs of disease and getting timely advice and treatment.

Animals can suffer from diseases which are caused by pathogens contaminating the feed or substances in their feed, or the way that feed is given to them. The major types of feed-related diseases are:

- Diarrhoea caused by an abrupt change in feed type.
- Digestive disorders caused by feeds which have large amounts of starch or other non-structural (i.e. non-fibre) carbohydrates, often accompanied by inadequate fibre, in the diets of horses, sheep, goats and cattle.
- Poisoning by pathogens present on or in the feed, e.g. prions, pathogenic bacteria, and moulds which grow on feeds and produce toxins (Chapter 12).
- Poisoning by secondary substances which are produced by plants to protect themselves from insects and other predators (including browsing animals) and which are either poisonous to animals or adversely affect the quality of their products (Chapter 12).

Digestive tract disorders

Rumen bloat (ruminal tympany) occurs when the gas which is produced in the rumen cannot escape. A large amount of CO_2 and CH_4 is produced in the rumen. This gas is released through the oesophagus by eructation ('belching'), and during this process moves from the gas cap above the rumen liquor in the dorsal rumen, through the cardiac sphincter at the distal end (bottom) of the oesophagus, and up through the oesophagus to the mouth. If there is any blockage, either in the oesophagus or at the cardiac sphincter, then gas cannot escape and accumulates in the rumen (Fig. 13.1).

Bloated animals may die from suffocation when the expanded rumen presses on the diaphragm and prevents breathing. Bloat also puts a strain on the heart because it restricts the flow of venous blood returning to the heart.

'Free gas' or obstructive bloat: This is the simplest type of bloating although it is relatively uncommon.

The oesophagus can be blocked by a piece of unchewed feed lodging there, or by swelling in tissue around the oesophagus.

Ruminal stasis (lack of movement in the muscles of the rumen) will also cause bloating, because there are no rumen movements to increase the volume around the cardia and to force gas from the gas cap above the rumen liquor through the cardiac sphincter into the oesophagus. Bloat caused by rumen stasis is common in cows suffering from acute acidosis as rumen movements stop when the pH falls to less than about 5.5.

Frothy bloat: This form of bloat prevents gas escaping by covering the cardiac sphincter with foam, and by trapping gas in stable bubbles which do not move up the oesophagus. It occurs when animals consume pastures rich in lucerne (alfalfa) and clovers. High concentrations of soluble proteins and saponins in the pasture promote foam formation by trapping gas within the rumen fluid (Majak *et al.*, 1995). Bloat is rare when animals are grazing tropical legumes because the soluble proteins in those plants are bound by tannins. The minimum condensed tannin concentration which appears to

DOI: 10.1079/9781786394453.0013

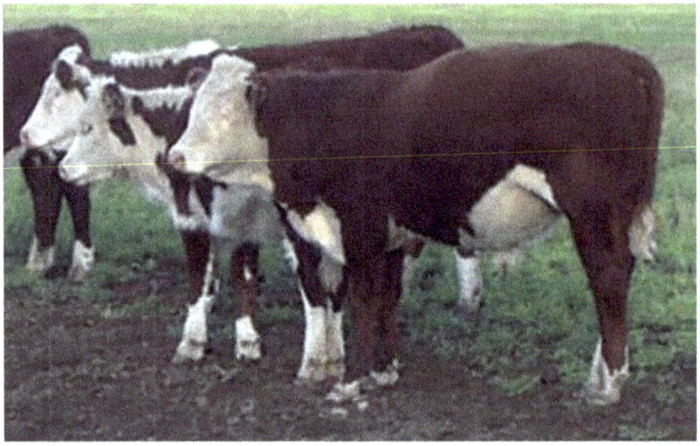

Fig. 13.1. A Hereford steer with bloat – the left flank is distended over the bloated rumen. (From Bailey, 2014; reproduced with permission.)

protect against bloat is 5 g/kg dry matter (DM) (Barry and McNabb, 1999).

Bloat occurs occasionally in animals eating grain-rich rations in feedlots. *Streptococcus bovis*, a bacterium which proliferates in the rumens of animals eating starch-rich rations, can produce a slime that forms a stable foam (Cheng *et al.*, 1998) which can trap rumen gas.

Factors that influence the occurrene of frothy bloat in grazing and lot-fed animals include:

- Higher levels of CH_4 production increase the risk of bloat because CH_4 is not water soluble.
- Pectin-rich legumes may increase the rates of fermentation and gas production.
- Animals that secrete more saliva are less prone to bloating. Cattle eating a concentrate-rich (and thus fibre-poor) feed secrete less saliva than those eating a roughage ration.

A bloat event can occur very quickly, within a few hours of an animal eating the bloating feed. Animals must be treated immediately or there is a risk that they will die. Emergency treatments include drenching with a detergent or vegetable oil, or in extreme cases by making an incision into the flank and releasing the gas. In some cases we will have to bail out the foam to release pressure in the rumen. The incision is best made with a trochar and cannula, but in the absence of these, the next best alternative is a sharp knife. Try to stop rumen liquor from getting into the peritoneal cavity and get veterinary help to repair the wound.

Methods of controlling frothy bloat include:

- Grazing management – by restricting access to immature, rapidly-growing legume-rich pastures.
- Oil and detergents – these reduce the surface tension of the rumen liquor and reduce the foam's stability. Oils can be given as feed supplements or by spraying them onto the pasture. Detergents can be given as liquid drenches, or in supplement blocks, or in the drinking water.
- Antibiotics such as monensin reduce methane production. They can be given from slow-release capsules or by including them in a feed supplement.

Impaction: Can occur in the ruminant stomach, the equine colon, and the bird's crop. The mass of impacted feed cannot flow from the impacted organ into the lower digestive tract and this reduces gastro-intestinal movements, interferes with water re-absorption from the digestive tract, and stops the animal from eating any more feed.

When a ruminant eats a feed which is very fibrous and difficult to digest, the mass of indigestible material can accumulate in the rumen, omasum or abomasum. Sand and gravel impaction occurs when animals eat silage or other feeds which are heavily contaminated with these materials. Impaction through eating plastic, twine and other similar material also occurs. Birds can suffer from an impacted crop if they eat long pieces of fibre such as long grass, or pieces of plastic or twine.

The progress of rumen impaction is described in this extract from a case report of Boer goats suffering from the effects of eating *Ficus esquiroliana* in

China (Zhai *et al.*, 2013) '… listlessness, less rumination, or no rumination. The goats subsequently exhibited ruminal impaction and ruminal tympany, before finally showing increased salivation, difficulty in breathing, no breathing, and/or death.' Impacted animals also suffer from metabolic alkalosis and dehydration.

Rumen impaction can occur as a separate disorder, or as a sequel to abomasal impaction. Note that digesta caught between the leaves of the omasum is usually quite dry. This is normal and should not be confused with omasal impaction.

Constipation in pigs: This is often a symptom of an underlying disease but can occur if the animal's water intake is restricted or if the diet has too little fibre.

Constipation occurs in newly farrowed sows if they have not replaced the body water lost during farrowing or if they have been confined for a long period. Constipated sows eat less feed and may suffer from enterotoxaemia. All types of pigs will show constipation as a symptom of water deprivation.

Colic in horses is a disorder of the large intestine, usually the colon, which causes pain (University of Minnesota Extension, 2018). Colic which is related to feeding can be caused by impaction by indigestible feed or the production of excessive amounts of gas during microbial fermentation. Colic is often caused by teeth problems which reduce the amount and effectiveness of chewing and thus lead to swallowing long pieces of roughage, or by feeding very dry feed without supplying enough water to drink.

How to prevent impaction and constipation: We can reduce the likelihood of an animal suffering from these disorders by:

- Making sure that they have adequate water (Chapter 2).
- Providing ruminants with an adequate amount of physically effective fibre (peNDF; Chapter 1).
- Keeping materials such as twine and netting (hay bale wrapping), plastic bags, and similar material out of the reach of inquisitive or hungry animals.
- Avoid feeding ruminants roughages which are difficult to digest or to chew. This type of material includes very mature cereal straw, and fodder tree browse (e.g. gliricidia, *Gliricidia sepium*; leucaena, *Leucaena leucocephala*; mulga, *Acacia aneura*) which contains amounts of large, lignified twigs. The risk of impaction from this type of material is high when we are using a 'cut-and-carry' feeding method, or hungry animals are given access to fodder trees such as mulga trees during droughts. Refer also to Chapter 6.
- Make sure that horses' teeth are in good condition so that they can chew their feed effectively (watch for 'quidding' – pieces of partly chewed feed are lost from the mouth).
- Avoid including sand, soil or gravel in feed. This can happen if a front-end loader is used to collect silage from a gravel- or earth-floored silage pit.

Nutritional diarrhoea (scours): Diarrhoea is a condition where the faeces are very liquid (loose). The condition is caused by a failure to adequately reabsorb water which has been secreted into the intestine. Most diarrhoea in neonatal animals is caused by pathogens (bacteria, viruses and cryptosporidia), and in adults the causes are often bacterial and/or viral diseases and internal parasites. But in some cases, in both young and adult animals, diarrhoea is caused by poor feeding management.

The main risk in diarrhoea is dehydration and loss of electrolytes. A secondary problem is that an affected animal absorbs less nutrients.

In order to protect young animals against scours caused by disease organisms, we should make sure that they get enough colostrum. Calves should be fed 4 L of fresh colostrum within 4 hours of birth (Meganck *et al.*, 2014).

For young ruminants fed artificial milk replacers, the most common causes of nutritional scours are:

- Overfeeding: a calf should be fed 10% of its live weight daily, and this should be given in 1 or 2 feeds each day, depending on its age and live weight.
- Rapidly changing feed type: calves will scour if their feed is changed rapidly; an example is an abrupt change from milk replacer to whole milk.
- Feeding low-quality milk replacers which do not form clots in the abomasum. Whole cows' milk forms a clot in the abomasum when the casein protein is attacked by chymosin. The liquid fraction left after clotting is called whey and consists of the whey proteins (mainly globulins), lactose, minerals and water. The casein and fat clot allows the main constituents in milk to be nearly completely digested because their exit from the abomasum is delayed. Some low-quality milk replacers use whey powder, or protein sources

such as soybean and fish meals, with added starch to make up the energy deficiency left when the milk fat is removed. These ingredients do not clot and the liquid digesta moves quickly through the digestive tract and forms liquid faeces.
- Sugar or molasses in the feed: the calf does not have an intrinsic enzyme which can digest sucrose.

Young pigs (neonates and newly-weaned) can suffer nutritional scours because of (Rhouma, 2017):

- Flow of undigested solid feed to the large intestine and which encourages the growth of pathogenic bacteria.
- Lack of Fe – common in neonatal pigs unless they have been given a ferrous Fe injection.
- Transient low feed intake which affects the intestinal epithelium.

Foals can suffer from scours (Dunkel, 2008):

- If they are fed a milk replacer which is reconstituted either too concentrated or too dilute.
- When they begin to sample solid feed and begin to establish a microbial population in their large intestine. This form of scouring is short-lived and has little effect on the foal's health.
- Irritation of the digestive tract by sand or other abrasive material.

In adult animals of all types, nutritional diarrhoea is caused by:

- a rapid change in feed type;
- feed with a high moisture content – e.g. some immature temperate grasses have as little as 10% DM and 90% water;
- deficiencies of Cu and Se; or
- some plant poisons.

Ways of preventing diarrhoea: Good feeding practice and good animal management will reduce the incidence of nutritional scours. This will involve:

- Reducing the stress caused by changing social groups, e.g. when young animals are re-allocated to a different pen and/or pen mates.
- Avoiding exposing animals to environment stresses, e.g. cold, damp conditions.
- Making any changes in feed type gradually, e.g. mixing the new feed with the old so that the change from 100% old to 100% new is done over 4 or 5 days, or more if the change is as marked as in adapting pasture-fed cattle to a feedlot ration.
- Watching piglets just after birth and at weaning and making any feed changes slowly. This will mean introducing suckling piglets to a starter ration or the weaner ration before they are weaned.
- Making sure that feeds are not contaminated by moulds, *Salmonella*, sand or dirt, etc.

Rumen acidosis, hyperkeratosis, rumenitis and liver abscess

These are a complex of conditions which occur in cattle, sheep, goats and other ruminant animals when the feed contains large amounts of a rapidly-fermented substance like starch or soluble sugars. Animals that are at risk are lot-fed beef cattle and sheep when they are fed diets with up to 80% grain, dairy cattle fed total mixed rations containing concentrates, and sheep and cattle grazing root crops such as brassicas or fodder beet.

What happens when a ruminant is fed an uncontrolled starch-rich diet: When a ruminant is fed a diet which is rich in starch or soluble sugars, volatile fatty acids are produced as micro-organisms ferment these carbohydrates and the rumen pH falls rapidly from its usual 6.5–7.5 (in animals eating roughage) to about 5.5. The sequence of events is shown in Fig. 13.2.

Those bacteria which produce lactic acid as an end-product of starch fermentation proliferate as the pH falls. Lactic acid is a stronger acid than the VFA, and is less easily absorbed, and so the pH of the rumen falls even more.

The decline in rumen pH to 5.5 or less (i.e. increasing acidity) has several consequences:

- All protozoa die at pH less than 5.0 and so the rumen loses the ability of these organisms to store starch granules away from bacterial digestion. The rumen thus loses the rate-limiting effect of the protozoa on starch fermentation.
- Rumen movements (contractions of the muscles in the rumen wall and muscular pillars) stop. This affects feed intake and can contribute to bloating (see above).
- Acid conditions in the rumen predispose to hyperkeratosis and rumenitis.
- Lactic acid is absorbed from the rumen and lowers the animal's blood pH.

Rumen acidosis: When a ruminant becomes overloaded with H^+ ions, the fine control of blood pH is overcome (Beef Cattle Research Council, 2019). Blood pH is closely controlled to pH 7.4 ± 0.03, and if the pH moves outside this range there can be serious consequences to the way that cells function, caused by structural changes in cell proteins.

Acute acidosis presents with lack of rumen movements, animals off feed (not eating), lethargy, increased heart and respiration rates, diarrhoea, animals going down, and death which occurs 1 to 3 days after the ingestion of the grain 'dose'. The condition is described by RAGFAR (2007). Death as a result of acute acidosis happens because rumen acids are absorbed into the blood and overcome the animal's ability to control its blood pH. Thus the rumen acidosis becomes a generalized metabolic acidosis. This happens through the sequence of events shown in Fig. 13.3.

In addition, acid conditions in the rumen may cause the *stratum corneum* (see below) to completely slough off, and the rumen papillae to regress (Steele *et al.*, 2009).

Subacute rumen acidosis (SARA) is a common disorder of dairy cattle that are fed grain-rich diets to promote high milk production (Morgante, 2009). It occurs when animals suffer repeated periods when the rumen pH falls to about 5.8. Subacute acidosis does not present with the symptoms described above for acute acidosis, although feed intake and growth are reduced, and the animal may be lame and/or have diarrhoea. What is not

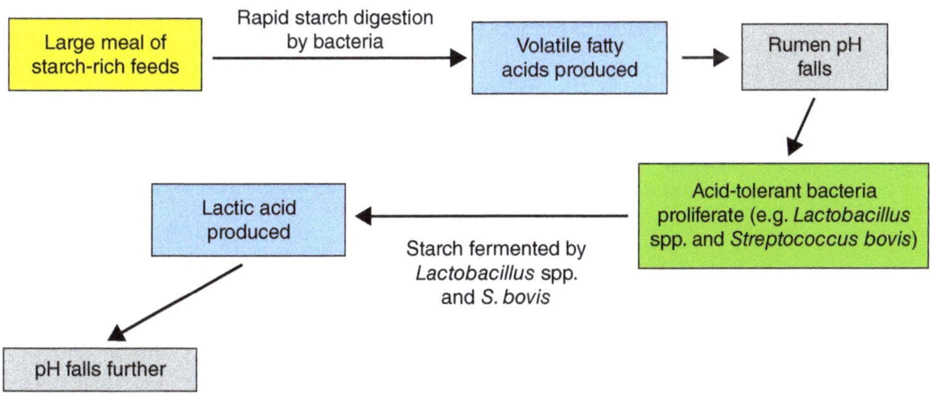

Fig. 13.2. The sequence of events which lead from eating a starch-rich meal to the rumen pH falling to low levels. (Copyright: Gordon McL. Dryden.)

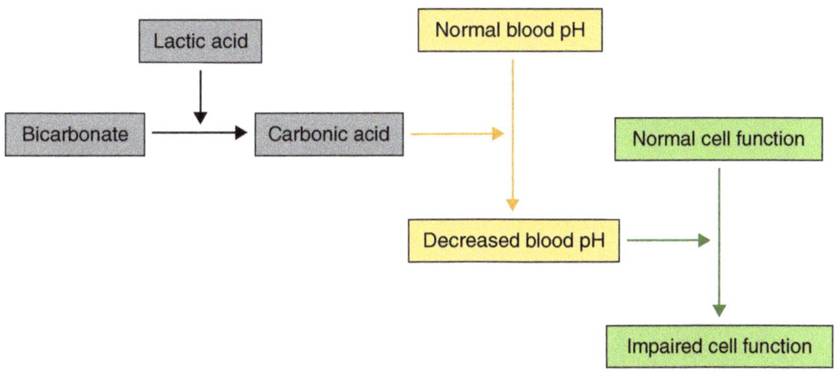

Fig. 13.3. The sequence of events in metabolic acidosis, a consequence of acute rumen acidosis. (Copyright: Gordon McL. Dryden.)

obvious, though, is that damage is being done to the rumen wall (Zhao *et al.*, 2018).

Hyperkeratosis and liver abscess: These disorders are consequences of acid conditions in the rumen and low dietary peNDF (Chapter 1) and are often found in cattle eating typical feedlot diets.

The rumen wall has an accumulation of dead keratinized cells several cells thick on its inside surface and exposed to the rumen liquor. This is called the *stratum corneum* (Fig. 13.4). These cells are continually being scraped off by the action of fibrous pieces of feed. If the feed has very little peNDF, then the cells in the *stratum corneum* accumulate and the layer becomes very thick, causing hyperkeratosis. Hyperkeratosis, together with the effect of acid conditions in the rumen, weakens the *stratum corneum* and gaps open up between the epithelial cells (Steele *et al.*, 2009). This can lead to rumenitis and ulcers forming in the wall (Fig. 13.5a). Weakening of the rumen wall allows bacteria to pass through, enter the hepatic vein (which carries absorbed nutrients from the rumen to the liver) and lodge in the liver causing liver abscesses (Fig. 13.5b).

Managing grain-rich ration feeding for ruminant animals

Ruminants have evolved to use diets that contain large amounts of plant fibre. When we feed them a ration which has a large amount of starch-rich ingredients, and consequently usually a low content of fibrous ingredients, we expose the animal to a real risk of metabolic disease. To reduce the likelihood of metabolic problems when cattle and sheep are fed the grain-rich diets which are typical of

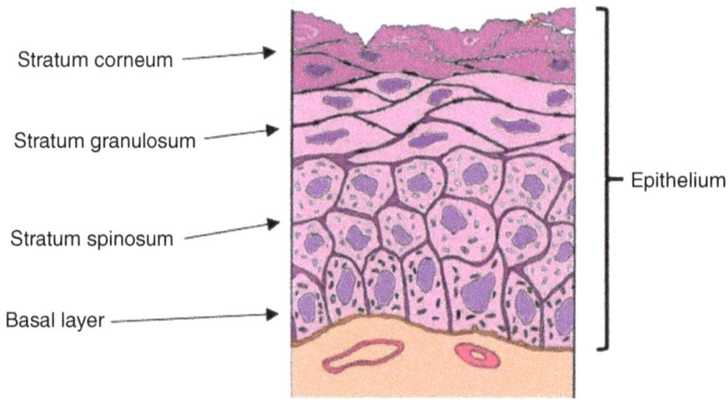

Fig. 13.4. Diagrammatic cross-section of the rumen epithelium (adapted from Steele *et al.*, 2016; reproduced with permission.)

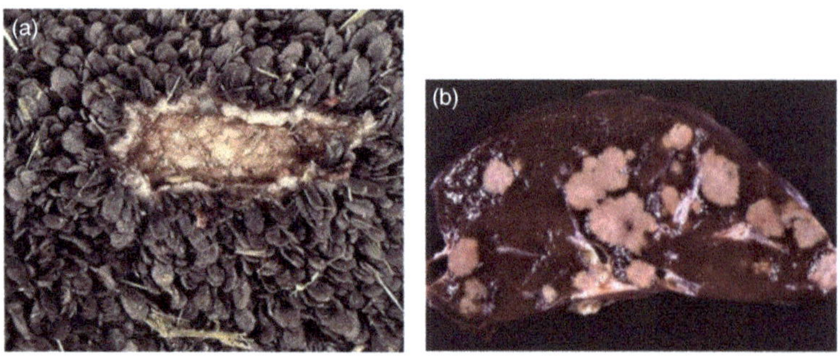

Fig. 13.5. (a) Ulcer in the rumen wall. (From Noah's Arkive, undated; reproduced with permission.) **(b)** Liver abscesses. (From Nation, in Noah's Arkive, undated; reproduced with permission.)

lot-fed beef and mutton production, and some dairy total mixed rations, we must be careful to set up conditions in the rumen which will protect the animal, as far as we can do this.

There are three things that will help to provide this protection:

- Increase the number of starch-fermenting bacteria, e.g. *Ruminobacter amylophilus*, *Butyrivibrio fibrisolvens* and *Streptococcus bovis*, and those bacteria which ferment lactic acid, e.g. *Selenomonas ruminantium* subsp. *Lactilytica* and *Megasphaera elsdenii*.
- Increase the numbers of protozoa – especially *Ophryoscolex* spp. In an adapted animal, protozoa act as rate limiters for starch digestion because they ingest whole starch granules and protect these from bacterial fermentation.
- Allow time for rumen papillae to grow as this helps to maintain high rates of VFA absorption.

By using appropriate feeding management, we can carefully adapt animals to a grain-rich diet. The most important thing is to make any change in feed composition gradually; this includes changes in the type of concentrates, as well as the amount of concentrates. It is best to use a step-by-step introduction to a new diet (Fig. 13.6). A gradual, stepwise (not continuous) change-over will help to accustom the animal to the taste, smell and physical feel of the new feed, and give time for the rumen microbial population to adapt to the new feed.

We should avoid feeding diets with more than about 40% grain to sheep and lactating dairy cattle. Sheep are less tolerant of starch-rich feeds than cattle, and dairy cattle need digestible plant fibre to promote acetic acid production by their rumen bacteria to maintain their milk fat content.

Careless feeding of cereal grains is the most common cause of rumen diseases, but be careful when feeding grain legumes such as chickpeas, peas, lentils and fava beans as these are also starch-rich feeds.

The following management practices will also help to control the rumen pH, and thus to maintain active bacterial and protozoal populations, as shown in Fig. 13.7:

- Provide physically effective fibre (peNDF; Chapter 1). This ensures that the animal ruminates and thus secretes volumes of saliva which contains phosphate and carbonate buffers. Fibre particles must be larger than about 2 mm otherwise they will pass out of the rumen without any need for chewing, but they should not be longer than about 5 cm in a mixed roughage/concentrate feed because long particles can be separated from the rest of the diet and not eaten.
- Try to avoid periods when the animal is unable to eat because the feed trough or bunk is empty, or because feed has been spoiled by heat or water (e.g. rain or snow). Use a diet with a higher roughage content when bringing cattle back on to feed after a period when their intake of a grain-rich ration has been limited, even if they have been previously adapted to this type of diet.

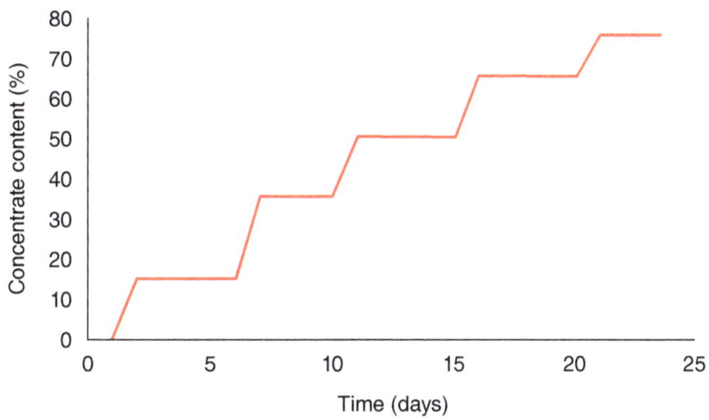

Fig. 13.6. A suggested method of introducing a new diet composition; changing from a complete roughage diet for cattle to a diet with 75% concentrate and 25% roughage. (Copyright: Gordon McL. Dryden.)

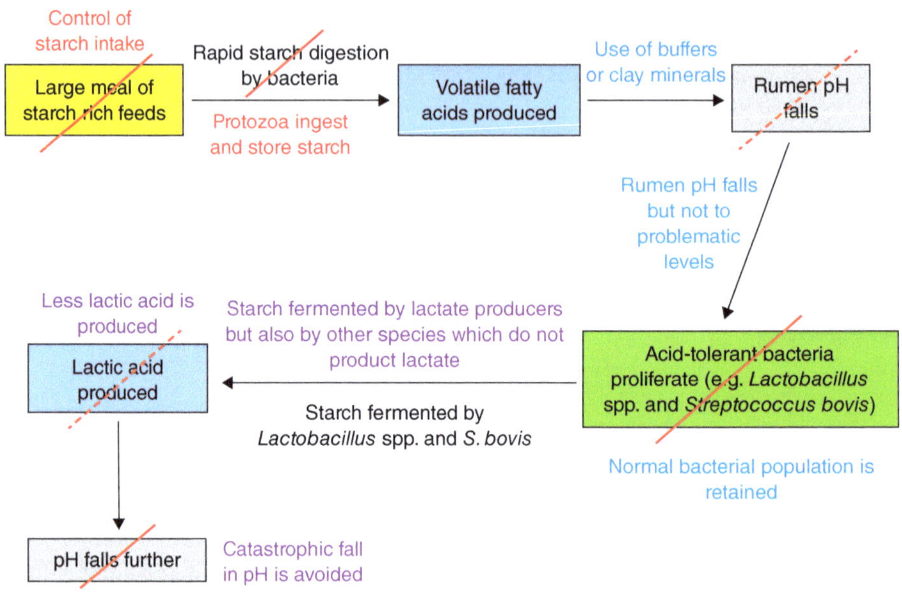

Fig. 13.7. The effects of controlling starch intake and using rumen buffers or clay minerals on rumen pH. (Copyright: Gordon McL. Dryden.)

- Consider using feed additives such as sodium bicarbonate, or clay minerals (e.g. vermiculite and bentonite) (Chapter 11). Do not use bicarbonate additives in diets for transition cows.
- Ionophores (e.g. monensin, lasalocid, narasin and salinomycin) also reduce the risk of acidosis by selectively targeting the lactic acid producing bacteria – *S. bovis* and *Lactobacillus* spp. We could also consider feeding virginiamycin, an antibiotic which kills lactate-producing bacteria. But note that the use of any antibiotic in animal feeding risks developing antibiotic-resistant strains of that organism and reduces the effectiveness of the antibiotic for treating diseases (Chapter 11).

Laminitis

Laminitis or founder is a condition where the soft tissue under the hard hoof wall becomes inflamed and swells. It is very painful. The condition in cattle is similar to that in equines but bleeding and abscesses under the claws are also seen. Laminitis occurs in an acute form and a chronic form.

Laminitis has several different causes. Many cases have a nutritional or metabolic basis, and it can be associated with metritis (an inflammation of the uterus wall following bacterial infection after foaling) or caused by physical injury (e.g. a lame animal standing with most of its weight on one leg for a time).

What is the cause of metabolic laminitis, and is it a stand-alone disorder? The answer to the second question is probably 'No', it is not a stand-alone disease, it is a symptom of another, underlying problem (Patterson-Kane *et al.*, 2018).

It is quite difficult to answer the first question, but what appears to be the case is described here. When starch is digested in the small intestine, glucose is released and is absorbed into the blood. High levels of blood glucose stimulate insulin secretion and so we have two possible causative factors: high blood insulin and high blood glucose. Both of these reduce the permeability of small blood vessels and so the toe of the hoof becomes starved of nutrients and the cells in the laminae die. Another possibility is that insulin affects the way that the laminae cells adhere to each other. This leads to the separation of the laminae along the white line. Some horses suffer from equine metabolic syndrome which makes them resistant (or unable to respond) to insulin. Because the blood glucose levels in these horses stay high (cells do not absorb glucose in response to insulin signals) and because the pancreas secretes even more insulin in response to the persistently high blood glucose, we get a situation which triggers laminitis. But note that the exact way in which high insulin levels may cause laminitis is not yet known.

Acute nutritional laminitis: This type of laminitis typically occurs 12 to 18 hours after a large amount of grain was eaten. The coronet and hoof are warmer than normal and affected animals are in severe pain, and they show the symptoms of anxiety, trembling and increased breathing rate. They do not want to walk, have a bounding digital pulse and may have a raised temperature. The front feet are more commonly involved, and horses may stand with their weight on their hind legs so as to relieve pressure on the front hooves. If all feet are affected the animal will lie for long periods.

Two serious consequences can occur as a result of severe laminitis. The third phalanx (the pedal bone) may rotate after the laminae separate. This can occur rapidly, within 72 hours in some cases. Rotation is caused by the pull of the deep flexor tendon and the weight of the horse on the phalanges, and the third phalanx turns towards and perhaps through the sole of the hoof. In severe cases of laminitis, the whole hoof wall may shed.

Acute laminitis progresses rapidly once it manifests itself, and palliative measures must be undertaken if we think that founder may occur. This should be done before the symptoms are evident. It is difficult to treat laminitis and we will need veterinary advice.

Chronic laminitis: This is a succession of subacute episodes of laminitis. In these cases, the hooves of affected animals show a series of rings which indicate at what stages in the growth of the hoof wall the laminitis occurred. Laminitis often occurs in the fore-feet and horses will adopt a typical stance with their weight off the front of their hooves. If the laminitis continues for some time the front of the hooves grows out like a 'slipper'.

Grain founder: This acute form of the disease is the most common in intensively managed horses and lot-fed beef cattle. It is caused by uncontrolled access to larger than usual amounts of grain. It is difficult to say what amount will cause laminitis because this depends on how well adapted the horse or cow is to its diet. The grains most often involved are wheat, maize (corn) and barley. Oats do not often cause founder in horses – they do contain starch, but in lower amounts than other grains (Chapter 6).

Horses digest starch in their small intestine. In cattle, much of the eaten starch is fermented to VFA in the rumen but if a large amount is consumed some passes intact into the small intestine where it is digested in the same way as occurs in the horse. In both situations the blood glucose level rises and precipitates the sequence of events described above.

To avoid grain founder, the most important thing is to prevent animals from suddenly engorging themselves on starch-rich feed. We can do this by keeping horses' grain and concentrate feed storages secure, and by slowly making any changes to a ration that contains grains.

Grass founder: This form of the disorder occurs when pasture-fed horses eat grasses which have high levels of either starch (in tropical species grasses) or soluble sugars (sucrose and others; in most temperate species).

Horses which contract grass founder are often obese, and the condition might be due to insulin resistance which accompanies obesity.

We can prevent, or at least reduce the likelihood of, grass founder by controlling the intake of sugars and/or starch, and by stopping the horse from getting over-fat by limiting its available energy intake. To do this with stabled (hand-fed) horses, we can:

- reduce the amount of feed horses are given to eat;
- feed mature dry roughage such as grass hay, but avoid cereal hays because these may contain developing seeds; and
- enforce exercise in horses which are inclined to be sedentary.

It is much more difficult to control feeding by grazing horses, but these are possible strategies:

- Use a muzzle: a device which fits around the horse's nose and mouth and prevents them from eating large amounts, although many horses (and donkeys) are adept at getting rid of these.
- Limit the time the horse is allowed to graze by confining it to a bare yard for part of the day.
- If possible, stop the horse from grazing grass which is likely to have high sugar or starch levels, e.g. restricting access to grass in the afternoon, or during overcast and cold days, when starch and sugars in the leaves are at their highest levels.

- Reduce the amount of pasture available to each horse by adding other animals, e.g. horses, cattle or sheep, to increase the stocking rate. Be sure that these animals are all accustomed to each other.

Oesophageal and gastric ulcers

Stomach ulcers occur frequently in adult (weaned) pigs and horses. The condition is very prevalent in horses, with studies suggesting that between 55% and 95% of intensively housed horses are affected. The disorder is also reported in pasture-fed horses. The incidence can be more than 60% in growing pigs. The condition is found most often in animals that are fed grain-rich, finely ground (milled) feeds. This includes horses being prepared for racing and other sports, and of course most commercial piggeries confine pigs in pens where they are fed grain-rich, often pelleted, diets. The relevance of pelleting is that cereal grains are ground finely before they are pelleted, and it is this small particle size that appears to be a principal cause of ulcer development.

Pigs and horses both have a part of their stomach, near the cardiac sphincter, which is non-glandular, and it is here where the ulcers form (Fig. 13.8). In serious cases, ulcers also develop in the lower oesophagus and proximal duodenum.

Ulcers form when the non-glandular squamous mucosa of the *saccus caecus* is exposed to acid. Hydrochloric acid is produced in the fundic part of the stomach – it is needed to activate the protein-digesting enzyme pepsin, which is also secreted from glands in this part of the stomach. The fundus and pyloric parts are protected by secreted mucus and bicarbonate, and the mucosal cells there repair quickly, but this is not the case with the *saccus caecus* mucosa.

Feeding very fine feed particles (<700 μm or 0.7 mm) which leave the stomach rapidly, and intermittent feeding which allows the stomach to partly empty, can expose the gastric mucosa and predispose the animal to ulcers. *Helicobacter* spp. bacteria (the same genus as is implicated in human gastric ulcers) has been identified in both horse and pig stomachs and may be involved in ulceration.

The effects of gastric ulcers: Horses are generally unwell and have acute and recurrent colic, diarrhoea, a rough hair coat and poor appetite. They lose weight and body condition, and their performance is compromised.

Pigs have a poor appetite, are pale and may have blood in their faeces due to internal haemorrhaging, experience stomach pain and grind their teeth, may vomit, become weak and may be found dead.

Preventing gastric ulcers: We can reduce the likelihood of an animal developing this condition by good feeding management (Lester *et al.*, 2008; Iowa State University, 2020). This can include:

- Using feeds which have a particle size larger than 700 μm. However, this will usually mean changing the feed from pellets to mash. This is acceptable for horses that are individually fed and where the feeding programme can be closely supervised, but pellets have several benefits in the group feeding of pigs. They allow the trace and minor components of the diet – minerals,

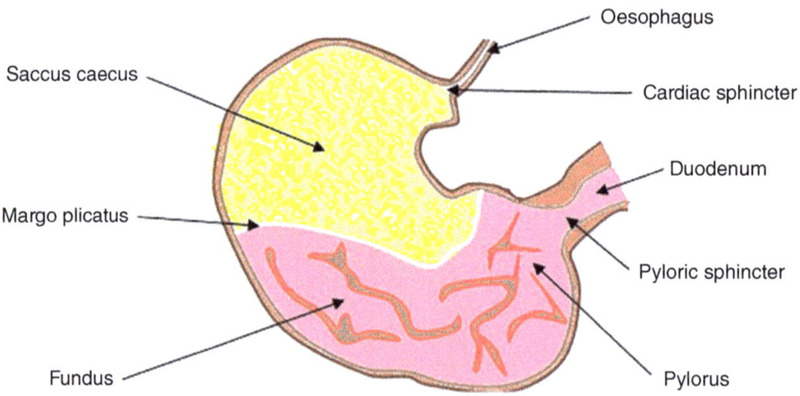

Fig. 13.8. A diagrammatic longitudinal section of a horse's stomach. (Copyright: Gordon McL. Dryden.)

vitamins, medications – to be mixed and retained in the diet in the concentrations that are required for optimum pig performance. In addition, pigs grow faster and sometimes more economically when their feed is pelleted.

- Making sure that horses and pigs always have feed available to them, as far as that is practicable. Horses continuously secrete HCl into their stomachs even when they are not eating. This exposes an empty stomach to a greater risk of ulceration. Horses which are often transported, e.g. from their stable to a training track, have a much higher incidence of ulcers. This could be because they have several periods without feed. Pigs can experience feed shortages if the feed conveying system breaks down.
- Avoiding stressful situations. Animals usually find transport stressful and they are usually not fed during transport unless they are unloaded for rest periods. Introducing new animals into a group upsets the social order and can put animals off their feed. Not all social situations are adverse – horses which have contact with others generally have fewer ulcers.
- Feeding pigs diets with at least 5% crude fibre. While too much fibre in a pig diet will dilute the available nutrients because plant fibre is not as well digested as the other feed constituents, too little fibre will allow rapid gastric emptying which exposes the mucosa to HCl secreted from the parietal cells in the fundus of the stomach.

Urea poisoning

Ruminant animals are often fed urea, an organic N-containing substance which rumen bacteria can use as a source of N. Methods of feeding urea to cattle are described in Chapter 16.

The advantage of urea is that it is a much cheaper source of ruminally available N than most protein meals. Its disadvantages are that it is unpalatable (but this can be masked by mixing it with ingredients such as molasses) and that it can poison ruminant animals if they eat too large a dose.

When urea enters the rumen, it is rapidly converted to NH_3 and CO_2 by the action of microbial urease. This happens quickly – urea is usually completely hydrolysed within 2 or 3 hours of being eaten. The amount of NH_3-N that can be incorporated by the rumen bacteria into amino acids depends on the amount of available carbohydrate and minerals in the rumen at that time. When urea contributes NH_3 in amounts that exceed the amount that can be assimilated by the rumen bacteria, excess NH_3 diffuses across the rumen wall into the animal's blood.

Free NH_3 is poisonous so it is transported in the blood to the liver where it is converted back to urea. Most of the urea circulating in the blood is then excreted in urine. Urea poisoning occurs when the amount of NH_3 in the blood is above that which can be detoxified by the liver; this NH_3 will pass through the blood/brain barrier.

Urea poisoning occurs rapidly, as quickly as 10 to 60 minutes after a toxic amount has been eaten. The symptoms of urea poisoning in cattle are (Parkes and Shilton, 2019):

- the cow appears to be aggressive;
- severe stomach pain, indicated by twitching of ears and facial muscles, grinding of the teeth;
- rapid, laboured breathing;
- frequent urination;
- bloating, and frothing at the mouth;
- muscular tremors, difficulty walking, weakness and then collapse; and
- violent struggling just before death.

The toxic dose of urea varies considerably between individual animals. Fat animals are more susceptible than leaner ones at the same live weight, and animals that have been carefully introduced to urea are more resistant. Given this, it is difficult to make a quantitative recommendation, but 30 g urea/100 kg live weight (about 120 g per day for a 400 kg steer) fed in a single dose may kill. The usual dose rates for a urea supplement are between 30 and 60 g/day for grass-fed cattle, up to 1% of a beef cattle feedlot ration (or about 100 g/day), and about 10 g/day for sheep.

Urea is not fed to horses, even though urea is hydrolysed by the bacteria in the horse's large intestine and the N from absorbed ammonia can be incorporated into protein. However, this does not occur in large enough amounts to make a significant contribution to the horse's N balance (Martin *et al.*, 1996). Of more concern are the possible adverse effects of urea. Horses which suffer from urea poisoning show neurological symptoms, e.g. head pressing and staggering. These cases are rare, and horses have to eat a very large amount of urea to cause them. Nevertheless, we should be watchful, and remember that horses grazing in the same paddock as cattle may investigate urea/molasses supplements.

References

Bailey, G. (2014). *Bloat in cattle and sheep*. PrimeFact 416, 3rd edn. Sydney, NSW: Dept. Primary Industries. Available at: www.dpi.nsw.gov.au/__data/assets/pdf_file/0009/111411/Bloat-in-cattle-and-sheep.pdf (accessed 30 December 2020).

Barry, T.N. and McNabb, W.C. (1999). The implications of condensed tannins on the nutritive value of temperate forages fed to ruminants. *British Journal of Nutrition* 81(4): 263–272.

Beef Cattle Research Council (2019). *Acidosis*. Available at: www.beefresearch.ca/research-topic.cfm/acidosis-63 (accessed 30 December 2020).

Cheng, K.J., McAllister, T.A., Popp, J.D., Hristov, A.N., Mir, Z. and Shin, H.T. (1998). A review of bloat in feedlot cattle. *Journal of Animal Science* 76(1): 299–308.

Dunkel, B. (2008). Diagnosis and treatment of non-infectious and infectious foal diarrhoea. *Pferdeheilkunde* 24 (4): 529–539.

Iowa State University (2020). *Ulceration of the Pars Oesophagea (Gastric Ulcers; Ulcers)*. Available from: www.vetmed.iastate.edu/vdpam/FSVD/swine/index-diseases/gastric-ulcers (accessed 30 December 2020).

Lester, G.D., Robertson, I. and Secombe, C. (2008). *Risk Factors for Gastric Ulceration in Thoroughbred Racehorses*. RIRDC Publ No 08/061. Available at: www.agrifutures.com.au/product/risk-factors-for-gastric-ulceration-in-thoroughbred-racehorses/ (accessed 30 December 2020).

Majak, W., Hall, J.W. and McCaughey, W.P. (1995). Pasture management strategies for reducing the risk of legume bloat in cattle. *Journal of Animal Science* 73(5): 1493–1498.

Martin, R.G., McMeniman, N.P., Norton, B.W. and Dowsett, K.F. (1996). Utilization of endogenous and dietary urea in the large intestine of the mature horse. *British Journal of Nutrition* 76(3): 373–386.

Meganck, V., Hoflack, G. and Opsomer, G. (2014). Advances in prevention and therapy of neonatal dairy calf diarrhoea: a systematical review with emphasis on colostrum management and fluid therapy. *Acta Veterinaria Scandinavica* 56:75–82.

Morgante, M. (2009). Blood gas analyses, ruminal and blood pH, urine and faecal pH in dairy cows during subacute ruminal acidosis. *Comparative Clinical Pathology* 18: 229–232.

Noah's Arkive (undated). *Image F27734. Healed rumen ulcer*. Available at: https://noahsarkive.cldavis.org/cgi-bin/show_image_info_detail.cgi?image=F27734 (accessed 30 December 2020).

Nation, P. (undated). Image F04081. *Liver necrotic hepatitis, Fusobacterium necrophorum*. Noah's Arkive. Available at: https://noahsarkive.cldavis.org/cgi-bin/show_image_info_detail.cgi?image=F04081 (accessed 30 December 2020).

Parkes, H. and Shilton, C. (2019). *Urea poisoning in cattle*. AgNote No. K46. Darwin, NT: Department of Primary Industry and Resources. Available at: https://dpir.nt.gov.au/__data/assets/pdf_file/0003/233058/796.pdf (accessed 30 December 2020).

Patterson-Kane, J.C., Karikoski, N.P. and McGowan, C.M. (2018). Paradigm shifts in understanding equine laminitis. *The Veterinary Journal* 231: 33–40.

Reference Advisory Group on Fermentative Acidosis of Ruminants (RAGFAR) (2007). *Ruminal Acidosis – Aetiopathogenesis, Prevention and Treatment*. Australian Veterinary Association, Sydney, Australia. Available at: www.researchgate.net/publication/279748378_Ruminal_Acidosis_-_aetiopathogenesis_prevention_and_treatment_A_review_for_veterinarians_and_nutritional_professionals (accessed 30 December 2020).

Rhouma, M. (2017). Post weaning diarrhea in pigs: risk factors and non-colistin-based control strategies. *Acta Veterinaria Scandinavica* 59: 31.

Steele, M.A., AlZahal, O., Hook, S.E., Croom, J. and McBride, B.W. (2009). Ruminal acidosis and the rapid onset of ruminal parakeratosis in a mature dairy cow: a case report. *Acta Veterinaria Scandinavica* 51: 39.

Steele, M.A., Penner, G.B., Chaucheyras-Durand, F. and Guan, L.L. (2016). Development and physiology of the rumen and the lower gut: Targets for improving gut health. *Journal of Dairy Science* 99(6): 4955–4966.

University of Minnesota Extension (2018). *Colic in your horse*. Available at: www.extension.umn.edu/horse-health/colic-your-horse (accessed 30 December 2020).

Zhai, S.-L. Wen, X.-H., Luo, M.-L., Lv, D.-H. and Wei, W.K. (2013). Ruminal impaction due to *Ficus esquiroliana* Levl. in Boer goats. *Springerplus* 2: 608.

Zhao, C., Liu, G., Li, X., Guan, Y., Wang, Y., Yuan, X., Sun, G., Wang, Z. and Li, X. (2018). Inflammatory mechanism of rumenitis in dairy cows with subacute ruminal acidosis. *BMC Veterinary Research* 14: 135.

14 Grazing behaviour – diet selection and pasture intake

The nutritional environment of grazing animals

Grazing animals exist in an environment which has varied climate, landform, soil type, and pasture composition and structure characteristics. This 'spatial' dimension is affected by 'temporal' factors – changes in time which vary from long-term to short-term effects.

These spatial and temporal factors get greatest expression when animals are managed extensively. Extensive grazing management is where animals are put into a (generally large) area and left there for several months. Stocking rates for this kind of management are low to very low, e.g. 1.1 adult beef cow/ha (about 0.4 adult/acre) in New Zealand North Island hill country, 1 adult dry cow/4 ha in Manitoba grasslands, to 10 adult dry cattle /km^2 in arid northern Australia. In these environments, grazing management is by set stocking and continuous grazing (see Chapter 15).

Spatial scales vary from very large to very small (O'Reagain and Schwartz, 1995). They are:

- Region or biome: large tracts which are distinguished by different climate, soil and vegetation types, e.g. northern Australian pastoral regions, Mediterranean grasslands, African savannas, American prairies or the Eurasian steppe.
- Landscape: areas of different types of vegetation within different topographies, e.g. hill slopes (shaded or sunny), creek banks, fertile valleys, eroded hill tops, wooded areas, and so on (Fig. 14.1). Farms occupy one or more landscapes, depending on how large they are and how varied are the plant communities within them.

Animals have their home ranges within landscapes. These are places where a herd or flock lives and finds its feed, water and shelter. 'Home range' is defined by Burt (1943; cited by Powell and Mitchell, 2012) as 'That area traversed by an individual in its normal activities of food gathering, mating, and caring for young.' The size of a home range is influenced by topography, vegetation type and quality (larger in times of low vegetation availability), season, availability of water, and climatic conditions (in droughts, home ranges contract with animals remaining close to permanent water sources).

Different species and breeds have different sized home ranges, and some individuals explore more widely than others. Animals often divide into separate groups of breeding females with offspring and a few dominant males, and young male groups; these have different home ranges. Reported home ranges for cattle vary from 100 to 400 ha (measured on Spanish pastures; Lazo, 1995; Perez *et al.*, 2017) to 500 ha (in a 2800 ha semi-arid region in Zimbabwe; Zengeya *et al.*, 2011). Sheep may have several home ranges, which will change depending on the season. These home ranges can be modified by feed supply, social structure and size of the social group. The home ranges of goats vary from about 1.5 km^2 in places where water and feed are plentiful, to as much as 375 km^2 in arid regions. Males have a larger home range than females (Parkes *et al.*, 1996). Home ranges for wild horses vary from 50 to 90 km^2 in size (Wilson *et al.*, 1992). Groups of young males are more mobile and tend to move to areas where the water supply is less reliable. They may require water only once per day in summer and every second day in winter.

- Patch: the size of a grazing patch varies from as little as 5 m^2 to as much as 100 m^2, i.e. from a single plant or small group of similar plants to a paddock of sown pasture, an area around a watering point, or an area of avoidance near urine and manure patches. Illius and Hodgson (1996) define a grazing patch as 'an area over which the instantaneous intake rate is fairly constant'. Figure 14.2(a) shows examples of grazing patches. The cattle graze at those patches where they have to expend the least amount of energy in finding and prehending feed and/or where they can find new, green leaves.

DOI: 10.1079/9781786394453.0014

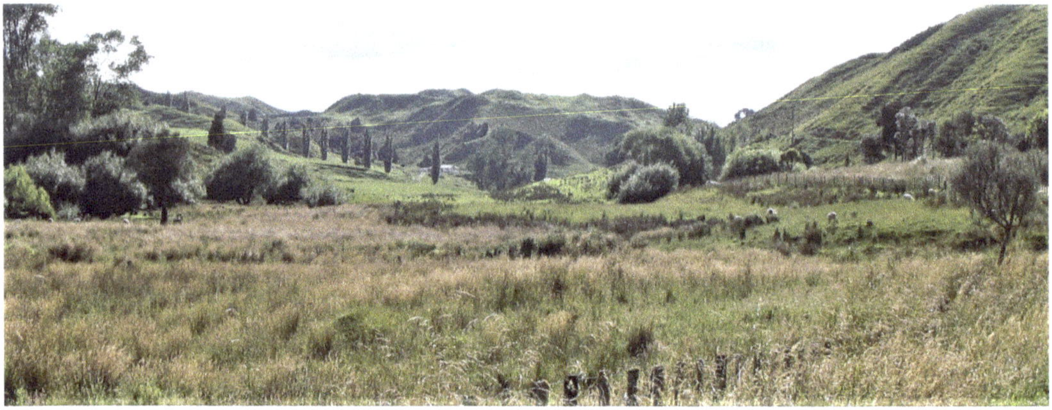

Fig. 14.1. Spatial grazing habitat scales – an example of a grazing landscape. (Copyright: Gordon McL. Dryden.)

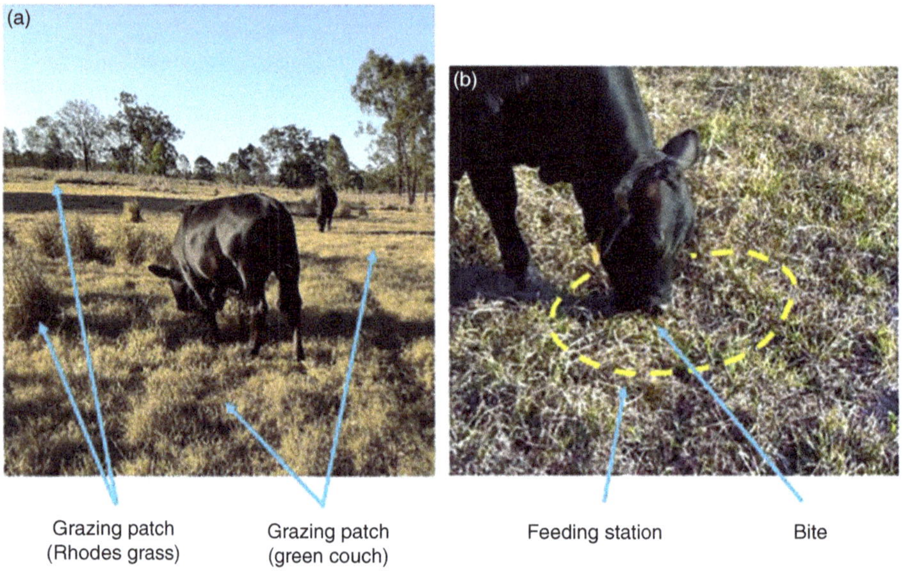

Fig. 14.2. Brangus heifers grazing a mature grass pasture. **(a)** The pasture consists of green couch (*Cynodon dactylon*) with areas of taller clumps of mature Pioneer Rhodes grass (*Chloris gayana*); each plant type comprises a different grazing patch. The cattle concentrate on green couch, although they seek out new green Rhodes grass leaves which are hidden within the dry, stemmy tussocks. **(b)** The feeding station is about 0.5 m^2; each bite concentrates on the shorter green grass, avoiding the longer dry, over-mature clumps. (Copyright: Gordon McL. Dryden.)

- Feeding station and bite: a feeding station (Fig. 14.2b) is the piece of a patch which the animal grazes while standing without moving more than a pace or two. There may be several feeding stations within a grazing patch. At the minimum, a grazing station consists of a single piece of plant material which is prehended, i.e. a 'grazing bite'. This can be a single leaf or several leaves, a piece of stem, or a flower or a seed head.

Landform factors which affect the choice of grazing location are described by Bailey *et al.* (1996) and Hinch (1999). Each of these factors operates at a different spatial scale:

- Topography: animals will graze according to the effects that sunlight and slope have on pasture composition and quality; and on their own comfort, e.g. in cold climates animals prefer the sunny face.
- Vegetation: quality and quantity of vegetation influence the movement of animals to their most preferred plant groupings. Grazing animals will select nutrient-rich sites more frequently than less productive sites. Cattle, horses and sheep are able to identify and remember grazing patches which have a rich supply of preferred feed.
- Water: the distance that animals are prepared to graze away from water differs between species and individuals. Under extensive grazing management this determines the size of the grazing area that is available to each animal. The concept of 'effective grazing area' is discussed in Chapter 15.

Temporal scales vary from very long to short. There are several ways that we can think about change over time, but it is useful to consider the time scales over which the nutritional environment may change. For example:

- Era- or decade-long changes in climate or weather patterns (e.g. global warming), and long-term changes in soil type and/or fertility. These changes influence the species composition and nutritional quality of pastures.
- Changes which occur over several years: the species composition of a pasture can change between years because of the effects of grazing pressure on preferred plants during continuous stocking, or changes in weather on a similar time scale, or because we have replaced the pasture with something different. Similarly, we have changes in growth rate and body composition, and thus nutrient requirements, over an animal's lifetime.
- Medium-term changes in pasture quality and animal performance which occur over weeks or months include changes in plant chemical composition, morphology and stage of maturity (vegetative, seed-set, maturation) which all change with changing seasons, i.e. over several months. These changes can occur during rotational or cell grazing, or over irrigation cycles. On a similar time scale, we have changes in pregnancy and lactation and consequent changes in nutrient requirements.
- Short-term changes: the chemical composition of individual plants can change within a day, e.g. changes in water, starch or oxalate contents from morning to evening.

Depending on the time scale we are considering, temporal changes are driven by weather, climate, soil fertility, plant metabolism (responding to the environment), animal physiological status (responding to our management) or the interactions between the grazing animal and the pastures it eats.

Foraging behaviour – how animals interact with their grazing environment

Foraging behaviour determines the feed intake and nutritional status of grazing animals. Foraging is influenced by:

- Pasture morphology: the shape and structure of the pasture, especially its height and density. Pastures which are made up of different grasses and legumes have different structures. Tropical pastures often contain tall and open plants, especially if the main components are grasses which have a tussock growth form. On the other hand, pastures which consist of temperate species (such as annual ryegrass pastures) are shorter and denser.
- Nutrient stratification: the location of nutrient-rich leaves within the sward.
- Stage of maturity of the plants in the pasture, which determines the pasture's nutritive value (see Chapter 15).
- Plant defences: the presence and amount of tannins and other plant defences against grazing.
- Animal physiology: effects of lactation and pregnancy on nutrient requirements and voluntary intake.
- Animal factors affecting feed intake: mouth shape and size, bite mass, biting rate and diet selection.
- Animal 'personality': effects of genotype, experience, learning, and social dominance on foraging behaviour (Garcia *et al.*, 2020).
- Herbage allowance: the amount of pasture allocated to each animal as influenced by stocking rate, pre-determined pasture utilization rate or the required residual dry matter (DM), or time allowed for grazing.

The interrelationships between these things are illustrated in Fig. 14.3.

Optimal foraging: Animals select grazing patches and feeding stations which give the best return on the energy invested in grazing. They try to find grazing sites where the pasture is dense, not too short or too long, and relatively immature. If they are browsing, they try to find browse which has no thorns and is low in tannins. If they can manage to find sites which have all of these characteristics, they will maximize their nutrient intake at minimum energy cost for grazing. This behaviour is called 'optimal foraging'.

Genotype influences grazing behaviour: There are grazing behaviours which are characteristic of different species (e.g. sheep, cattle, horses, goats) and breeds, and most members of these animal classes share these characteristics. For example, Merino sheep form flocks when grazing, whereas British breed sheep forage more individually and form flocks less often (Elliott, 1996), and Highland cattle are less selective in choosing pasture plants than more productive breeds (Pauler *et al.*, 2020).

Individual animals respond in a variety of ways to their environment and to the other animals that they live with (Neave *et al.*, 2018), and these personality characteristics impact on how they use grazing lands. Overall, these can be categorized as 'fear or reactivity', 'sociability' and 'exploratory' personalities.

'Exploratory' animals investigate more of a new environment and are more likely to move away from others in the flock as they do this. This behaviour helps them to find new grazing patches and to investigate new feeds and may be responsible for preferences shown for different localities (e.g. flat or hilly ground), and the different distances that individual cattle in rangelands will graze away from water (Chapter 15). Sociable animals tend to remain in groups and this can limit their access to high-quality grazing patches.

In non-grazing environments, 'exploratory' behaviour may be expressed in a greater willingness to adapt to a novel environment. For example, to sample concentrate feed supplements, adapt from pasture to a feedlot, or when dairy heifers are introduced to machine milking.

Animal personality is responsible for the differences between fast ('fearful' or 'reactive' animals) and slow eaters (more dominant animals), and various social behaviours such as leader/follower, learning, and so on.

These behaviours are consistent for each individual, although they can change when the animal is faced with management controls such as a high

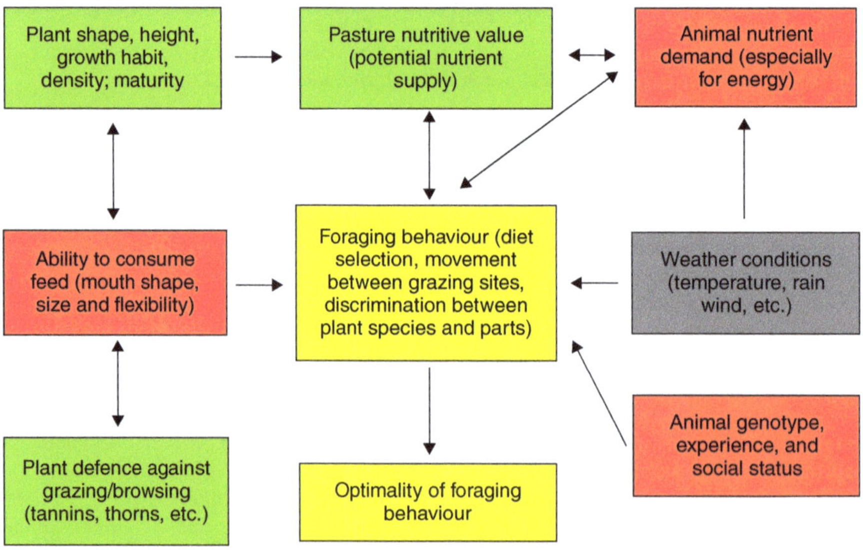

Fig. 14.3. The environmental, plant and animal factors which influence foraging behaviour. (Copyright: Gordon McL. Dryden.)

stocking rate, provision of supplements, rotational (or cell) grazing systems, changed herbage allowance, etc.

Some cattle personality characteristics are moderately heritable and so can be selected for (Garcia *et al.*, 2020). However, we need to be careful about this because animals, especially beef and dairy cattle, are exposed to several different environments in the course of their productive life and a behaviour which fits them for one situation may not be appropriate for another.

Feed intake by grazing animals

Factors affecting pasture intake: The interrelationships between pasture condition and grazing behaviour, and their effects on pasture intake, are summarized in Fig. 14.4.

Grazing animals have different types of biting/chewing action: Grazing (or prehension) bites by ruminants are made when plant material is collected by the tongue, drawn into the mouth and compressed against the dental pad with the tongue and lower incisors. The mouthful is then cut from the rest of the plant by jerking the head sideways and upwards. Sheep and goats also use their lips in prehension, while horses use lips and upper and lower teeth (see Chapter 3).

Chewing movements are then used to reduce the prehended feed into smaller particles and to form it into a bolus before swallowing. As well as helping to form a bolus, chewing breaks the plant cell walls so that the cell contents are released (Dryden *et al.*, 1995).

Further particle comminution occurs during rumination, which occurs when ruminant animals are resting from grazing. Rumination also releases cell contents, but its main effect is to reduce the particle size of undigested plant fibre and further expose cell walls to microbial digestion in the rumen. Rumination bites are not part of the feed prehension process. Horses and other non-ruminant herbivores make only grazing and bolus-forming bites.

Grazing bite mass has a major influence on feed intake: Bite mass, which is the weight of feed prehended in each mouthful, is the main factor which influences the daily feed intake of grazing animals. In each prehension bite grazing cattle consume 0.35–0.6 g of DM, and sheep 0.05–0.25 g DM, under optimum conditions. Cattle and sheep can

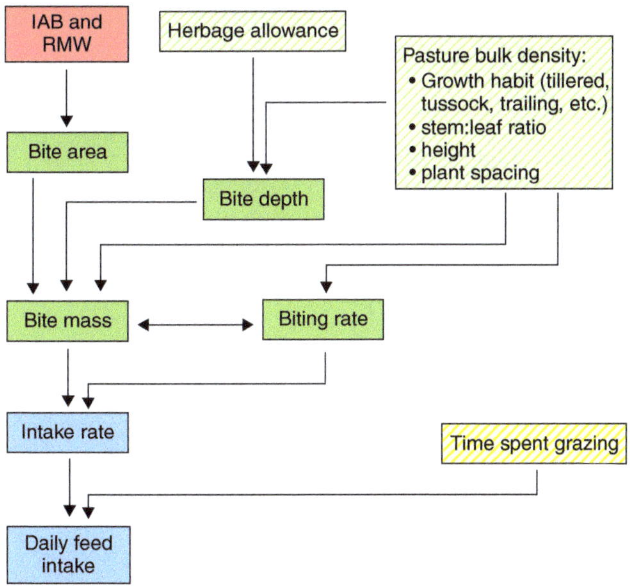

Fig. 14.4. Interrelationships between mouth shape (incisor arcade breadth, IAB, and relative muzzle width, RMW), grazing behaviour, pasture factors, time spent grazing, herbage allowance and feed intake. (Hatched boxes are those factors which can be influenced by management.) (Copyright: Gordon McL. Dryden.)

make 50 000 or more grazing bites in a day, but they make as few as 10 000 bites under less than optimum conditions. A 600 kg dairy cow producing 15 L of milk daily eats about 16.5 kg of DM each day (see Chapter 7); at a bite mass of 0.5 g DM this animal must make 33 000 prehension bites each day.

Mouth shape and size affect the size of grazing bites: There are four measurements of mouth shape and size which relate to the size of grazing bites (Fig. 14.5). These are the muzzle width (MW, the distance between the outer corners of the mouth), the incisor arcade breadth (IAB, the distance between the outer edges of the 4th incisors), the palatal width (PW, the distance between the molars), and the relative muzzle width (RMW = PW/MW). Animals with larger RMW can take larger bites, but they may not be able to select the composition of the bite as effectively as animals with narrower muzzles. Bite mass is also influenced by the depth of the mouth cavity.

Pasture composition and structure influence bite mass: Pasture species differ in their morphology, and in turn, pastures which are made up of different grasses and legumes differ in their density and structure. The grazing animal's feed intake is influenced by these characteristics of the pasture, principally through their effects on the animal's bite mass.

Pasture characteristics which reduce bite mass are:

- low pasture bulk density;
- trailing growth habit;
- plant maturity – due to a combination of increasing stem length and lignification (Chapter 15); and
- resistance to grazing due to the increasing stem content of ungrazed material, and/or to the generally higher stem:leaf ratio and fibre content of tall (often C4; see Chapter 15) plant species.

Bite mass may increase with increasing tiller (leaf) length and pasture height (Fig. 14.6), but there are varying responses to this (Moser and Jennings, 2007; Hirata *et al.*, 2011). As grasses become taller, the leaves are more widely spaced (the plant bulk density decreases) and this can make it difficult for grazing animals to prehend a full mouthful. On the other hand, bite mass is greater if the pasture consists of a sward of tall but densely packed leaves. Cattle grazing tall plants (e.g. forage maize (forage corn)) start eating at the lower part of the plant and progress upwards, and they can prehend one or more leaves at a time. Horses and sheep prefer shorter swards, but for cattle a tall sward gives the greatest ease of prehension and therefore the most efficient grazing.

Biting rate and grazing time: Biting rate is the number of prehension bites taken per hour. The time to take a bite includes the time it takes both to prehend the feed at the feeding station and to prepare a bolus of feed to be swallowed, and we could add the time it takes to walk to a new feeding station to search for and select feed. Note that 'biting rate' does not include the time or activity spent in ruminating.

Grazing time is the time spent harvesting feed. It does not include the time spent ruminating or resting, and some definitions exclude the time taken to find new grazing patches.

In general, both grazing time and biting rate decrease with increasing sward height, while bolus formation chewing and rumination chewing increase (Laca *et al.*, 1994; O'Reagain and McMeniman, 2002). Large bite masses may be associated with lower biting rates because either the bolus takes longer to be processed and swallowed, or the animal more easily meets its energy requirement from the larger bites.

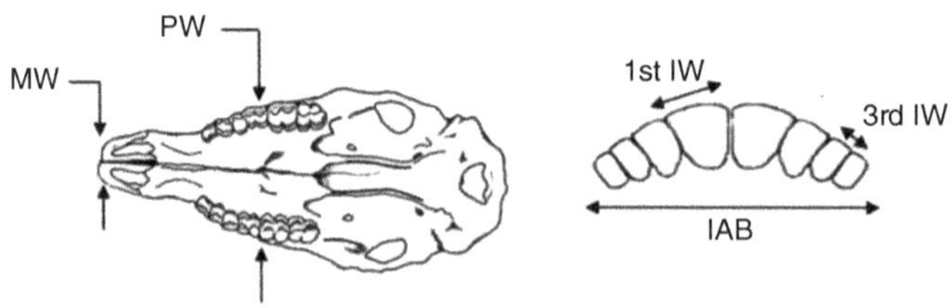

Fig. 14.5. Measurements of mouth and tooth morphology: muzzle width (MW) and palatal width (PW); the diagram shows the upper jaw. Incisor width (IW) and incisor arcade breadth (IAB); bottom jaw. (Adapted from Dryden, 2008; reproduced by permission.)

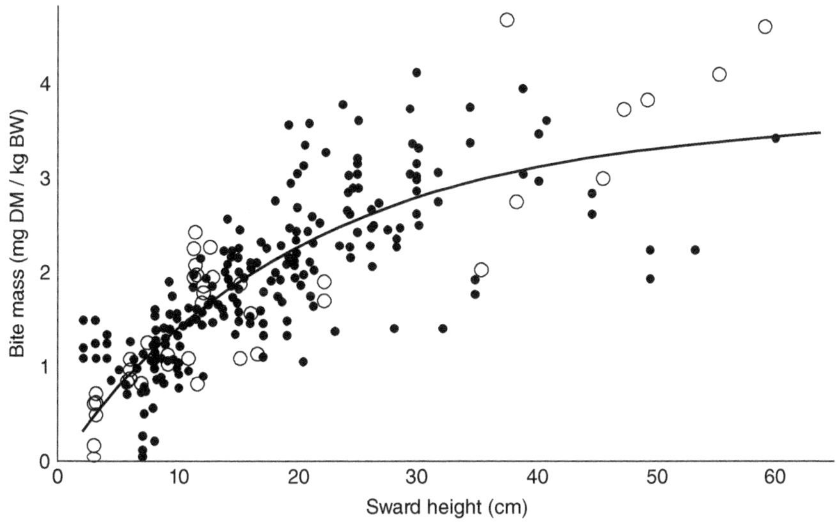

Fig. 14.6. Relationships between sward height and bite mass (small ruminants, open circles; cattle, closed circles). (From Boval and Sauvant, 2019; reproduced with permission.)

Consistently, grazing time and biting rate increase if animals are in sparse pastures, although in very sparse pastures animals may simply give up grazing.

Management can modify grazing behaviour: If grazing time is restricted by the time taken by twice-daily milking, or by high daytime temperatures, or when competition for feed works against maximizing bite mass, animals compensate by increasing their biting rate and moving more quickly between feeding stations. For example, when access to pasture is restricted by rotational grazing and/or milking, cows eat more quickly and their feed intake rate increases when they are released to pasture after the afternoon milking. While bite mass declines with reduced pasture DM availability or herbage allowance (Fig. 14.7), biting rate increases to try to maintain DM intake and satisfy the animal's hunger (Barrett *et al.*, 2001).

Herbage allowance: The amount of feed a grazing animal eats can be controlled by altering its herbage allowance, i.e. the daily amount of pasture DM that we allocate to each animal (Fig. 14.7). Herbage allowance is controlled by allowing grazing to a pre-determined pasture height or residual DM (see Chapter 15), or by adjusting the stocking rate (Chapter 15) or the size of the paddock or grazing strip, or the allowed grazing time.

Diet selection and its effect on nutrient intake and pasture quality

Grazing animals do not behave like lawnmowers. One of their most important interactions with pasture is diet selection, because this impacts on the animal's intake of nutrients and can affect the species composition of pastures.

Selection, palatability and preference ranking: Diet selection is the preference that an animal shows for certain plants or plant parts. We can say that a plant is chosen over another because the animal finds it to be more palatable. 'Palatability' implies that different feeds belong in a fixed hierarchy of desirability, but this is not correct. Because feed choices change in different circumstances it is better to talk of 'preference ranking' than 'palatability'.

Although animals generally prefer the more nutritious parts of pastures, preference does not necessarily equate to nutritive value and a less-preferred plant species can be just as nutritious as a preferred one.

Plant factors which influence feed choice: Grazing animals prefer to eat plants that are rich in available nutrients, especially energy and protein. Accordingly, they prefer to eat young, green leaf which they prefer over older green leaf or green stem. Dry leaves and stems are not preferred and may remain ungrazed even if they are the only material in the

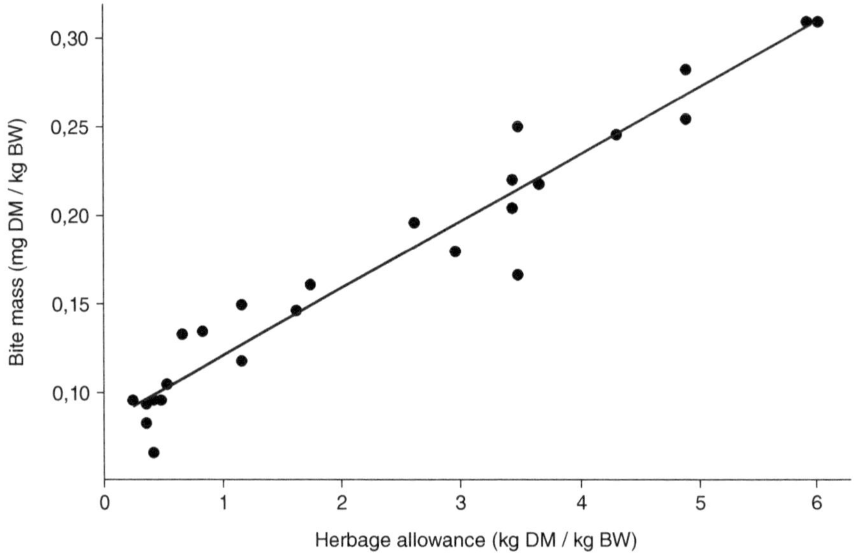

Fig. 14.7. The relationship between herbage allowance and pasture intake. (From Boval and Sauvant, 2019; reproduced with permission.)

pasture. Animals actively seek plants that require less chewing, i.e. that are less fibrous.

Preference is also affected by plant characteristics such as:

- Structure and shape, e.g. stem:leaf ratio; trailing, tillering or tussock growth habits; pasture density, etc.
- Maturity, which affects the plant's protein, mineral, non-structural carbohydrate and fibre contents.
- The presence of secondary substances and other plant defences against grazing or browsing.

Pasture species composition and the amount of feed on offer also influence selection. Preference rankings change with changes in pasture species composition over different seasons, and the range of accepted plants becomes much wider in droughts and when the more highly preferred plants have been removed from the pasture. We can see this illustrated by the grazing preferences of sheep in northern Australian rangelands (Fig. 14.8). Sheep greatly prefer Mitchell grass (*Astrebla* spp.) and avoid Flinders grass (*Iseilema* spp.) which they eat only when it is immature. Much of their nutrition comes from annual plants (grasses and legumes) which make up a very small part of the pasture (shown as 'other' in Fig. 14.8).

Animal factors which affect diet selection include (Lynch *et al.*, 1992):

- Species and breed differences: smaller animals are more selective than larger ones. This is because mouth and digestive tract sizes scale directly with body size (W) while energy requirements scale with metabolic size ($W^{0.75}$; Chapter 8). This means that the maintenance energy requirement of an adult is lower in proportion to its capacity to consume feed than is the case with young animals.
- The animal's nutrient demand: animals which have a high demand for nutrients may graze less selectively than less productive animals of a similar size. Male cattle grow faster, and thus have higher nutrient requirements, than female cattle of the same age, and they have a wider range of plant species preferences. As well, lactating females have a higher nutrient demand and graze less selectively than non-lactating animals.
- Animal age: animals of different classes (e.g. calves, heifers, cows) eat diets with different nutrient contents, e.g. calves and heifers consistently selected diets with more protein than those eaten by steers and cows, except when the pasture had only low levels of protein (Grings *et al.*, 2001). Age differences may reflect the effect of

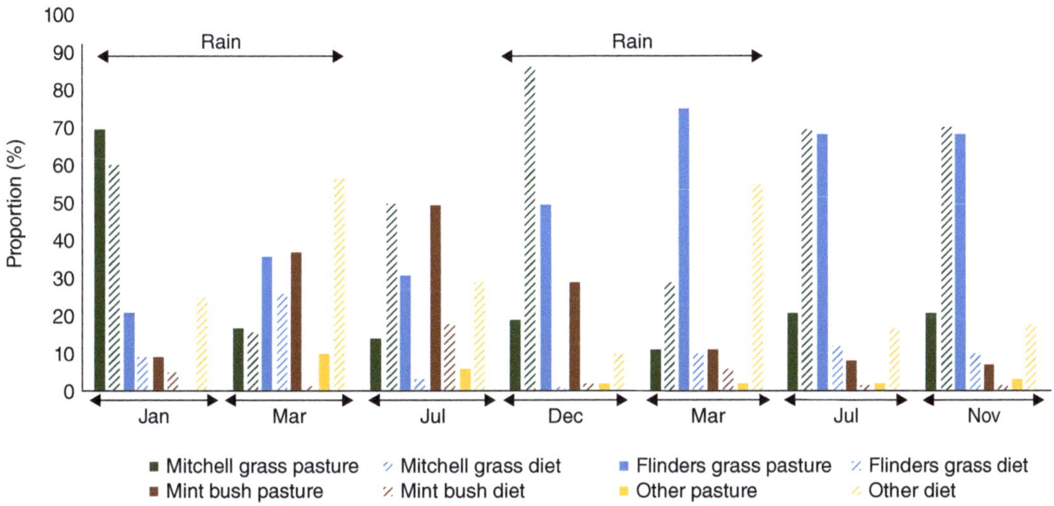

Fig. 14.8. Seasonal changes in diet selection by sheep grazing a Mitchell grass pasture in northern Australia as a result of changing pasture species composition between seasons. Solid bars show the proportions of plant species in the pasture, hatched bars show the proportions of plants in oesophageal extrusa (i.e. the diet). Mint bush is *Streptoglossa adscendens*. (Data from Lorimer, 1978; reproduced with permission.)

different body size (see above), and young animals are able to select higher-quality diets because they have narrower muzzles than older animals.

- Previous experience of the pasture: naïve animals consume different diets than animals which are experienced, or which have learnt from experienced animals. Learning involves knowing where different plant species occur, the taste, smell and feel of plants, and how the animal feels after it has eaten them (see below). In this regard, 'fearful' animals are less likely to explore the pasture and sample novel plants. Grazing animals appear to have an excellent memory for the location of preferred feeds and become very proficient at finding their preferred feed.

Different abilities to prehend the selected diet lead to differences in the quality of the selected diet: Sheep have a relatively narrow muzzle so they can select with great accuracy. Sheep actively select green, leafy material; they can select individual grass tillers and can graze close to the soil. They select strongly for the plants that they prefer and avoid others (O'Reagain and McMeniman, 2002). This highly selective behaviour is illustrated by an experiment by Lynch *et al.* (1992) who found that sheep which were offered a high-quality grass/clover pasture selected for grass leaf and avoided clover, grass stem or dead material. The sheep grazed within 0–4 cm from the ground where 95% of the green leaf was located. These workers showed that sheep could select a single species as 80% of their diet during a period when the species was only 1% of the herbage available. This ability to graze selectively allows sheep to generally select a higher quality (i.e. less fibrous) diet than either goats or cattle grazing the same pasture (Norton *et al.*, 1990).

The diet of sheep in arid rangelands is variable. Grasses are usually the most preferred species, although forbs are eaten more in wet times, and shrubs in dry conditions (Dawson and Ellis, 1994). The grass species selected by sheep under extensive management tends to reflect the relative abundance of these species in the pasture, although some species are strongly selected or avoided (see Fig. 14.8).

Cattle have an uncleft upper lip and a broad dental arcade, which means that they cannot manipulate individual plants or plant parts to the same degree as sheep, goats or horses. Nevertheless, the relatively broad and inflexible mouth of cattle does not prevent them from selecting young, green plant material in preference to dry material because they use their long tongues to prehend plant material. Cattle generally harvest grasses and legumes but can browse on shrubs and trees, although their mouth parts are not well designed for this.

Cattle show grazing patch selectivity and prefer to graze tall, dense, dark-green pastures, and will graze in riparian areas or pasture regrowth after burning (Hinch, 1999). In sward pastures, cattle first graze the upper strata, where the concentration of leaf is highest (Ison *et al.*, 2019) and reject plants growing near faeces or urine patches.

Goats eat a wide variety of plants. They can eat foliage, twigs, bark, flowers, plant litter, seeds, fungi and roots (Parkes *et al.*, 1996). Goats eat both ground storey plants and browse species; browse is preferred over grass and forbs, although they select more actively growing grass during the wetter seasons. They eat more browse than sheep, partly because of a greater preference for some of these species and also because they browse higher (up to 2 m) so more of the palatable trees and shrubs in their range are accessible to them.

Horses are grazers; in natural conditions their main diet component is grass, although they will consume roots, bark, buds and fruit. They use sight to orientate themselves in the paddock, and smell and touch to identify the species and parts of the plant that they want to eat. Horses may use their feet to manipulate feed into a suitable consistency for eating.

Horses prefer grass to browse, and shorter grass to long, rank grass – they graze and re-graze preferred patches and by doing this they produce and maintain patches of short grass in areas of tall pasture. They select the most preferred plant species before moving to less palatable species. They may select within a single plant, e.g. eating only the top leaves of the taller (10–20 cm) grasses, and also selecting seed heads.

Diet composition is affected by stocking rate and social ranking: Dominant animals tend to monopolize their preferred grazing patches while subordinate animals graze lower quality patches. When competition for feed is increased by increased stocking rate (e.g. goats; Wan *et al.*, 2018) there is less discrimination between plant species and more time spent grazing.

Why do animals choose to eat certain foods and not others, and how do they learn about their environment? There are three behaviours which appear to strongly influence dietary preferences:

- Neophobia: fear of the new, preference for staying with the known. Animals which are inherently more fearful are more likely to be wary of novel feeds, while less fearful individuals will explore their environment (e.g. a new paddock) and find quality feed patches.
- Post-ingestive feedback: learning about the consequences of eating particular feeds. How the animal feels after it has eaten a particular feed is a very important source of information and is discussed below.
- Imitating their mothers or others in the herd: learning and memory inform activities such as the selection of grazing patches and the plants within these, the location of watering points, and how to use feeding equipment (troughs, hay racks and urea dispensers).

Although not proven, it seems reasonable to assume that these behaviours have become established because they contribute to the survival of genotypes which find highly nutritious foods the most acceptable. Taste, odour (smell) and nutrient content (probably experienced through post-ingestive feedback) are important factors which influence feed choice (Roura and Navarro, 2018).

Post-ingestive feedback: Animals learn about their nutritional environment by a form of operant conditioning called post-ingestive feedback (Provenza, 1996). Operant conditioning is when an animal consciously behaves in a certain way because of the consequences of doing or of not doing that action.

Animals learn by experiencing the good or bad effects of eating particular plants and they associate these effects with the plant's smell, taste and texture. The by-products of microbial fermentation (i.e. volatile fatty acids) are quickly absorbed from the rumen and provide a rapid indication of the nutritional value of food and help to modify the animal's liking for that particular flavour (Villalba and Provenza, 1997). Negative experiences can make animals reluctant to eat certain plants. This has been shown in sheep which reject feeds that make them ill and they remember this negative effect (Thorhallsdotter *et al.*, 1987). By contrast, animals develop preferences for the flavours of familiar foods that they have associated with the positive post-ingestive effects of nutrient intake. For example, we can get sheep to eat unpalatable feeds like gliricidia leaf by getting them to associate gliricidia with the positive feedback they get from eating a protein meal (Karda, 2000).

Dietary preferences and dietary overlap: When different types of animals graze the same pasture there is often some similarity about their preferences for the plants in the pasture. This dietary overlap must be taken into account when we set stocking rates.

If there is no overlap, then we can treat the part of the pasture that each animal type prefers as separate feed sources. If the preferred diets do overlap (e.g. annual grasses in Fig. 14.9), then there will be competition for these components which can result in over-grazing.

What is the effect of diet selection on the animal's nutrient intake? Selective grazing results in animals consuming a diet which is of better nutritional quality than the total plant material on offer (Fig. 14.10 and Table 14.1). This outcome of selective grazing is essential in maintaining life and productivity

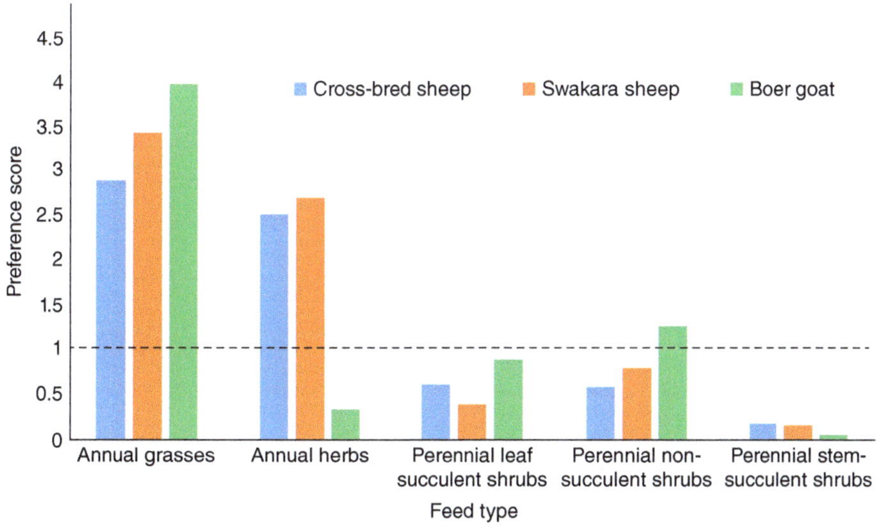

Fig. 14.9. Examples of the preference rankings of different animal types and different degrees of overlap in the selected diets of goats and sheep grazing grass and shrub vegetation in the succulent Karoo in the winter rainfall period. Bars above the dotted line indicate positive preference for the plant type, below the line indicate rejection of the plant type. (Drawn from data in Schroeder *et al.*, 2019; used with permission. Copyright: Gordon McL. Dryden.)

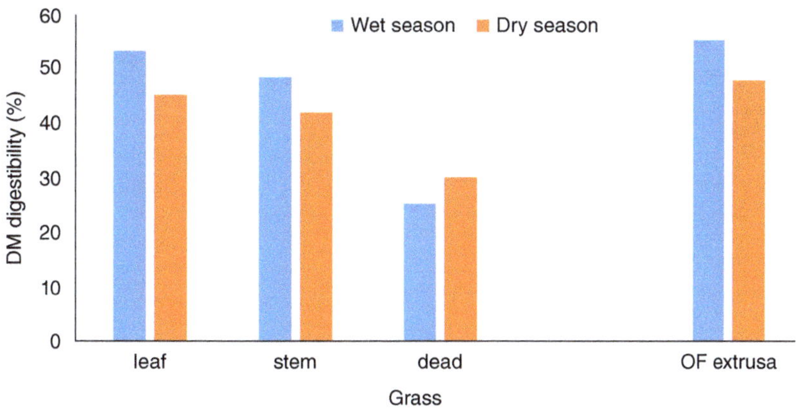

Fig. 14.10. Seasonal differences in diets selected by sheep grazing an *Andropogon gayanus* pasture in Colombia as indicated by the composition of extrusa collected from oesophageal fistulae (OF). The high dry matter (DM) digestibility of the eaten diet illustrates the preference of sheep for leaf rather than stem and dead material. (From Bohnert *et al.*, 1986; reproduced with permission.)

Table 14.1. Nutritive value of pastures and diets selected by grazing sheep. (From Douglas *et al.*, 1995; reproduced with permission.)

Constituent	Birdsfoot trefoil (*Lotus corniculatus*)	Mixture (trefoil and lucerne)	Lucerne (*Medicago sativa*)
Total N (g/kg DM)			
Offered	26.2	35.7	32.5
Selected	40.2	47.3	47.2
Acid detergent fibre (g/kg DM)			
Offered	356	277	286
Selected	205	160	163
Neutral detergent fibre (g/kg/DM)			
Offered	446	389	413
Selected	255	238	247
Organic matter digestibility (%)			
Offered	66.8	72.3	71.5
Selected	81.1	85.7	85.2

in rangelands, where the whole-plant protein and P contents, and digestibilities of native grasses, can fall to 3–5% protein and 0.05% P (DM basis) and DM digestibilities to 40% or less. These levels are below even the maintenance requirements of cattle, let alone the requirements of pregnant cows which have to find adequate nutrient intakes from unproductive pastures during the dry season.

Diet selection and animal health: Apart from the positive effects of diet selection on nutrient intake, there are also some positive effects on health. Sheep that are infected with internal parasites (e.g. barber's pole worm, *Haemonchus contortus*) are able to detect the effect of feeds containing substances that kill the parasites and will quickly alter their diet to include more feeds of that type (Poli *et al.*, 2018; and see Chapter 12).

Animals avoid toxic plants if they can recognize them. Animals which have grown up with toxic plants in their environment learn about them when they eat them in small amounts and experience some of the adverse effects. However, animals do not always avoid plants which will harm them. An example is horses eating grasses such as kikuyu (*Pennisetum clandestinum*) or *Setaria* spp., which contain amounts of oxalic acid which bind Ca and cause the disease osteodystrophia fibrosa (or 'bighead'; see Chapter 12). Sometimes animals cannot avoid eating poisonous plant material – an example is when dust formed from dry, mature *Pimelea* spp. leaves get mixed with pasture grasses and is eaten or inhaled. *Pimelea* causes the often fatal 'St. George disease' in cattle in northern Australia.

A synthesis – using knowledge about grazing behaviour in the practical management of cattle, sheep and horses

In order to effectively manage our farm, we need to understand the landscape in detail. This means that we know how vegetation (pasture species, weeds, potentially poisonous plants, browse trees, etc.) is distributed, where water points are accessible, and how soil type affects the nutritive value of pasture. Further, we must also know how the nutritional environment changes between seasons and years, so that we can provide, as far as possible, feed of adequate availability and quality.

Vegetation type and quality, soil type, topography (slope, aspect, hilliness), latitude and weather conditions all influence how far animals will travel, and their distribution at both a landscape and a grazing patch level.

Manage for pastures or animals or both? We can either manage to maintain healthy, productive pastures and get even grazing use over the whole paddock or farm, or we can manage to get best animal performance. These two objectives are different and require different approaches. However, pasture is our basic resource while animal products provide our income, so we have to try to optimize both of these.

Good pasture management means that we have to control grazing at both large and small spatial scales. Over-grazing can be a major issue with animals under extensive management. If animals consistently re-visit areas of their home range perhaps to re-graze new growth or prefer to graze sunny faces or areas with particular plants, then they are likely to overgraze these patches with the consequent loss of the preferred species. On the other hand, shady hill faces, very steep slopes, heavily wooded areas, areas with less preferred pasture species, and those parts of the landscape which are distant from watering points, are likely to be less utilized.

While animals identify preferred grazing patches at a landscape scale, we get areas of concentrated use even in small paddocks. 'Attaining more even use within paddocks should therefore be viewed as a separate management objective, requiring different techniques, to obtaining more effective use of the landscape as a whole' (Hunt *et al.*, 2007).

To spread pasture usage as evenly as possible we should carefully plan paddock sizes and fencing alignment. Fences can be both physical and 'virtual' (CSIRO, 2019; Lomax *et al.*, 2019). In addition, we can control grazing by strategically placing water points (see Chapter 15) and supplement feeding stations, including salt licks, in under-used areas. Fencing, water and supplement station placement will influence grazing at both landscape and grazing patch scales.

On the other hand, we will often get best animal performance if they are allowed to graze selectively in an environment which contains a range of different pasture species. The greater variety of plants provides better overall nutrition, and perhaps relieves the boredom experienced when animals always have to eat the same plants.

The most valuable pastures species for extensive grazing management are those which are palatable,

Table 14.2. Management practices and their effects on landscape use and animal performance. (Adapted from Bailey, 2005; reproduced with permission.)

Management practice	Effect on the habitat	Effect on animals	Expected change in grazing distribution
Water point placement	Horizontal and vertical distances between water and grazing patches will be reduced	Less energy expended in moving between water and grazing; more grazing area available	More even distribution of grazing over the landscape
Installing tracks	Better access to parts of the landscape which are otherwise difficult to get to	Less effort needed to get to otherwise inaccessible grazing	Increased use of the landscape
Fencing	More even grazing pressure over the whole landscape	Animals are required to use otherwise less-preferred sites	Animals are confined to certain areas and excluded from others
Burning and fertilizing pasture	Fertilization or grass regrowth after burning improves pasture nutritional value; burning removes litter, changes pasture species, but removes potentially usable feed	Nutrient content of consumed feed improves	Animals are attracted to new plant growth, or to growth which is nutritionally enriched by fertilization
Placement of supplement feeding stations	May increase the grazing pressure at these sites	Nutrient supplements may encourage greater use of low-quality pasture; improved animal performance	Animals are attracted to grazing areas near these stations
Animal species or breed selection	May change the preference ranking of pasture species and thus pasture species composition	Improved animal performance because of improved habitat use	Better adapted animals will use more of the landscape
Choice of grazing system	More intensive systems give more even use of the habitat	Performance may be reduced by requiring most of the pasture to be eaten (see Chapter 15)	Distribution, and thus pasture use, is controlled by the manager

perennial and productive – these are called '3P' species (Chapter 15). Identifying these plants is a first task for good animal management in extensive regions.

With careful management we can use information about how animals find, select and eat pasture to optimize our management of both animals and pastures. We should:

- Give young animals preferential treatment. They need high-quality feed because they have higher nutrient requirements in relation to their size than older animals (except for lactating females), and also for the relationships between mouth size, nutrient requirements and body size described above. Ways of providing good feed to young animals are described in Chapters 15 and 17.
- Mix naïve animals with experienced stock, where this is appropriate. Young animals usually learn from their mothers about the pastoral environment – how to recognize highly ranked pasture species and the mechanisms of grazing; but they will also learn from experienced animals of their own age.
- Be familiar with animals' diet preferences and how this behaviour will, over time, affect the pasture species composition. Be aware that preferences will change with seasons, as the species composition of the pasture changes.
- Be able to recognize, and to incorporate into pastures, the local 3P plant species. If possible, avoid developing plant monocultures when planting pastures or over-sowing into an established pasture.
- Provide animals with dense, young pasture (this will probably not be possible during dry or cold seasons) and try to match pasture height to the preferences of cattle, sheep and horses. Where possible, and under careful control, let animals develop the pasture profile that suits them but note that this behaviour will be inconsistent with the uniform use of pasture and the persistence of preferred species.
- Consider how to subdivide the landscape – separate sunny and shaded hill faces into different paddocks, give access to a variety of pasture species, and encourage animals to graze the whole pasture by providing tracks, bridges or culverts, and carefully placing water points and supplement feeders.

Several other ways of managing grazing and pastures are suggested in Table 14.2.

References

Bailey, D.W. (2005). Identification and creation of optimum habitat conditions for livestock. *Rangeland Ecology and Management* 58(2): 109–118.

Bailey, D.W., Gross, J.E., Laca, E.A., Rittenhouse, L.R., Coughenour, M.B., Swift, D.M. and Sims, P.L. (1996). Mechanisms that result in large herbivores' grazing distribution patterns. *Journal of Range Management* 49: 386–400.

Barrett, P.D., Laidlaw, A.S., Mayne, C.S. and Christie, H. (2001). Pattern of herbage intake rate and bite dimensions of rotationally grazed dairy cows as sward height declines. *Grass and Forage Science* 56(4): 362–373.

Bohnert, E., Lascano, C. and Wenige, J.H. (1986). Botanical and chemical composition of the diet selected by fistulated steers under grazing on improved grass-legume pastures in the tropical savannas of Colombia. 2. Chemical composition of forage available and selected. *Journal of Animal Breeding and Genetics* 103: 69–79.

Boval, M. and Sauvant, D. (2019). Ingestive behaviour of grazing ruminants: meta-analysis of the components of bite mass. *Animal Feed Science and Technology* 251: 96–111.

Burt, W.H. (1943). Territoriality and home range concepts as applied to mammals. *Journal of Mammalogy* 24: 346–352.

CSIRO (2019). *Case study. Virtual fencing*. Available at: www.csiro.au/en/Research/AF/Areas/Livestock/Virtual-fencing (accessed 30 December 2020).

Dawson, T.J. and Ellis, B.A. (1994). Diets of mammalian herbivores in Australian arid shrublands: seasonal effects on overlap between red kangaroos, sheep and rabbits and on dietary niche breadths and electivities. *Journal of Arid Environments* 26: 257–271.

Douglas, G.B., Wang, Y., Waghorn, G.C., Barry, T.N., Purchas, R.W., Foote, A.G. and Wilson, G.F. (1995). Liveweight gain and wool production of sheep grazing *Lotus corniculatus* and lucerne (*Medicago sativa*). *New Zealand Journal of Agricultural Research* 38(1): 95–104.

Dryden, G.McL. (2008). *Animal Nutrition Science*. Wallingford, UK: CAB International.

Dryden, G.McL., Stafford, K.J., Waghorn, G.C. and Barry, T.N. (1995). Comminution of roughages by red deer (*Cervus elaphus*) during the prehension of feed. *Journal of Agricultural Science* 125(3): 407–414.

Elliott, M. (1996). *Sheep Production*. Castlemaine, Victoria, Australia: Richard Lee Publishing.

García, C.A.M., Maxwell, T.M.R., Hickford, J. and Gregorini, P. (2020). On the search for grazing personalities: from individual to collective behaviors. *Frontiers of Veterinary Science* 7: article 74.

Grings, E.E., Short, R.E., Haferkamp, M.R. and Heitschmidt, R.K. (2001). Animal age and sex effects on diets of grazing cattle. *Journal of Range Management* 54(1): 77–81.

Hinch, G.N. (1999). Spatial behaviour of grazing livestock and the memory of food position. *Recent Advances in Animal Nutrition in Australia* 15: 193–200.

Hirata, M., Tanikawa, T. and Tobisa, M. (2011). Quantifying short-term foraging behavior of cattle grazing a tall grass: A preliminary study with maize. *Livestock Science* 138(1–3): 220–228.

Hunt, L.P., Petty, S., Cowley, R., Fisher, A., Ash, A.J. and MacDonald, N. (2007). Factors affecting the management of cattle grazing distribution in northern Australia: preliminary observations on the effect of paddock size and water points. *Rangeland Journal* 29(2): 169–179.

Illius, A.W. and Hodgson, J. (1996). In Hodgson, J. and Illius, A.W. (eds), *Ecology and Management of Grazing Systems*. Wallingford, UK: CAB International.

Ison, K.A.D., Barber, D.G., Benvenutti, M.A., Kleinitz, N., Mayer, D. and Poppi, D.P. (2019). Defoliation dynamics, pasture intake and milk production of dairy cows grazing lucerne pastures in a partial mixed-ration system. *Animal Production Science* 60(1): 175–179.

Karda, I.W. (2000). *Feeding Value for Sheep of the Leaf of Gliricidia sepium and Leucaena leucocephala cv. Tarramba*. PhD thesis, School of Animal Studies, The University of Queensland.

Laca, E.A., Ungar, E.D. and Demment, M.W. (1994). Mechanisms of handling time and intake rate of a large mammalian grazer. *Applied Animal Behaviour Science* 39(1): 3–19.

Lazo, A. (1995). Ranging behaviour of feral cattle (*Bos taurus*) in Doiiana National Park, S.W. Spain. *Journal of Zoology, London* 236: 359–369.

Lomax, S., Colusso, P. and Clark, C.E.F. (2019). Does virtual fencing work for grazing dairy cattle? *Animals* 9(7): 429.

Lorimer, M.S. (1978). Forage selection studies 1. The botanical composition of forage selected by sheep grazing *Astrebla* spp. pasture in north-west Queensland. *Tropical Grasslands* 12(2): 97–108.

Lynch, J.J., Hinch, G.N. and Adams, D.B. (1992). *The Behaviour of Sheep: Biological Principles and Implications for Production*. Wallingford, UK: CAB International and Melbourne: CSIRO Publishing.

Moser, L.E. and Jennings, J.A. (2007). Grass and legume structure and morphology. In: Barnes, R.F., Nelson, C.J., Moore, K.J. and Collins, M. (eds), *Forages. The science of grassland agriculture*. Ames, Iowa, USA: Blackwell Publishing, pp. 15–35.

Neave, H.W., Weary D.M. and von Keyserlingk, M.A.G. (2018). Review: Individual variability in feeding behaviour of domesticated ruminants. *Animal* 12(S2): s419–s430.

Norton, B.W., Kennedy, P.J. and Hales, J.W. (1990). Grazing management studies in Australian cashmere goats. 3. Effect of season on the selection of diet by cattle, sheep and goats from two tropical grass-legume pastures. *Australian Journal of Experimental Agriculture* 30: 783–788.

O'Reagain, P.J. and McMeniman, N.P. (2002). Nutrition of sheep under rangeland conditions. In Freer, M. and Dove, H. (eds), *Sheep Nutrition*. Wallingford, UK: CAB International, pp. 263–284.

O'Reagain, P.J. and Schwartz, J. (1995). Dietary selection and foraging strategies of animals on rangeland. Coping with spatial and temporal variability. In Journet, M. *et al.* (eds), *Recent Developments in the Nutrition of Herbivores*. Paris, France: INRA, pp. 407–424.

Parkes, J., Henzell, R. and Pickles, G. (1996). *Managing Vertebrate Pests: Feral Goats*. Canberra: Australian Government Publishing Service, pp. 22–23.

Pauler, C.M., Isselstein, J., Suter, M., Berard, J., Braunbeck, T. and Schneider, M.K. (2020). Choosy grazers: Influence of plant traits on forage selection by three cattle breeds. *Functional Ecology* 34(5): 980–992.

Perez, J.M.L., de la Varga, M.E.A., Garcia, J.J. and Lacasa, V.R.G. (2017). Monitoring Lidia cattle with GPS-GPRS technology; a study on grazing behaviour and spatial distribution. *Veterinaria Mexico* 4(4). DOI: dx.doi.org/10.21753/vmoa.4.4.405

Poli, C.H.E.C., Thornton-Kurth, K.J., Legako, J.F., Bremm, C., Hampel, V.S., Hall, J., Ipharraguerre, I.R. and Villalba, J.J. (2018). Self-selection of plant bioactive compounds by sheep in response to challenge infection with *Haemonchus contortus*. *Physiology & Behavior* 194: 302–310.

Powell, R.A. and Mitchell, M.S. (2012). What is a home range? *Journal of Mammalogy* 93(4): 948–958.

Provenza, F.D. (1996). Familiarity and novelty in animal diets: implications for management. *Proceedings of the Australian Society of Animal Production* 21: 12–16.

Roura, E. and Navarro, M. (2018). Physiological and metabolic control of diet selection. *Animal Production Science* 58: 613–626.

Schroeder, A., Samuels, M.I., Swarts, M., Morris, C., Cupido, C.F. and Engelbrecht, A. (2019). Diet selection and preference of small ruminants during drought conditions in a dryland pastoral system in South Africa. *Small Ruminant Research* 176: 17–23.

Thorhallsdotter, A.G., Provenza, F.D. and Balph, D.F. (1987). Food aversion learning in lambs with or without a mother: discrimination, novelty and persistence. *Applied Animal Behavioural Science* 18: 327–340.

Villalba, J.J. and Provenza, F.D. (1997). Preference for wheat straw by lambs conditioned with intraruminal infusions of starch. *British Journal of Nutrition* 77: 287–297.

Wan, L.Q., Liu, K.S., Wu, W., Li, J.S., Zhao, T.C., Shao, X.Q., He, F., Lv, H. and Li, X.L. (2018). Effect of stocking rate on grazing behaviour and diet selection of goats on cultivated pasture. *Journal of Agricultural Science* 156(7): 914–921.

Wilson, G., Dexter, N., O'Brien, P. and Bomford, M. (1992). *Pest Animals in Australia. A Survey of Introduced Wild Animals*. Kenthurst, NSW: Bureau of Rural Resources and Kangaroo Press, pp. 8–38.

Zengeya, F., Murwira, A. and de Garine-Wiechatitsky, M. (2011). An IKONOS-based comparison of methods to estimate cattle home ranges in a semi-arid landscape of southern Africa. *International Journal of Remote Sensing* 32(22): 7805–7826.

15 Grazing management

Introduction

Grasses, legumes and forbs:

- Grasses are members of the *Poaceae* (*Gramineae*) family. They are monocotyledonous plants (monocots; their seeds have a single cotyledon – the first leaf which grows after the seed germinates). They have elongated leaves which grow from a crown or a stem, and their stems are hollow except at the nodes. They resist grazing by animals because their growing points are hidden at the base of the plant.
- Legumes are dicots and are members of the *Fabiaceae* (*Leguminosae*) family. These plants have broad leaves and pith-filled stems. They have a symbiotic bacterium, *Rhizobium*, which grows in nodules formed on the plant's roots. The rhizobia synthesize NH_3 from gaseous N_2 and this is used as the starting material for amino acid and protein synthesis. Consequently, legumes have characteristically higher protein contents than non-legumes.
- Forbs are flowering plants other than grasses, although the term is not usually applied to legumes.

Perennials and annuals: Annual plants produce seeds at the end of their growing season and just after this the plant dies; they persist by regrowing from seed in the next growing season. Perennials become dormant in cold or dry seasons and then regrow when conditions improve; they also produce seeds towards the end of each growing period.

Perennial grasses have a well-developed root system which helps maintain soil stability, and they provide sustainable pastures that maintain land condition. The most desirable perennials for grazing are the '3P' grasses; these are perennial (long-lived), palatable and productive.

Climate and pasture: Climate influences plant growth and nutritive value through the effects of:

- temperature;
- rainfall (amount of soil moisture); and
- day length (amount of solar radiation).

There are many different climate types, and these are described in the Köppen–Geiger climate classification system (Kottek *et al.*, 2006; Beck *et al.*, 2018). We can divide grasses into tropical (C4 or panicoid) and temperate (C3 or festucoid) types (see below), and this classification tells us which grow best in which climate, i.e. hot/warm or cool/cold regions.

When we consider how our climate determines the types of pasture we can grow, and the seasonal changes in pasture quantity and quality, we need to think about:

- The average temperatures throughout the year, and how these change with seasons or at different times of the year in those places where seasons are not markedly different.
- How much rain falls, and in what seasons and how reliably we can expect rain: some regions have four distinctly different seasons, while others may have only two – a wet and a dry season – and in others rainfall is quite constant over the whole of the year.
- How day length changes over the year: this is determined by latitude; tropics have only small changes in day length, while high latitudes have much greater variations between summer and winter.

C3 and C4 grasses

Types of photosynthesis: C3 and C4 grasses use different pathways to introduce CO_2 into their photosynthetic reactions (Gowik and Westhoff, 2011). C3

DOI: 10.1079/9781786394453.0015

grasses carry out photosynthesis in chloroplasts in their mesophyll cells. They incorporate atmospheric CO_2 which has entered the mesophyll cells through the stomata directly into 3-phosphoglyceric acid and this 3-C molecule (hence the name 'C3 photosynthesis') is used as the starting point for the Calvin cycle (the photosynthesis reactions which synthesize glucose and other sugars). C4 grasses can close their stomata to reduce water loss from the mesophyll tissue, but this restricts CO_2 entry. To counter this, the C4 grasses use oxaloacetic acid (a 4-C molecule) as a way of trapping CO_2 which has entered the mesophyll cells and then moving it into the chloroplasts in their bundle sheath cells. This allows a more efficient harvesting of CO_2.

The chemistry of plant tissues: The plant's tissues (epidermis, mesophyll, vascular tissue and sclerenchyma) are made up of cells which have a tough cell wall, a watery cytoplasm and various cell organelles. As far as a grazing animal's nutrition is concerned the important things are:

- The composition of the cell wall – mostly long-chain polysaccharides, with lignin, some protein and (in some cells) a small amount of waxes (Chapter 4).
- The proportion of cell contents to cell wall, because the cell contents are almost completely digestible while the digestibility of the cell wall varies.

The main cell wall constituents are long-chain carbohydrates: pectins, celluloses and hemicelluloses. These are the plant's 'structural' carbohydrates. The 'non-structural' carbohydrates are starches and sugars which are found in the cell contents. The other major cell wall constituent is lignin; this cannot be digested by animals or most micro-organisms, and so the amount of it in the cell wall determines the digestibility of that cell component and thus the whole plant (Chapter 4, Fig. 4.1).

Leaf anatomy and plant digestibility: The important nutritional difference between C3 and C4 grasses is in the amount of fibrous tissue that these plants have in their leaves. The characteristically large (about 10% units) differences in the digestibilities of C4 and C3 grasses are related to this. The main leaf tissues are illustrated in Fig. 15.1. They are:

- Epidermis (both upper and lower): single layers of cells which have a waxy (and indigestible) cuticle on the outside surface. The epidermis also has stomata which allow the passage of gases and water.
- Mesophyll: in C3 plants these cells contain the chloroplasts where photosynthesis takes place. They are large, thin-walled, non-lignified cells.
- Vascular tissue: this contains the xylem vessels, which are heavily lignified; phloem, made up of small, non-lignified cells; and the cells of the vascular bundle sheath(s) where photosynthesis occurs in C4 plants.
- Sclerenchyma: small, heavily lignified cells which form a rib running the length of the leaf and which support it so that the leaf blade is exposed to a maximum amount of light.

The most fibrous, and indigestible, plant tissues are the vascular bundles (which transport water and nutrients through the plant) and the sclerenchyma. Tissues such as the epidermis, mesophyll and phloem are less lignified and thus more digestible. The large difference in the proportions of mesophyll and vascular tissue (Table 15.1) is responsible for the difference in the digestibility of C3 and C4 grass species (Table 15.2), and the greater resistance to both chewing and rumen microbial degradation of C4 grasses.

The nutritive value of pastures

Pasture quality is determined by:

- the amount of forage available for grazing;
- the nutritive value of the forage – especially its digestibility, and protein and mineral contents;
- the acceptability of the pasture components to the grazing animal; and
- the way in which the pasture structure influences diet selection and feed prehension.

These factors are, in turn, influenced by:

- differences between C3 and C4 grasses, and legumes, in their nutritive value and plant structure;
- soil fertility, especially the N, and P and trace mineral contents; and soil moisture; and
- changes in plant structure, growth rate, digestibility, and protein and mineral contents which are associated with seasonal changes in day length, rainfall and temperature.

Morphological and physiological differences between plant species: There are characteristic differences in nutritive value between C3 and C4

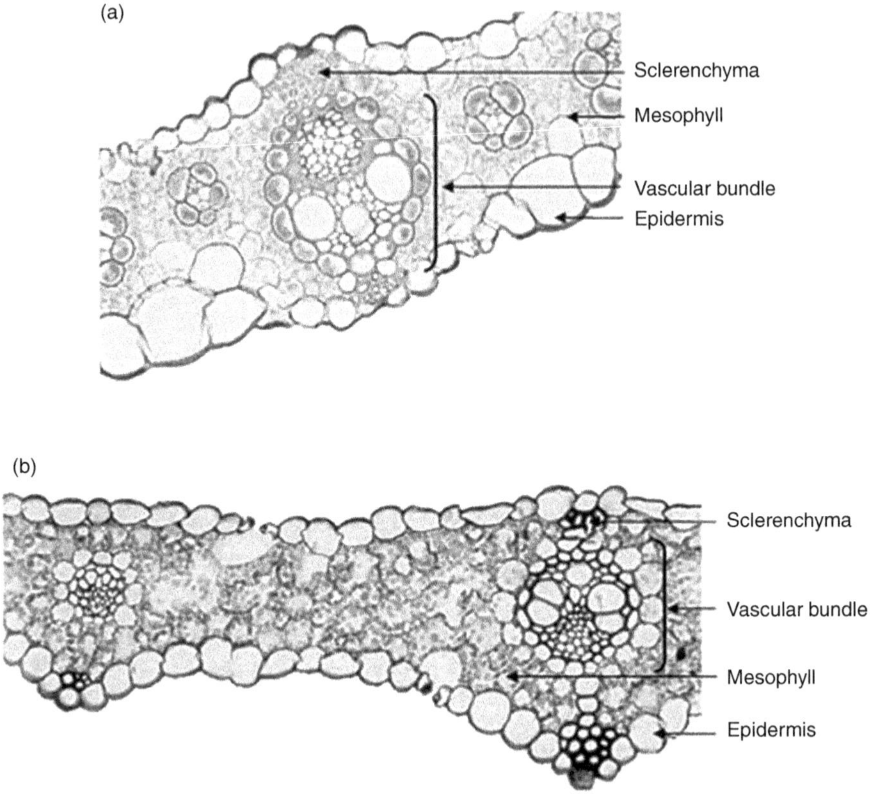

Fig. 15.1. Micrographs of cross-sections of leaves from **(a)** *Zea mays* (C4; tropical) and **(b)** *Bromus willdenowii* (C3; temperate) monocot plants, showing typical C3 and C4 (Krantz) anatomies. C3 plants have 15 or more mesophyll cells between adjacent vascular bundles, while C4 plants have only 2 to 5 mesophyll cells. (From Dryden, 2008; reproduced with permission.)

grasses, and between grasses and legumes. These differences are related to:

- whether plants are annuals or perennials;
- the start and length of the growing season;
- growth habit, e.g. erect (tussock or bunch) or trailing, tillering or stoloniferous;
- dry matter production, i.e. the rate and amount of plant growth;
- the characteristic stem:leaf ratio, in both the individual plants and the pasture; and
- stem and leaf anatomy, and how this affects the amount of fibre (cell wall constituents) in the plant and consequently its digestibility (Table 15.2).

Pastures reflect the structure of their constituent plants. For example, tropical pastures often contain tall and open plants, especially if the main components are grasses which have a tussock growth form. These grasses are upright with leaves interspersed between stem and dead material. This makes it difficult for livestock to prehend large amounts of leaf (O'Reagain and McMeniman, 2002), principally through effects on the animal's bite size (Chapter 14). Temperate species (such as annual ryegrass pastures) have a tillering growth habit and form a uniform, leafy, dense sward which is easily harvested.

Pasture nutritive value is affected by climate and altitude: Tropical grasses grown in hot climates grow quickly, and flower and mature quickly (Norton, 1981). Pastures grown in cooler environments remain in a vegetative state longer, with accompanying higher protein and energy contents. The nutritive value of grasses changes with altitude,

Table 15.1. Proportions of leaf tissues in selected grasses. (From Akin and Burdick, 1975; reproduced with permission.)

Grass species	Mesophyll + phloem	Epidermis + bundle sheath	Lignified vascular tissue
C4 grasses			
Coastal bermudagrass	31	55	14
Coastcross-1 bermudagrass	27	56	17
Pensacola bahiagrass	55	36	9
C3 grasses			
Kentucky-31 tall fescue	62	27	11
Clair timothy	56	31	12
Smooth bromegrass	56	26	19

Table 15.2. Proportions of tissues in *Panicum* (*Megathyrsus*) spp. grass leaves, and correlations between tissue types and dry matter digestibility and content of cell wall constituents. The *Panicum* genus includes species which have a C3 or C4 anatomy, and some which have an intermediate (C3/4) structure. (From Wilson *et al.*, 1983; reproduced with permission.)

	Proportions (%)			Correlations	
Leaf tissue type	C3	C3/4	C4	DM digestibility	Cell wall constituents
Mesophyll	66	48	43	0.62	–0.76
Bundle sheath cells	10	18	20	–0.67	0.69
Vascular tissue	3	6	8	–0.53	0.66
Epidermis	22	26	27	–0.23	0.44
Sclerenchyma	0.5	2	2	–0.29	0.51

e.g. for *Dactylis glomerata* the fibre content, and concentrations of Ca, P and other minerals, are lowest at high altitudes (Tenikecier and Ates, 2019).

Differences between C4 and C3 grasses, and legumes:

- C3 grasses have a longer growing season than C4 grasses.
- C4 grasses use N more efficiently than C3 grasses.
- C4 grasses have higher potential dry matter (DM) yields than C3 grasses.
- C3 grasses and legumes tend to have less fibre (NDF) and higher metabolizable energy (ME) contents than C4 grasses.
- Legumes generally have more protein than grasses (illustrated in Fig. 15.2).

The effects of these characteristics on animal factors are illustrated in data reported by Archimède *et al.* (2018) who observed lower DM intakes, digestibilities and passage rates of undigested feed from the rumen (particle turnover rates) of cattle eating C4 grass compared to C3 grass. These differences relate to the higher fibre (74% versus 61% NDF; 7.4 versus 6.1% lignin) and lower protein contents (12 and 8% versus 13 and 8%) of the C4 grass in that experiment (Fig. 15.3).

Soil type and fertilization: Pasture protein and mineral contents are strongly influenced by soil fertility, and by any fertilizers that we use to improve this.

N fertilizers, e.g. urea, aqueous or anhydrous ammonia, or animal manure, are often used to improve plant growth rates and protein contents. The actual response depends on the:

- type of pasture plants;
- amount of N applied – we can expect a plateau in response, influenced by rainfall;
- rainfall and temperature, which allow the plant to use the added N; and
- soil type, which affects how the added N is retained in the soil or taken up by the plant.

These things are illustrated in work done by Cowan *et al.* (1995; Fig. 15.4) with Callide Rhodes grass (*Chloris gayana*, cv. Callide). In this study, after 3 years of N application, the soil pH was

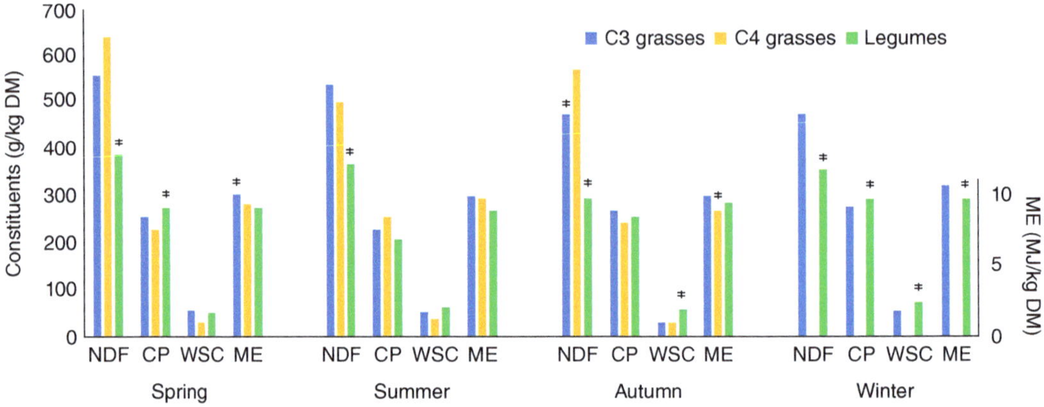

Fig. 15.2. Cell wall (neutral detergent fibre, NDF), protein (CP), water-soluble carbohydrate (WSC) and metabolizable energy (ME) contents of C3, C4 grasses and legumes grown in southern Australia. Asterisks indicate significantly different ($P<0.05$) means. The lower ME content of legumes in winter is probably due to their lower hemicellulose and higher lignin contents. (Drawn from data in Fulkerson *et al.*, 2007; reproduced with permission.)

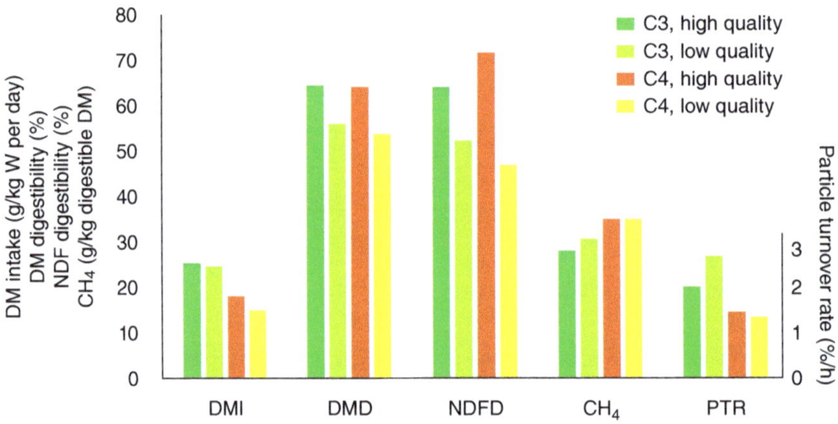

Fig. 15.3. Differences in the nutritive values of C3 (*Dactylis glomerata* and *Festuca* spp.) and C4 (*Dichanthium* spp.) grasses. C3 and C4 species differ in dry matter intake (DMI), dry matter digestibility (DMD), NDF digestibility (NDFD), methane production (CH_4) and the turnover rate of undigested feed particles (PTR). (Drawn from data in Archimède, *et al.*, 2018; reproduced with permission.)

reduced by up to 1.6 units (from the initial pH =7.5), pasture growth improved in those years when rainfall allowed this, the amount of litter increased, and the plant structure changed from tussocky to stoloniferous at high N applications.

Phosphatic fertilizers are commonly used to improve low soil P levels and to enhance legume production which in turn produces more N for grass growth. However, the economics of P fertilization depends on having adequate rainfall to allow the plant to make use of the extra P, correct soil pH, and other minerals available from the soil.

Other minerals are provided through fertilization where these are required and where economic pasture and/or animal responses can be obtained. Lime provides Ca and improves the pH of acid soils, and gypsum provides Ca and S. Trace minerals are used in some in regions either to promote pasture growth, e.g. Cu and B, or to prevent a potential deficiency in animals which will eat the pasture, e.g. Co and Se.

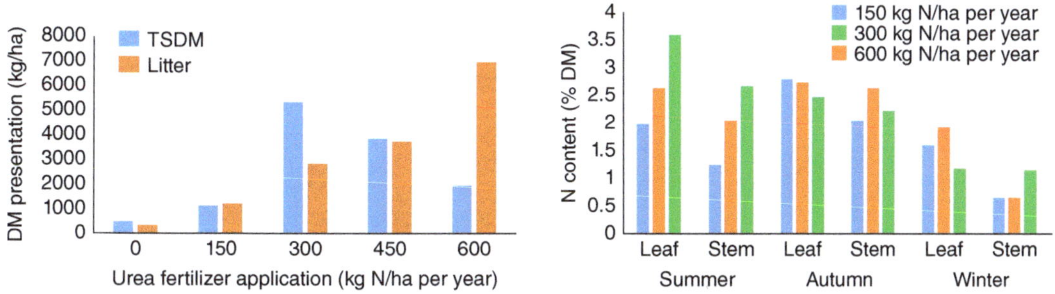

Fig. 15.4. Responses of Callide Rhodes grass to N fertilization (the rainy season is in summer and early autumn (fall) when about 70% of the annual rainfall occurs). TSDM is total standing dry matter (excluding leaf litter). (Drawn from selected data in Cowan *et al.*, 1995; reproduced with permission.)

Some minerals, such as Se and Co, are essential nutrients for animals but are not needed for plant metabolism (although Co is needed by the rhizobia which fix N). Pastures may not show any effects of low soil Co or Se contents, but they will not support animal production. Trace mineral deficiencies are widespread, and they include Co-deficient pastures in southern Australia, parts of New Zealand and the southeast Atlantic coast of the USA, Cu deficient (or where soils have excess Mo) regions of New Zealand, Australia and many areas of North America, and regions of low soil Se content in North America, South Africa, Europe and other countries. Animals grazing these pastures must be supplemented with the deficient mineral; options include fertilizers enriched with Co, Cu or Se, or rumen boluses, or drenches and injections (Chapter 16).

Seasonal and plant maturity changes in the nutritive value of pasture: The response to seasonal changes in day length, rainfall and temperature determines whether the plant grows vegetatively (i.e. produces leaves) or becomes mature and produces a seed head.

As the plant moves through its annual vegetative and reproductive phases its nutritive value first increases as leaves grow, and then declines as the leaves and stems become lower in protein, non-structural carbohydrate and mineral contents. This is because in both annuals and perennials, seed production is accompanied by the transfer of nutrients from the vegetative plant into the seeds, and perennials withdraw nutrients from their leaves and store these in the crown and roots to support the growth of new leaves from the crown in the next growing season. This maturing is associated with more cell wall lignification and a decrease in the ratio of leaf to stem.

Figure 15.5 illustrates seasonal changes in a northern Australian perennial *Themeda/Chrysopogon/Sorghum* pasture. The pasture begins to grow when effective rain (about 50 mm in this region) has fallen after the start of the wet season, rapidly reaches its maximum protein and P contents, and then almost as rapidly these fall to low values as nutrients are translocated into the crown and roots, and dead leaves are leached.

There are similar changes in the nutritive value of C3 and C4 grasses and white clover (Fig. 15.6) in an eastern Australian subtropical region where rain mostly falls between February and June. The ME content of these pastures fell when they began to flower and set seed. This is illustrated by the decline in ME content of biennial ryegrass in October/November when almost all of the tillers became reproductive. The ME decline shown in Fig. 15.6a was accompanied by an almost 50% increase in NDF content.

Changes in the species composition of pastures reflect the ways in which the individual species respond to seasonal and between-year changes in rainfall and temperature, competition from other plant species, and grazing. Examples are the responses of a perennial ryegrass/white clover pasture in subtropical coastal Australia (Fig. 15.6b), and Mitchell grass pastures in northern Australia (Table 15.3). These changes not only influence the nutritive value of the pasture (especially if grasses are replaced by legumes or herbs), but they also influence the grazing animal's diet.

Grazing systems

Grazing systems are ways of managing the access of animals to pasture, and they influence the way

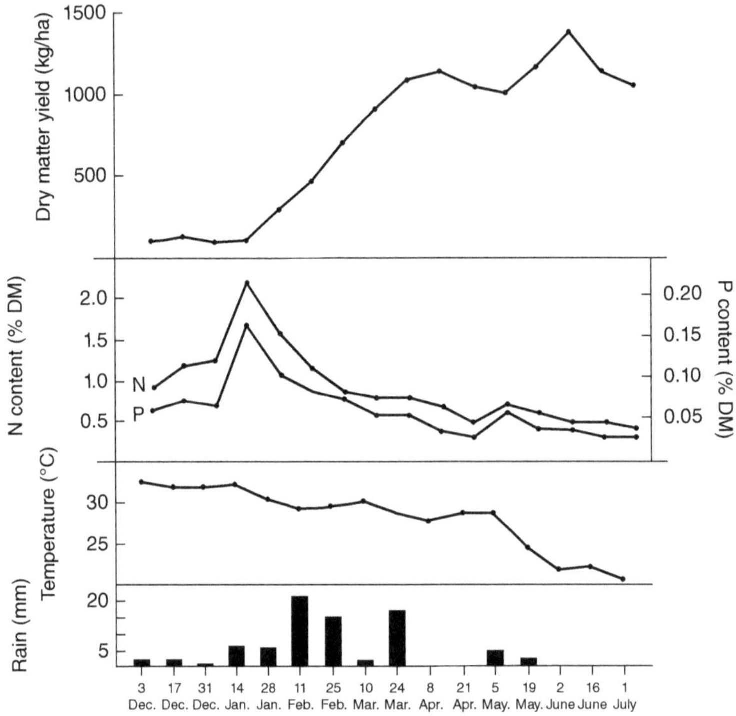

Fig. 15.5. Seasonal changes in the growth and nutrient content of a Northern Australian native rangeland pasture. (Adapted from Norman, 1963; reproduced with permission.)

that animals use pasture and how pastures respond to this use.

Continuous grazing: This is a method where animals are allocated to a pasture and remain there for a substantial period, e.g. a season, a year, or longer. Set stocking is a form of continuous grazing where the number and class of animals remains unchanged. Under continuous grazing we find that:

- Animals perform well, provided that there are no feed gaps and that the stocking rate (SR) does not exceed the seasonal carrying capacity.
- Animals are able to express their feed preferences, within the limits imposed by the seasonal growth of annual plants, and the gradual loss of preferred species due to selective grazing.
- Pastures suffer the effects of continuous preferential grazing, i.e. the selection and removal of preferred plant species leading to their eventual loss from the pasture and replacement by less acceptable species.
- Management is simple; however, animals may be left with little supervision and this is not usually an advantage.

Cell and rotational grazing: These are both ways of moving animals around a sequence of paddocks, allowing time between visits to a particular paddock for the pasture to regrow before being grazed again. Cell grazing (also called 'time-controlled grazing') usually refers to larger-scale, semi-rangeland rotations, while rotational grazing refers to the repeated use of smaller-scale, intensively managed swards.

The aim is to make animals eat most of the total standing DM (TSDM; defined below), and so improve the 'efficiency' of pasture use. As a result, both methods apply much higher utilization rates (UR; see below) than are recommended for continuous grazing. However, plants must not be grazed so far down their profile that regrowth is impaired, because the rotation programme can be easily and irretrievably upset if the next paddock or cell is not ready for grazing when it is required.

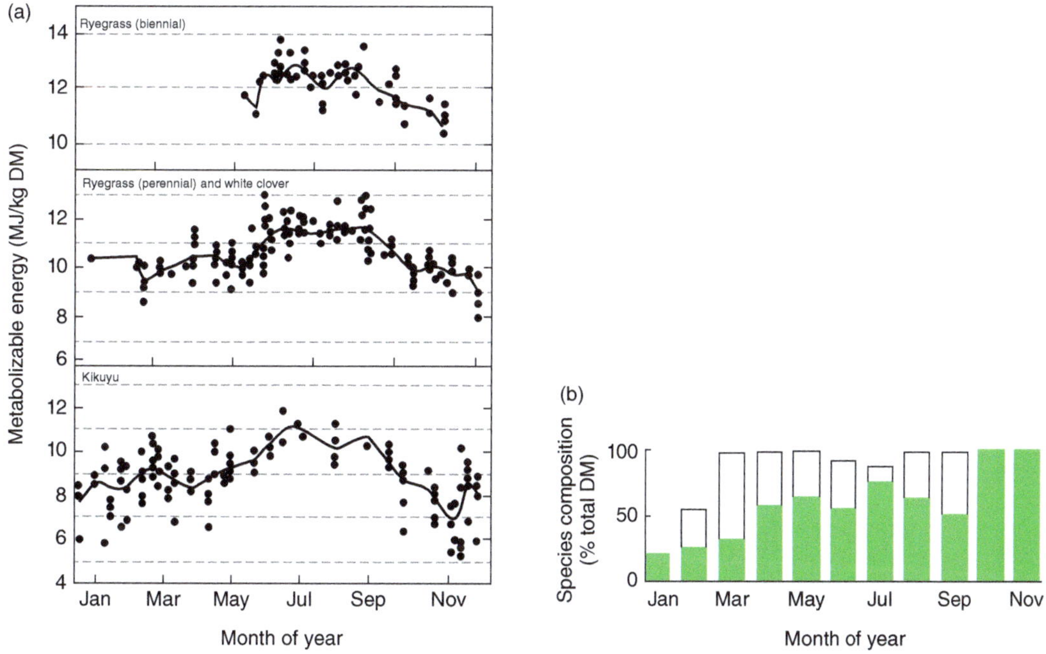

Fig. 15.6. Seasonal changes in pasture nutritive value. **(a)** Patterns of metabolizable energy content in (top to bottom) biennial ryegrass (*Lolium multiflorum*) (C3), perennial ryegrass (C3) and white clover (*Lolium perenne/ Trifolium repens*), and kikuyu (*Pennisetum clandestinum*) (C4) pastures in subtropical Australia. The shorter run of data for biennial ryegrass reflects its shorter growing season, as it does not tolerate hot summer temperatures. **(b)** Pasture species composition: green bars are perennial ryegrass; white bars are white clover. (From Fulkerson *et al*., 1998; reproduced with permission.)

Table 15.3. Seasonal changes in the species composition of Mitchell grass pastures. Changes between seasons are due to seasonality of rainfall (in this region, most rain falls in summer – December to February) and temperature. The between-year differences are caused by different amounts and seasonality of rainfall, and variations in seasonal temperature. (From Lorimer, 1978; reproduced by permission).

	Pasture species composition (%)			
Time of year	Mitchell grass	Flinders grass	Mint bush	Other species
Year 1				
January	70	21	9	0
March	17	36	37	10
July	14	31	50	6
December	19	50	29	2
Year 2				
March	11	76	11	2
July	21	69	8	2
November	21	69	7	3
March	29	53	3	15

Overall, the performance of animals under cell grazing and continuous stocking is similar (Briske *et al.*, 2008), and cell grazing gives more uniform pasture use than continuous grazing.

A form of rotational grazing used in rangeland management is to spell (not graze) parts of the farm during the growing season. This allows plants to recover from previous grazing pressure and is beneficial for preferred species which may be particularly affected by selective grazing.

Cell grazing can be a component of regenerative agriculture (Gosnell *et al.*, 2020).

Strip or 'break' grazing: This method involves a highly intensive management of grazing on high-quality pasture or forage crop. Animals are allocated each day, or perhaps twice a day, a new strip or 'break' of pasture. Access is controlled by temporary electric fencing – always one in front of the strip and sometimes another at the back to prevent access to previously grazed areas. When these fences are installed, we must take care to make sure that animals still have access to water and shelter.

Like other forms of rotational grazing, strip grazing maximizes the efficiency of pasture use.

Leaders and followers: Different animal classes have different nutrient requirements. Typically, calves, lambs, kids and foals need feed with higher ME and protein contents than older livestock. We can provide this by allowing young stock to graze a paddock before older animals are given access to the same pasture. The young stock are, therefore, the leaders, and the older stock the followers. Because young animals are smaller, they eat less than adults and will graze the paddock lightly. Even though they will remove the most nutritious material, pasture of sufficient quality is left for the older animals which follow.

Mixed grazing: This is when animals of different species, typically sheep and beef cattle, are allocated to the same pasture at the same time. Mixed grazing has several results, for example improved individual sheep productivity (wool and live weight gain) of up to 25% and individual cattle growth of up to 10%, compared to when these animals are grazed alone (Walker, 1994; d'Alexis *et al.*, 2014). There are similar trends in production per hectare, although these are less than the improvements in individual animal production.

Horses and sheep prefer to graze short pasture while cattle find it easier to prehend longer/taller swards. Accordingly, mixed grazing by cattle and either sheep or horses should give a more uniform use of pasture. There is little evidence that these species have different plant species preferences and none that they prefer different parts of the sward – i.e. green leaf versus green stem versus mature forage. However, sheep may use pasture growing near cattle manure which is avoided by cattle.

Cut-and-carry: This management system is not a grazing method but is often used in small-holdings as an alternative to grazing. The animals are kept in pens or tethered and so confined to a small grazing space. These animals rely entirely on their owner for feed and water.

Feeds used in cut-and-carry systems are often pasture or conserved forage (hay or silage), or fodder trees. The major risk in this method is that in our desire to reduce the cost of feeding or to make feed reserves stretch as far as possible, we:

- do not give our animals enough feed;
- give feed with less than the required nutritive value; or
- when feeding fodder trees, we harvest woody stems as well as leaves – this reduces the nutritive value of the feed and is likely to cause rumen or omasal impaction (Chapter 13), with usually fatal consequences.

Grazing management – assessing pasture yield, growth and quality

Yield, growth and quality assessments: Pasture yield (or pasture mass) is the amount of forage material above the ground; it can be the whole DM or exclude the bases of pasture plants and any dead litter. It is referred to as TSDM, or dry matter presentation yield, or feed on offer, or average pasture cover. Pasture yield is measured in kg DM/ha or lb DM/ac (1 lb/ac = 1.122 kg/ha, 1 kg/ha = 0.893 lb/ac).

The amount of TSDM present in an intensively managed sward pasture can be estimated fairly easily by using rising plate meters (DairyNZ, 2008), capacitance or ultrasonic meters, or by visual estimation. If necessary (and especially with visual inspection), these methods can be calibrated by cutting, drying and weighing the forage obtained from a series of quadrats (usually 25 × 25 cm or 50 × 50 cm).

In rangelands and other extensive farming situations it is very difficult to look at every part of the farm, and pastures comprised of tussock grasses are more difficult to measure than swards. In these situations, TSDM can be estimated more conveniently by photo comparisons, pasture height ruler, lasers, and drone or satellite imagery (MLA, 2008; Kallenbach, 2015; Schaefer and Lamb, 2016).

Pasture growth is the amount of forage material (including leaves, tillers, stems, stolons, flower heads and seed heads) which accrues above the ground as the plant grows. Growth is expressed as kg DM/ha per day (or lb DM/ac per day). Future pasture growth can be predicted by plant growth mathematical models which use expected temperature, soil moisture (rainfall) and solar radiation values as inputs. Forecasts of ambient temperature and soil moisture in the coming seasons can be obtained from historical weather records, and weather predictions can be made from climate data such as the Indian Ocean Dipole, the Southern Oscillation Index, and the El Niño and La Niña effects in the southern hemisphere, and the Northern Hemisphere Annular Mode, North Atlantic Oscillation and Aleutian Low in the northern hemisphere.

Pasture quality is greatly influenced by its maturity, which can be judged by eye – look for stem thickness, and the development of flowers, early seed development (boot stage) and seedheads from which the seeds have been lost (over-ripe). Alternatively, the quality of the selected diet can be predicted by faecal near-infrared reflectance spectroscopy (discussed in Chapter 16) or estimated from satellite data (see below).

Satellite remote sensing vegetation indexes: These are numbers which rate the quantity and greenness of vegetation, based on the amounts of radiation which are received and reflected from objects on the Earth's surface. The Normalized Difference Vegetation Index (NDVI) is the most commonly used index. Index values range between –1 and +1; values below +0.1 indicate water or bare ground while higher values indicate 'greenness' or photosynthetic activity (Meneses-Tovar, 2011/2012). Greenness indicates how much vegetation mass there is, and its stage of maturity and health.

Satellite data only approximately estimate the available ME because the relationships between vegetation indexes and plant biomass or photosynthetic activity are not perfect. This is because the NDVI data can be compromised by changing sun angles, topography (especially hilly country), atmospheric conditions including rain, clouds or shadow, and the soil background (Matsushita *et al.*, 2007). Before they are made publicly available, the relationships between the NDVI values and the actual TSDM are checked for accuracy of prediction and repeatability over different seasons and years. Some providers claim high accuracies, with NDVI data explaining more than 85% of the variation in TSDM. Plant growth rate predictions may be much less accurate, explaining from 47% to 70% of the on-ground variation.

The usefulness of satellite information is influenced by:

- The degree of resolution, which ranges from 9 m^2 to 1 km^2.
- The correlation between satellite data and ground-truthing data (discussed above), including how this relationship changes at each end of the NDVI scale. *Pastures From Space* (LIC, 2021) predictions are most accurate when TSDM is <2000 kg/ha.
- How cloud cover is dealt with: providers deal with this in different ways, e.g. by not making predictions if the data indicates cloud cover, or by using the highest NDVI value recorded during a series of passes by the satellite.

There are several providers of this information. Two which are freely available are:

- *Pastures From Space* (PIRD, 2020b; LIC, 2021): this service gives estimates of present pasture biomass and estimates of future pasture growth rate. The service covers Australian rangeland and intensive pasture regions, and the dairying areas of New Zealand.
- *VegScape Vegetation Condition Explorer* (NASS, 2020): which reports current NDVI index values for the United States.

Pasture utilization rate

Pasture utilization rate (UR) is the proportion of the TSDM which we allow our animals to eat. Choosing an appropriate utilization rate is critical in managing grazing. An appropriate UR will ensure that animals will consume feed with an appropriate nutritive value and protect pastures from over-grazing.

Residual dry matter is a complementary concept. This is the amount (kg DM/ha) of forage DM which remains uneaten after animals are removed from the pasture. (Another, different, use of 'residual DM' is related to a concept used in selecting animals for efficient feed utilization; this is discussed in Chapter 7).

Over-grazing of pastures impacts on pasture and animal productivity: Over-grazing will:

- Impair the plants' ability to recover after grazing if they are grazed to the crown, i.e. the place in vegetative grasses where the growing point is located. This is particularly detrimental to pasture condition if rangeland pastures are grazed too hard during their early growth; it might take a year or more of spelling to return these pastures to reasonable condition. As well, rotationally grazed pastures must be able to regrow quickly.
- Remove plant material which would otherwise protect soils from erosion. Living plant material and dead litter reduce erosion by preventing rain drops from dislodging the soil and run-off water from washing it away.
- Remove the preferred plants and ultimately reduce the feeding value of the pasture because of excess growth of unpreferred plants.
- Force animals to graze into those strata of the pasture which have older leaves and stems, and are less nutritious (Fig. 15.7).

Grazing into the lower pasture strata impairs animal performance: A study by Ison *et al.* (2019; Fig. 15.8) illustrates what happens when dairy cows are forced to graze into the lower strata of pastures (in this case, a lucerne (alfalfa) pasture). They found that:

- Cows first graze across the paddock, eating the top, leafy layer. When this is all eaten, they then re-graze into the lower, more stemmy, strata. This behaviour is also found in beef cattle grazing tropical grass pastures.
- When cows reach the lower layers of the pasture their bite size and intake rate decreases because they then have to bite off, and chew, the more resistant plant stems.
- The time spent grazing falls when cows have to graze into the stemmy layer – they simply refuse to eat this material.
- Feed intake and milk production both fall as cows eat below the leafy top stratum.

Grazing behaviour can vary with different types of pasture. Figure 15.8 illustrates what happens

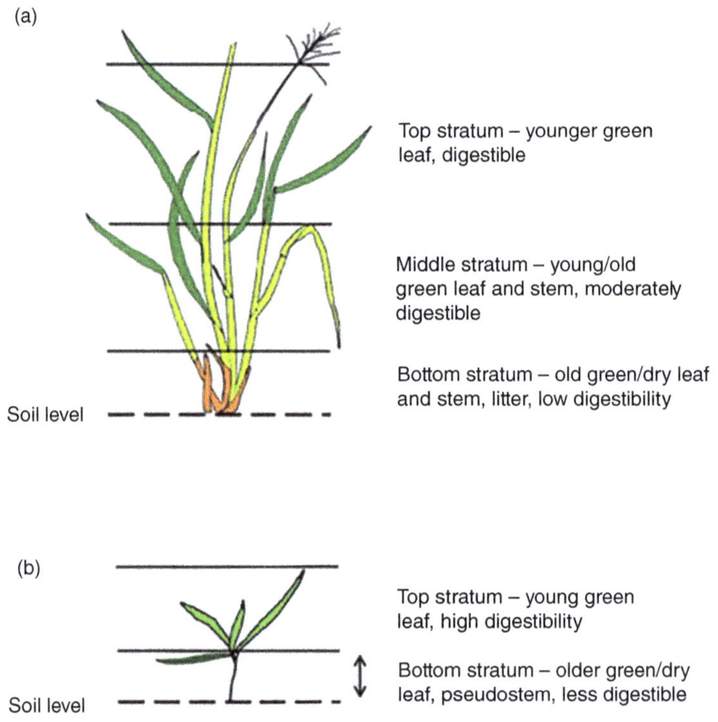

Fig. 15.7. Diagrams (not to scale) showing how the growth and structure of grasses results in nutrient stratification within the plant. **(a)** Green panic (*Megathyrsus* spp.); **(b)** ryegrass (*Lolium* spp.). (Copyright: Gordon McL. Dryden.)

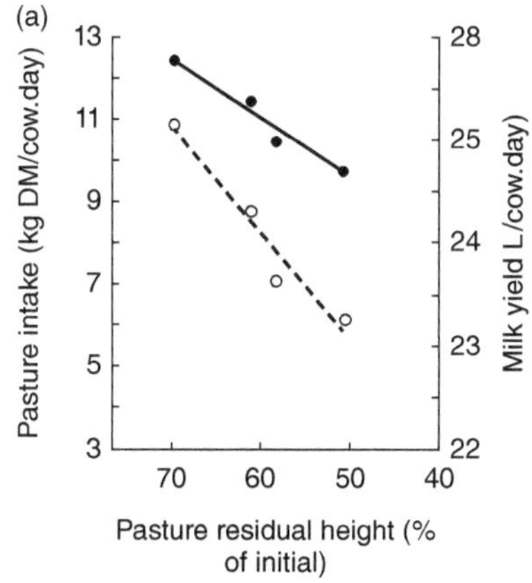

(b)

Characteristic	Treatments			
	1	2	3	4
Allocation (kg DM/cow per day)	30.6	20.6	14.8	10.8
Residual DM (% of initial)	69.7	61.1	58.2	50.7
NDF (% DM)	22.2	23.7	24.9	27.5
Protein (% DM)	30.2	30.3	29.5	27.8
ME (MJ/kg DM)	11.0	10.9	10.7	10.4
Grazing resistance (kg/100 cm^2)	43.8	53.7	59.4	72.8

Fig. 15.8. Grazing behaviour and effects on productivity (milk yield) when dairy cows are forced to eat into the lower strata of a lucerne (alfalfa) pasture. **(a)** Changes in milk yield (solid line) and dry matter intake (dotted line). **(b)** Changes in the nutritive value of the consumed pasture. All the trends in the table, except for protein content, are significant. (From Ison *et al.*, 2019; reproduced with permission.)

Table 15.4. Expected growth responses (based on NRC (2000) data) of Angus steers (275 kg live weight) grazing a Callide Rhodes grass pasture at differing utilization levels. The proportions of the plant in each stratum and the dry matter digestibilities and protein contents of each stratum are indicative only.

Stratum	Proportion of plant (%)	DM digest (%)	Protein (% DM)	DM intake (kg/day)	ME intake (MJ/day)	LWG (kg/day)
Top	15	65	16	7.8	82.3	1.5
Upper middle	20	60	13	7.0	68.5	0.9
Lower middle	25	55	10	5.9	48.9	0.5
Base	35	40	7	4.5	27.4	–0.3
Litter	5	30	3	3.3	14.8	–0.7

when animals graze plants which have a large and tough stem stratum. The performance of animals grazing plants which have less fibrous pseudostems, such as ryegrass, also falls as the pasture allocation is reduced, but this is more likely to be due to reduced feed intake than to changes in feed quality.

Table 15.4 illustrates the probable outcomes of lax, moderate and over-grazing of a subtropical C4 grass pasture. In these calculations, the animals are Angus steers weighing 275 kg. Their DM intakes are influenced by the feed DM digestibility (intakes are lower when digestibility is lower) and their ME requirement for maintenance is estimated to be 33–40 MJ/day, increasing as the efficiency of use of ME for maintenance declines with reducing pasture quality. In this example, 'lax' grazing animals eat the top stratum, 'moderate' grazing includes the middle strata, and 'heavy' or 'over' grazing includes material at the base of the plant.

We can see that in this example the steers will grow very well if they are asked to eat only the top 27%, but once we get to the base growth ceases and animals lose weight. From this analysis, we find that the maximum acceptable utilization rate for this pasture is about 60%, i.e. we can graze down to the lower middle stratum of this pasture if we consider that a growth rate of 500 g/day is acceptable.

Calculating carrying capacities and stocking rates

Carrying capacity is the number of animals which can be sustained on a given area over a season, a whole year or indefinitely. An alternative name is 'grazing capacity'. Implicit in this concept is that the pasture can withstand the grazing pressure exerted by this number of animals without deteriorating. Carrying capacity is measured in animals/ha or (in rangelands) animals/square kilometre (or often, the number of ha or km^2 which are required to sustain a single animal).

The carrying capacity of a farm is not constant. It is influenced by:

- the type of animal (e.g. milking cows, growing lambs or steers or heifers), the productivity which is expected of these, and seasonal changes in their nutrient requirements; and
- seasonal conditions throughout the year, as pasture growth and quality change with seasons and plant maturity.

We can estimate the annual carrying capacity of a farm with this formula:

$$\text{Carrying capacity (no. year)} = \frac{(\text{TSDM, kg / ha}) \times (\text{UR, decimal}) \times (\text{effective grazing area, ha})}{(\text{animal DM requirement, kg / year})}$$

This formula:

- assumes that all the required pasture DM is present at the start of the year;
- does not allow for any pasture growth, or change in pasture nutritive value throughout the year; and
- caters for only one type of animal and assumes a constant daily DM intake.

To be more accurate, we can base the calculation on animal ME requirements and the ME provided by the pasture [(TSDM, kg) × (ME content, MJ/kg DM)]. By allowing for monthly changes in ME availability and ME requirement we can further improve the prediction of carrying capacity.

Effective grazing area: Is the area of pasture which animals can or will graze. In many cases it is similar to the farm area, minus the area taken up by dams, forested areas, lanes and building sites, etc. The terms 'utilized agricultural area' used in the EU and 'effective farm area' used in New Zealand, are similar concepts.

The area of usable grazing is also limited by areas taken up by unpalatable plants, e.g. wiregrass (*Aristida* spp.) and barbed wire grass (*Cymbopogon refractus*) in northern Australia, crested wheatgrass (*Agropyron cristatum*) and cheat grass (*Bromus tectorum*) in the North American northern Great Plains, or alpine dock (*Rumex alpinus*) in Switzerland.

In rangelands and other extensive grazing areas, the effective grazing area is also determined by watering point (troughs, streams and dams) placement and it is the area that animals can reach when they graze out from these watering points (Fig. 15.9).

The distance that animals move varies with species, breed and individual. Beef cattle will walk up to 10 km from water, and Beattie (1956, cited by Lynch and Alexander 1973) reported a case where cattle were found 19 km from the nearest water. However, most cattle graze within 2–3 km of water, and visit water every day, or once every two days. Sheep walk up to 5 or 6 km per day and drink once or twice daily; they may not need drinking water if their pasture is immature with a low DM content, although it is not wise to rely on this.

Because of these behaviours, the pasture near watering points becomes overgrazed. Consequently, the feed intake of those animals which do not venture far from water becomes limited. Widely spaced watering points may lead cattle to drink less frequently. This is likely to reduce feed intake and thus animal performance.

While the cost of installing new watering points can be very high, there are some valuable production and environmental benefits. By reducing the distance between watering points (and therefore increasing the number of these) we reduce the energy demand for walking and thus have more nutrients available for production.

As well as these benefits for animals, we get greater flexibility in relation to grazing management – it is possible to spell areas of paddocks by closing (or turning off) a watering point so that animals will graze away from that and toward others. The ability to access new watering points also acts as a drought mitigation strategy in more extensive grazing enterprises.

Livestock equivalents: When we wish to determine a pasture's carrying capacity and we want this number to give a general overview of the number of animals we can sustainably stock on the paddock, it is best to use 'livestock equivalent' as the measure of animal nutrient demand rather than the

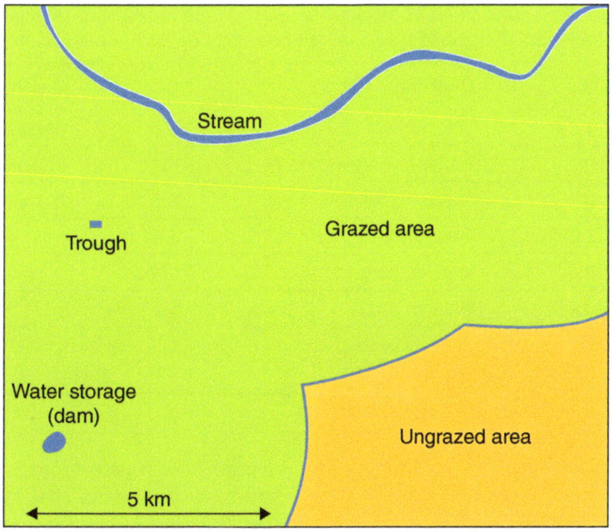

Fig. 15.9. A diagram showing how the availability of water can determine the effective grazing area of a large paddock (in this case for cattle which will walk 5 km from a watering point). (Copyright: Gordon McL. Dryden.)

expected DM intake (Chapter 7) or ME requirement (Chapter 8) of a particular type of animal.

There are several ways of expressing livestock equivalents. Each method uses a different type of animal as the reference, and they may compare either the DM or ME requirements of different classes of livestock. Equivalents which are based on the known ME requirement of the reference and comparison animals are more accurate than those based on assumed DM intakes.

Examples of livestock equivalents are:

- Livestock unit (LSU): the ME requirement of an adult dairy cow producing 3000 kg of milk in its lactation. Used in the EU (Eurostat, 2013).
- Dry stock equivalent (DSE): the ME required to maintain the live weight of a 2-year-old Merino sheep with a live weight of 45 or 50 kg (different authorities use different bases); the animal is 'dry', i.e. either a wether (castrated male) or a non-lactating, non-pregnant ewe. Used in Australia (PIRD, 2020a).
- Animal equivalent (AE): the ME requirement of a 450 kg *Bos taurus* steer at maintenance, 2.25 years of age, grazing on pasture with diet quality of 7.75 MJ ME/kg DM and walking 7 km/day. Used in Australia (MLA, 2018).
- Animal unit (AU): the annual DM intake of a 1000 lb (454 kg) live weight beef cow, assumed to eat 26 lb (11.8 kg) of DM/day; some definitions include a suckling calf. Used in North America (Waller *et al.*, 1986; Manitoba Agriculture, 2019).
- Stock unit (SU): annual feed requirement of a 'standard' 55 kg breeding ewe rearing a single lamb. Used in New Zealand (Beef + Lamb New Zealand, 2020). Table 15.5 gives the SU of different livestock classes.

Stocking rate (SR) is the number of animals which are allocated to a particular area of pasture. SR is measured in animals/ha or km^2. If we define SR in terms of livestock equivalents, then it is similar to the EU term 'grazing livestock density index':

$$\text{Stocking rate (no./ha)} = \frac{(\text{no. of livestock equivalents})}{(\text{effective grazing area, ha})}$$

Unless we are prepared to provide extra feed, the SR should not exceed the carrying capacity. If it does, we risk damaging the pasture because we will exceed the recommended UR, and risk over-grazing the pasture with the consequences for animal performance and pasture sustainability which are described above.

Table 15.5. Livestock equivalents, measured as stock units (SU), of different classes of animals in New Zealand. (From Beef + Lamb New Zealand, 2020; permission granted for re-use by Beef + Lamb New Zealand).

Sheep	SU	Beef cattle	SU	Dairy cattle	SU
Ewe with lamb	1.0	Weaner	3.5	Jersey (lactating)	6.5
Hogget or wether	0.7	Heifer (1.5 years)	4.4	Friesian (lactating)	8.5
Ram	0.8	Steer (2.5 years) or bull	5.5	Dairy bull	5.0
Goats	SU	Deer (red)	SU		
Yearling	0.5	Weaner stag	1.4		
Female	0.8	Weaner hind	1.2		
Buck	0.8	Hind (breeding) Stag (breeding)	1.9 2.2		

Pasture budgeting

Pasture budgeting is a way of planning pasture use over a defined period – a season or a year. It requires information on current TSDM and expected pasture growth, appropriate pasture UR or residual DM, and expected animal DM intakes.

Intensive pasture management with rotational grazing: To calculate the carrying capacity of pastures under intensive management, e.g. a perennial ryegrass (*Lolium perenne*) pasture under rotational grazing, we have to:

1. Decide on a suitable rotation length. This is the time that we expect it will take for enough pasture to grow between grazings for each paddock in the rotation to be able to be regrazed. The rotation length should optimize:

- Pasture regrowth – pastures must not be grazed below the plants' growing points, nor should we leave more than the desired residual DM as this will lead to poorer quality pasture as it regrows.
- Animal nutrient intake – we do not want to graze into the less nutritious strata (see above).

For ryegrass pastures, rotation lengths vary from about 21 to 25 days. This varies with season as the pasture growth rate varies – from about 20 to 140 kg DM/ha per day (in southern Australia; Reed *et al.*, 2011). During times of fast growth, reserve some paddocks for conserving as silage or hay for seasons when pasture supply does not meet the animals' requirements.

2. Decide on an appropriate residual DM; these vary with pasture species composition and animal type. If we estimate the residual DM from measures of pasture height after grazing, remember that the depth of the top, leafy stratum can vary across the paddock (Ison *et al.*, 2019) and we should monitor this. Recommended residuals for dairy cattle grazing ryegrass are between 1400 and 1600 kg DM/ha. This equates to a pasture height of about 5 cm and corresponds to the bottom stratum in Fig. 15.7(b).

3. Calculate the amount of pasture DM expected to be available ($TSDM_E$) in each paddock in the rotation. To do this, measure the current TSDM and add the amount of DM expected to grow between now and the next grazing:

$$TSDM_E\,(kg/ha) = \begin{bmatrix}(TSDM,\ kg/ha)+\\(added\ DM,\ kg/ha)\end{bmatrix} \times (area\ of\ the\ paddock,\ ha)$$

and where:
Added DM (kg/ha) = (DM growth rate, kg/ha per day) × (time until the paddock will be used, days)

4. Estimate the DM intake of the animals (Chapter 7), and calculate the carrying capacity (in animal days):

$$Carrying\ capacity = \frac{\begin{bmatrix}(TSDM_E,\ kg/ha)-\\(residual\ DM,\ kg/ha)\end{bmatrix} \times (paddock\ area,\ ha)}{(animal\ DM\ intake,\ kg/day)}$$

We have to base the whole-farm SR on the carrying capacity of a single paddock, not the total farm area, because we cannot graze those paddocks which are regrowing between leaving and entering the rotation.

Continuous grazing on rangeland pastures: These pastures present a more difficult problem than the intensive management example given above. First, it is fairly difficult to measure the TSDM in rangelands. Second, the growing season in rangelands can be quite short – as little as 4–8 weeks, and if we are using a grazing system which requires animals to be rotated around different paddocks this will fail when we reach the end of the growing season. And third, there is great variability in pasture growth and species composition between years because of variable rainfall and the effects of selective grazing.

Growing season and dormant season carrying capacities are very different for rangeland pastures, and we have to decide how to deal with this.

When a breeding herd or flock gets to the end of the pasture growing season and has grazed 15–30% of that season's growth (i.e. they have removed the utilizable pasture), we will have an amount of dry, standing DM remaining. Usually, we will continue to graze this pasture, often using a N supplement such as a urea/molasses lick (Chapter 16) to encourage animals to graze into the dry, dormant pasture. N and/or P supplements given to deficient cattle can increase DM intake by up to 30% (urea) or 100% (P). Forage budgets for rangeland pastures should take into account the increased grazing pressure resulting from the use of these supplements, and we must avoid over-grazing.

However, in other situations like extended dry periods (drought), or if our resources allow, we can/should:

- irrigate the pasture (if dormancy occurs solely because of moisture stress, and this option is practicable);
- give animals conserved feed such as hay, silage, or a forage crop, or give a cereal grain supplement;
- remove animals from the farm altogether, perhaps into a feedlot or to rented agistment; or
- sell the surplus animals.

It is more difficult to implement these strategies with a breeding, compared to a growing/finishing, enterprise because we cannot easily change the number of breeders and followers between seasons. It is desirable therefore to make decisions on carrying capacity towards the end of the growing ('wet') season when we can reasonably judge future pasture condition, and if possible before the breeding females are mated. Animal numbers need to be adjusted while stock are in good condition and have a good sale value.

Setting stocking rates in the rangelands: We can either use a strategic or tactical approach.

A strategic approach involves setting a SR which we can maintain indefinitely (except in droughts). We could adopt a SR which has been used by successful farmers in the district over the last 10 to 15 years, at least to get a starting point. Express actual stock numbers as livestock equivalents.

A tactical approach allows for other options (Ash *et al.*, 2000; O'Reagain *et al.*, 2018). We could, for example, calculate a SR for the next 12 months to apply from the end of the present growing season. To do this we will:

1. At the end of the growing (e.g. 'wet') season (point **A** in Fig. 15.10) estimate the TSDM (kg/ha) over the whole effective grazing area (EGA), taking account of different pasture and soil types, and watering point placement.
2. Decide on an appropriate pasture UR; this should vary with pasture species composition and maturity but will be between 15 and 30%, depending on climate, pasture and soil type. Apply this to the pasture present at the end of the wet season, and to new pasture growth.
3. Calculate the number of animals the farm can carry for the next year, this provides a substantial buffer against any failure of the next growing season:

$$\text{Carrying capacity (no.)} = \frac{(\text{TSDM, kg/ha}) \times (\text{UR, decimal}) \times (\text{EGA, ha})}{(\text{animal DM intake, kg/day}) \times (365\,\text{days})}$$

This gives a conservative, or 'dry season' SR, and some of the new pasture grown during the next growing ('wet') season will not be used. If our management system allows, we could increase the number of animals carried during the wet season by buying in stock, but we must not exceed the recommended UR. However, animal purchases at this time will be fairly expensive because there is a demand for restocking animals at the start of the new pasture growth season.

A second tactical option is to revise stock numbers at the start of the wet season (point **B** in Fig. 15.10). The calculation is the same as above, but we make a TSDM assessment at the end of the dry season and base our calculations on the expected wet season pasture growth. This option involves some risk because we have to predict pasture growth from climate data and a pasture growth model. We also have to be prepared to reduce stock numbers at the end of the wet season – a time when

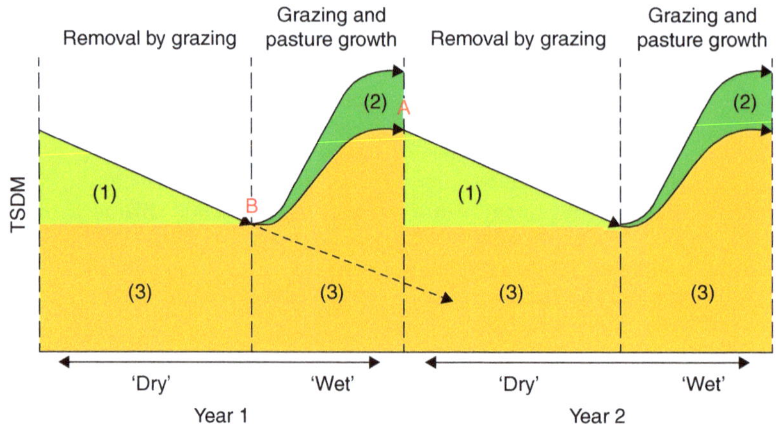

Fig. 15.10. A diagrammatic illustration of how the total standing dry matter (TSDM) of a dryland (rain-grown, non-irrigated) pasture can change with time. A and B are starting times for stocking rate calculations (see the text), (1) is pasture DM eaten during the dormant ('dry') season, (2) is pasture DM eaten during the growing ('wet') season, (3) is the residual DM. The dotted arrow is the TSDM projection if a growing season fails. (Copyright: Gordon McL. Dryden.)

sale prices for these animals, unless well finished, will be trending down. Stocking through the year at the growing season carrying capacity, or over-estimating the carrying capacity at any time, may work in the short term but will certainly crash at some time. A long-term grazing study in northern Australia (O'Reagain *et al.*, 2018) shows that heavy stocking:

- may be profitable in 'good' seasons but will be unprofitable in poor seasons;
- reduces management options and incurs greater costs (e.g. survival feeding) over the long term; and
- results in pasture and soil deterioration.

Feed-year plans

The productivity of grazing animals, and thus the profitability of grazing enterprises, depends on the amount and quality of pasture available for grazing throughout the year. Any period of limited pasture availability or nutritive value will restrict animal performance and will effectively impose a limit on the number, or type, of animals which can be carried.

It is essential to make a feed-year plan when we are starting in a new environment and we want to know how animal nutrient requirements and pasture productivities are expected to change over a sequence of different seasons. To do this, we must know the type of pasture (e.g. all grass, grass plus legume, fodder crop, browse shrubs) we have, and understand how these pastures grow in our environment.

When we design a feed-year plan we use pasture growth as the basic input. This cannot be changed, unless we are fortunate enough to be able to grow irrigated crops or special pastures. On the other hand, we may have some flexibility in planning a breeding calendar. Cattle breed throughout the year, and although most sheep breeds are short day breeders, by using Dorset or Merino breeds we can get sheep to breed outside the usual autumn (fall) period.

The basic approach: In this description, we will use cattle grazing on a native grass pasture in northern Australia as our example.

The first thing that we need to be clear about is the seasonal pattern of grass growth. Figs. 15.5 and 15.11 illustrate the changes in pasture growth and nutrient content of C4 grass pastures growing in a highly seasonal, summer rainfall dominant environment. Of course, similar changes occur in the DM yield and nutritive value of C3 grasses.

We can similarly plot the seasonal changes in a breeding cow's nutrient demand. It is convenient to use the ME requirement, although the seasonal changes in energy, protein and mineral requirements are slightly different. Fig. 15.12 is based on a calving pattern suitable for northern Australia – it shows how the milk production and conceptus (foetus plus placenta) weight change over the year.

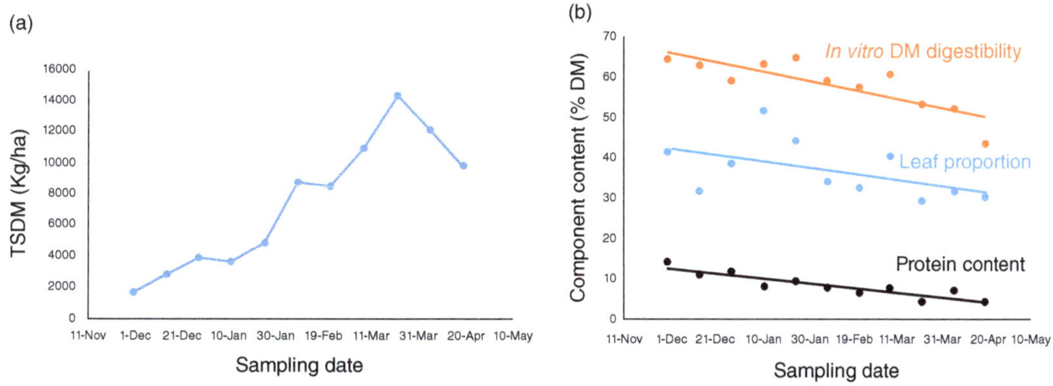

Fig. 15.11. Growth pattern of a typical tropical (C4) grass, a Callide Rhodes grass pasture growing in southern Queensland. **(a)** Total standing dry matter. **(b)** Leaf, dry matter digestibility and protein contents. (From Granzin, 2000; reproduced with permission.)

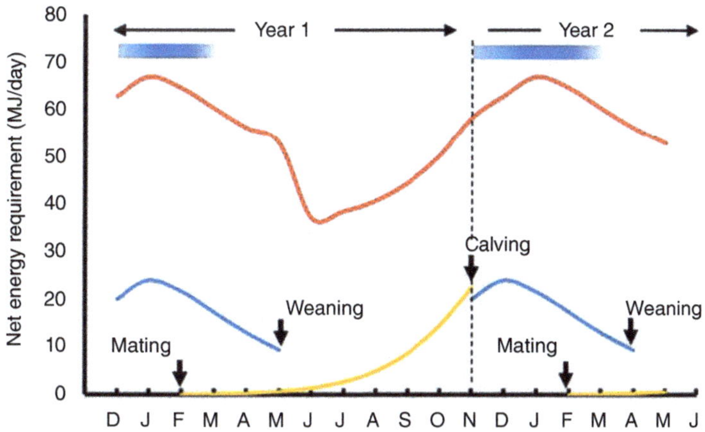

Fig. 15.12. Seasonal changes in the net energy requirements for maintenance (red line, drawn from data in NRC, 2000), milk production (blue line) and pregnancy (yellow line) of a mature beef cow calving a 40 kg calf, with a peak milk production of 8 kg/day and no change in live weight. Horizontal blue bars indicate the probability of rainfall. (Copyright: Gordon McL. Dryden.)

The dates are those which would be expected for a cow calving in the middle of the season.

When the effects of weather (temperature and rainfall) are included in the maintenance energy requirement, and account is taken of the need to make sure that the cow is in good nutritional condition at mating, we get the pattern of nutrient demand illustrated in Fig. 15.13.

'Feed gaps' are periods of the year when pasture fails to meet the animal's nutrient needs. The timing and duration of feed gaps are different for different animal classes and change between years mainly in response to rainfall variability. In Fig. 15.14 the seasonal changes in pasture ME availability (a composite of ME content and DM production) are compared with seasonal changes in nutrient demand.

By plotting the seasonal changes in ME requirements and pasture ME availability we can easily see when problems are likely to occur, and thus we can work out what to do to fix them. Solutions to the problem of low pasture supply in dry seasons could include sowing a special-purpose

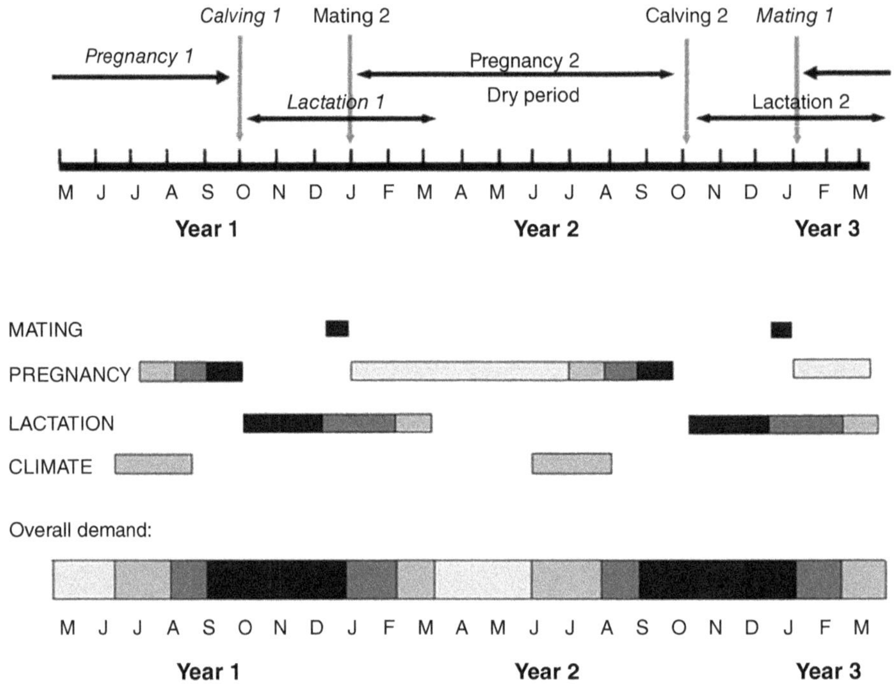

Fig. 15.13. Seasonal changes in the nutrient demand of breeding cows in northern Australia. The shading indicates the breeding cow's daily ME requirement changing from low (light shading) to high (dark shading). (Copyright: Gordon McL. Dryden.)

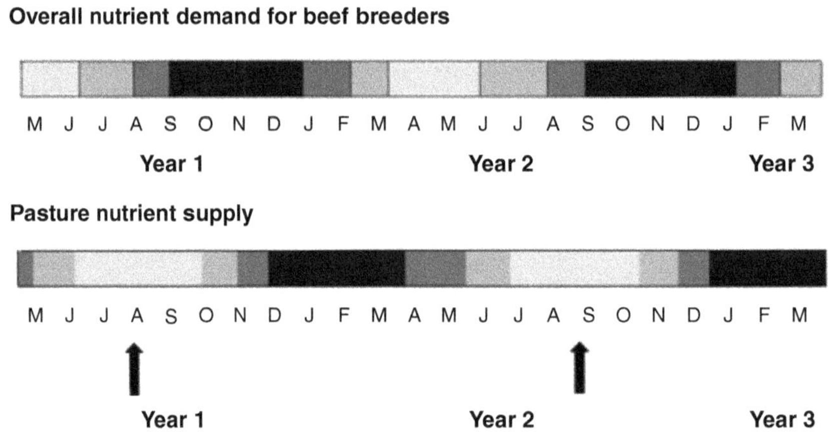

Fig. 15.14. Feed-year planning: plots of periods of high and low ME demand, and high and low pasture ME supply for breeding cattle in northern Australia. In this southern hemisphere environment, breeders experience feed gaps in late winter/early spring (indicated by arrows). (Copyright: Gordon McL. Dryden.)

pasture or forage crop if irrigation is possible or feeding a concentrate supplement or conserved pasture (hay or silage), or controlling mating so that cows calve (and thus lactate) nearer the time when good pasture growth is expected. Controlled mating is effective but it relies on paddock security (good fences) and mustering efficiency, which may be problematic in rangelands. In addition, managers must be prepared to alter grazing management, adjust stock numbers and alter calf weaning age, to either reduce the total animal nutrient demand or to adjust the timing of events so that they better fit the pattern of pasture nutrient supply. Early weaning is a practical option as it significantly reduces the energy demand on the breeder cow.

There is no 'best' solution – choose ones which are feasible on the farm in question, and which will give the most sustainable financial outcome.

References

Akin, D.E. and Burdick, D. (1975). Percentage of tissue types in tropical and temperate grass leaf blades and degradation of tissues by rumen microorganisms. *Crop Science* 15(5): 661–668.

Archimède, H., Rira, M., Eugène, M., Fleury, J., Lastel, M.L., Periacarpin, F., Silou-Etienne, T., Morgavi, D.P. and Doreau, M. (2018). Intake, total-tract digestibility and methane emissions of Texel and Blackbelly sheep fed C4 and C3 grasses tested simultaneously in a temperate and a tropical area. *Journal of Cleaner Production* 185: 455–463.

Ash, A., O'Reagain, P., Mckeon, G. and Stafford Smith, M. (2000). Managing climate variability in grazing enterprises: a case study of Dalrymple Shire, north-eastern Australia. In Hammer, G.L., Nicholls, N. and Mitchell, C. (eds), *Applications of Seasonal Climate Forecasting in Agricultural and Natural Ecosystems*. Atmospheric and Oceanographic Sciences Library, Springer Nature: Switzerland, pp 253–270.

d'Alexis, S., Sauvant, D. and Boval, M. (2014). Mixed grazing systems of sheep and cattle to improve liveweight gain: a quantitative review. *Journal of Agricultural Science* 152(4): 655–666.

Beattie, W.A. (1956). *A Survey of the Beef Cattle Industry of Australia*. CSIRO Bulletin No. 278.

Beck, H.E., Zimmermann, N.E., McVicar, T.R., Vergopolan, N., Berg, A. and Wood, E.F. (2018). Present and future Köppen-Geiger climate classification maps at 1-km resolution. *Nature Scientific Data*. DOI:10.1038/sdata.2018.214.

Beef + Lamb New Zealand (2020). *Benchmarking Tool*. Available at: www.beeflambnz.com/data-tools/benchmarking-tool (accessed 30 December 2020).

Briske, D.D., Derner, J.D., Brown, J.R., Fuhlendorf, S.D., Teague, W.R., Havstad, K.M., Gillen, R.L., Ash, A.J. and Willms, W.D. (2008). Rotational grazing on rangelands: reconciliation of perception and experimental evidence. *Rangeland Ecology and Management* 61: 3–17.

Cowan, R.T., Lowe, K.F., Ehrlich, W., Upton, P.C. and Bowdler, T.M. (1995). Nitrogen-fertilised grass in a subtropical dairy system. 1. Effect of level of nitrogen fertiliser on pasture yield and soil chemical characteristics. *Australian Journal of Experimental Agriculture* 35(2): 125–135.

DairyNZ (2008). *Farmfact 1-15 Using the Rising Plate Meter (RPM)*. Available at: www.dairynz.co.nz/publications/farmfacts/farm-management/farm-fact-1-15/ (accessed 30 December 2020).

Dryden, G.McL. (2008). *Animal Nutrition Science*. Wallingford, UK: CAB International.

Eurostat (2013). *Statistics explained. Glossary: Livestock unit (LSU)*. Available at: www.ec.europa.eu/eurostat/statistics-explained/index.php?title=Glossary:Livestock_unit_(LSU) (accessed 30 December 2020).

Fulkerson, W.J., Slack, K., Hennessy, D.W. and Hough, G.M. (1998). Nutrients in ryegrass (*Lolium* spp.), white clover (*Trifolium repens*) and kikuyu (*Pennisetum clandestinum*) pastures in relation to season and stage of regrowth in a subtropical environment. *Australian Journal of Experimental Agriculture* 38(3): 227–240.

Fulkerson, W.J., Neal, J.S., Clark, C.F., Horadagoda, A., Nandra, K.S. and Barchi, I. (2007). Nutritive value of forage species grown in the warm temperate climate of Australia for dairy cows: grasses and legumes. *Livestock Science* 107(2–3): 253–264.

Gosnell, H., Charnley, S. and Stanley, P. (2020). Climate change mitigation as a co-benefit of regenerative ranching: insights from Australia and the United States. *Interface Focus*, 10: 20200027. DOI: dx.doi.org/10.1098/rsfs.2020.0027.

Gowik, U. and Westhoff, P. (2011). The path from C_3 to C_4 photosynthesis. *Plant Physiology* 155(1): 56–63.

Granzin, B.C. (2000). *Improving the Nutrient Uptake of Dairy Cows Fed Rhodes Grass (Chloris gayana) Grown During Autumn in North-Eastern Australia*. PhD thesis, University of Queensland, Australia.

Ison, K.A.D., Barber, D.G., Benvenutti, M.A., Kleinitz, N., Mayer, D. and Poppi, D.P. (2019) Defoliation dynamics, pasture intake and milk production of dairy cows grazing lucerne pastures in a partial mixed-ration system. *Animal Production Science* 60(1): 175–179.

Kallenbach, R.L. (2015). Describing the dynamic: measuring and assessing the value of plants in the pasture. *Crop Science* 55(6): 2531–2539.

Kottek, M., Grieser, J., Beck, C., Rudolf, B. and Rubel, F. (2006): World Map of the Köppen-Geiger climate classification updated. *Meteorologische Zeitschrift* 15: 259–263.

Livestock Improvement Corporation (LIC) (2021). SPACE™. Available at: https://www.lic.co.nz/products-and-services/space/ (accessed 22 March 2021).
Lorimer, M.S. (1978). Forage selection studies 1. The botanical composition of forage selected by sheep grazing *Astrebla* spp. pasture in north-west Queensland. *Tropical Grasslands* 12(2) 97–108.
Lynch, J.J. and Alexander, G. (1973). *Animal behaviour and the pastoral industries*. In Alexander, G. and Williams, O.B. (eds), *The Pastoral Industries of Australia*. Sydney: Sydney University Press, pp. 317–400.
Manitoba Agriculture (2019). *Animal Unit Months, Stocking Rate and Carrying Capacity*. Available at: www.gov.mb.ca/agriculture/livestock/production/sheep/how-to-determine-stocking-rates-for-manitoba-pastures.html (accessed 30 December 2020).
Matsushita, B., Yang, W., Chen, J., Onda, Y. and Qiu, G. (2007). Sensitivity of the Enhanced Vegetation Index (EVI) and Normalized Difference Vegetation Index (NDVI) to topographic effects: a case study in high-density cypress forest. *Sensors (Basel)* 7(11): 2636–2651.
Meat and Livestock Australia (MLA) (2008). *Making More From Sheep. Module 7: Grow More Pasture.* Available at: www.makingmorefromsheep.com.au/grow-more-pasture/index.html (accessed 30 December 2020).
Meat and Livestock Australia (MLA) (2018). *Animal Equivalent Methodology*. Available at: www.mla.com.au/research-and-development/search-rd-reports/final-report-details/Productivity-On-Farm/Animal-Equivalent-Methodology-A-methodology-to-accurately-and-consistently-calculate-cattle-grazing-loads-in-northern-Australia/453 (accessed 30 December 2020).
Meneses-Tovar, C.L. (2011/2012). NDVI as indicator of degradation. *Unasylva* 238 62: 39–46.
National Agricultural Statistics Service (NASS) (2020). *VegScape. Vegetation Condition Explorer*. Available at: https://nassgeodata.gmu.edu/VegScape/ (accessed 30 December 2020).
National Research Council (NRC) (2000). *Nutrient Requirements of Beef Cattle*, 7th edn. Update. Washington, DC: National Academies Press. Available at: www.nap.edu/catalog/9791/nutrient-requirements-of-beef-cattle-seventh-revised-edition-update-2000 (accessed 9 January 2021).
Norman, M.J.T. (1963). The pattern of dry matter and nutrient content changes in native pastures at Katherine, NT. *Australian Journal of Experimental Agriculture and Animal Husbandry* 3(9): 119–124.
Norton, B.W. (1981). Differences between species in forage quality. In J.B. Hacker (ed.), *Nutritional Limits to Animal Production from Pastures*. Wallingford, UK: CAB International, pp. 89–110.
O'Reagain, P.J. and McMeniman, N.P. (2002). Nutrition of sheep under rangeland conditions. In M. Freer and H. Dove (eds), *Sheep Nutrition*. Wallingford, UK: CAB International, pp. 263–284.
O'Reagain, P.J., Bushelle, J., Pahl, L. and Scanlan, J.C. (2018). *Wambiana grazing trial Phase 3: stocking strategies for improving carrying capacity, land condition and biodiversity outcomes*. North Sydney, Australia: Meat and Livestock Australia. Available at: www.era.daf.qld.gov.au/id/eprint/6338/ (accessed 30 December 2020).
Primary Industries and Regional Development Western Australia (PIRD) (2020a). *Livestock comparisons for estimating grazing pressure in the rangelands*. Available at: www.agric.wa.gov.au/rangelands/livestock-comparisons-estimating-grazing-pressure-rangelands (accessed 30 December 2020).
Primary Industries and Regional Development Western Australia (PIRD) (2020b). *Understanding Pastures from Space for South West Western Australia*. Available at: https://www.agric.wa.gov.au/sheep/understanding-pastures-space-south-west-western-australia (accessed 30 December 2020).
Reed. K.F.M., Nie, Z.N., Walker, L.V. and Mace, W. (2011). Weather and pasture characteristics associated with outbreaks of perennial ryegrass toxicosis in Southern Australia. *Animal Production Science* 51(8): 738–752.
Schaefer, M.T. and Lamb, D.W.A (2016). Combination of plant NDVI and LiDAR measurements improve the estimation of pasture biomass in tall fescue (*Festuca arundinacea* var. Fletcher). *Remote Sensing* 8: 109.
Tenikecier, H.S. and Ates, E. (2019). Effect of altitude on morphological and nutritive characteristics of orchard grass (*Dactylis glomerata* L.) collected from natural flora of Ganos Mountain in Thrace region, Turkey. *Range Management and Agroforestry* 40(2): 286–292.
Walker, J.W. (1994). Multispecies grazing: the ecological advantage. *Sheep Research Journal Special Issue*: 52–64.
Waller, S.S., Moser, L.E. and Anderson, B. (1986). EC86-113. *A Guide for Planning and Analyzing a Year-Round Forage Program*. Historical Materials from University of Nebraska-Lincoln Extension. 1623. Available at: https://digitalcommons.unl.edu/extensionhist/1623/ (accessed 30 December 2020).
Wilson, J.R., Brown, R.H. and Windham, W.R. (1983). Influence of leaf anatomy on the dry matter digestibility of C_3, C_4, and C_3/C_4 intermediate types of *Panicum* species. *Crop Science* 23(1): 141–146.

16 Assessing nutritional status and nutrient supplements for grazing animals

Assessing the nutritional status of animals

Appearance and behaviour: We should have a good idea of the appearance and behaviour of a 'normal' animal – one that is productive and in good health. If there seems to be a problem, then look for:

- live weight or body condition score that are not as expected for an animal of that age and physiological state;
- lameness or other skeletal problems;
- hair condition, including hair loss and change in colour;
- feed intake: the animal is not eating, or is eating less than expected, or is eating sporadically;
- digestive function: the animal is not ruminating (for ruminants), there is evidence of diarrhoea or constipation, or of bloat or rumen impaction in ruminants, or of quidding (loss of partly chewed feed from the mouth) in horses; and
- penned animals (e.g. grower pigs or lot-fed cattle) showing evidence of competition for feed – dominant animals are aggressive towards others, or subordinate animals appear to avoid others, or there is evidence of tail biting in pigs.

Comparison with district animal performance: A sound knowledge of industry or local production norms will help to establish whether the enterprise is functioning well. This information will allow us to recognize abnormal animals and production levels, and so decide whether nutritional problems exist or not. Some farmers have overly optimistic ideas about the levels of performance which they feel they should achieve, while others may fail to recognize problems when they occur.

Target weights: If we can match the herd or flock average live weight against a specific target weight (e.g. mating live weights of 35 kg for a Border Leicester/Merino ewe, or 280 kg for a British breed heifer), it is possible to identify shortfalls in feed supply, either generally or at specific times of the year.

Response to nutrient supplementation: We may be able to confirm a nutrient deficiency by feeding a supplement and measuring the response. But there are two disadvantages to this approach:

- Animals can suffer from multiple nutrient deficiencies and are not likely to respond to a supplement of a single nutrient unless it is the limiting nutrient (Chapter 1). For example, grazing beef cattle may not respond to a P supplement when pasture is mature because ruminally available N (RAN) is likely to be the limiting nutrient. Similarly, a growing pig is not likely to respond (except by becoming over-fat) to an energy supplement if the limiting nutrient is available lysine.
- It takes a long time for animals to respond to a supplement in a way that we can easily see or measure.

Feed analysis and comparison with published feeding standards: Analyses of nutrient content, the presence or content of secondary substances (e.g. tannins, alkaloids), and the presence or content of contaminants (e.g. aflatoxins, insecticides, heavy metals, poisonous seeds) can give useful information as to why animals are not performing. Nutrient contents can be compared with established feeding standards (Chapter 8) for most types of domestic animals. These publications give recommended minimum nutrient contents for various classes of animal and are reliable guides to animals' nutrient requirements (with horses under high work levels and growing pigs in tropical regions being two possible exceptions). If a ration does not contain the recommended nutrient contents or has more than the recommended levels of secondary substances or contaminants, it is unlikely that the animals will perform satisfactorily.

DOI: 10.1079/9781786394453.0016

When collecting feed samples for analysis, it is important to get quantitative data, obtained by reliable sampling and testing methods, from a representative sample. If the problem seems to revolve around some contamination, then take a separate sample of the more heavily affected material.

Use a sampling spear (also called a 'probe' or 'trier') to sample the whole mass of the feed and collect enough to allow all the necessary tests to be carried out – contact the lab before sampling. As a guide (Grain Trade Australia, 2018), take these samples:

- Bagged feed: sample from every bag if fewer than 6 bags, every third bag if there are 6 to 30 bags (but sample at least 6 bags), otherwise from every fifth bag (but sample from at least 10 bags).
- Bulk feed: sample from three places for amounts up to 10 tonnes, add another sampling place for each additional 10 tonnes.

Record (on the package or a label fixed to it) the sample details, seal the sample to prevent loss of moisture, and keep the sample cool until it has been delivered to the lab.

Assessing body condition

Body condition scoring is one of the best methods of identifying the general nutritional status of an animal, and because it is done by visual assessment it is the easiest method to use. Several body condition scoring schemes are available for sheep (Jefferies, 1961; Russel *et al.*, 1969), *Bos taurus* dairy and beef cattle (Earle, 1976; Lowman *et al.*, 1976), *Bos indicus* beef cattle (Nicholson and Butterworth, 1986), *Bos javanicus* cattle (Soares and Dryden, 2011), goats (Ghosh *et al.*, 2019), horses (Carter *et al.*, 2009), pigs (PISC, 2009) and deer (Audigé *et al.*, 1998).

A body condition score (BCS) is a measure of the amount of soft tissue in an animal's body relative to the size of the animal's skeletal frame. It indicates the animal's energy status (fat animals have more soft tissue than thin ones) relative to the animal's age and size (frame size is a good indicator of age). One of the most significant benefits is that a BCS can be made on the live animal, and we do not have to pen or yard the animal or even touch it. BCS are repeatable provided that the scorer is experienced. However, there may be consistent differences between scorers.

BCS methods for sheep, goats, horses and beef cattle use a 5-point scale (although in some there are half-point intervals), and dairy systems usually use a 9- or 10-point scale.

All scales have ranks which range from severely emaciated (and possibly on the point of death) to over-fat. The description of these ranks is similar for all animals but avoid using a BCS system designed for a different animal type because each differs in terms of how their body composition (e.g. relative masses of internal and subcutaneous fat, and where fat is deposited) changes as their nutritional condition changes. The system for Bali cattle is given in Table 16.1 as an example.

BCS can be related to live weight, and if we know this relationship (Table 16.2), we can estimate the amount of metabolizable energy needed to grow an animal from one BCS to another (Table 16.3).

BCS also predict animal performance. Ovulation rates in sheep increase by 0.13 to 0.56 ova/BCS, and the post-partum anoestrus interval decreases in beef and dairy cattle as BCS increases (SCARM, 1990). Grainger *et al.* (1982) showed that BCS was positively associated with improved milk yield of dairy cattle in early lactation.

Methods for identifying mineral deficiencies

Symptoms of mineral deficiencies: Some mineral deficiencies have more-or-less specific symptoms. A selection of these is given in Table 16.4; note that some symptoms are common to deficiencies of several different minerals. Many nutrient deficiencies reduce feed intake and cause a general loss of productivity, but the affected animals show no specific symptoms.

Hypomagnesaemia (grass tetany) and hypocalcaemia (milk fever) are not included in Table 16.4 because they have a significant metabolic component, i.e. are not solely due to diet mineral deficiencies. Milk fever is a result of a greatly increased demand for Ca for colostrum synthesis and failure to regulate blood Ca levels because of poor absorption from the digestive tract and/or mobilization from bones, rather than a dietary Ca deficiency *per se*. Grass tetany is related to an inability to absorb sufficient Mg from the diet. Both conditions have multi-factorial origins – deficiencies and excesses of other minerals, especially Mg, P and K, are involved. PennState Extension (2016) and DairyNZ (2020) have more information on these diseases.

Table 16.1. An example body condition scoring system for Bali (*Bos javanicus*) cattle (from Soares and Dryden, 2011; reproduced with permission.)

BC 1	Hindquarters are flat, hollow or 'dished' at the top; shoulder bones are prominent and easy to see; the upper part of the neck below the vertebrae is fairly flat; the tailhead is very flat; vertebrae, ribs and hooks are very prominent; the dewlap is non-existent or very small
BC 2	Hindquarters are flat at the top; the shoulders are well covered with soft tissue; the neck is quite full with a distinctly rounded appearance; vertebrae, ribs and hooks are easily seen; tailhead is flat; dewlap is present
BC 3	Hindquarters are flat at the top; the shoulders are well covered with soft tissue; the neck is quite full with a distinctly rounded appearance; vertebrae and ribs can be seen but are covered with soft tissue; hooks are easily seen; the tailhead is essentially flat, with very slight rounding; the dewlap is present
BC 4	Hindquarters are flat or slightly rounded at the top; the shoulders are well covered with soft tissue; the neck is quite full with a distinctly rounded appearance; vertebrae can be seen only by looking closely (e.g. by looking obliquely at the animal and the processes are indicated by shadows); ribs can be seen but are covered with soft tissue; hooks can be easily seen; the tailhead is essentially flat, with very slight rounding; the dewlap is present
BC 5	Skin covering the legs is wrinkled; hindquarters are slightly rounded at the top, the hind legs below this area are very full; the shoulders and forequarters are very well covered with soft tissue; the neck is rounded and this extends below the top of the neck down the sides of the neck; neck wrinkles are apparent/present; vertebrae are covered by soft tissue and are not visible; the ribs can only be seen by close inspection; the hooks are covered with soft tissue, but are usually able to be seen; the tailhead has small mounds of soft tissue; the dewlap is large, especially near the brisket

Table 16.2. Regression of live weight (kg) on condition score (scale 0–5) of sheep, goats and beef cattle. (From CSIRO, 2007; reproduced with permission.)

Breed, sex and physiological state		Change in Lwt (kg/unit BCS)	R^2
Ewes (dry)			
Polwarth × South Aust. Merino:	Adult	6.3	0.27
	Maiden	7.3	0.28
Saxon Merino:	Adult	5.6	0.29
	Maiden	7.0	0.31
Scottish Blackface:	Adult	10.6	0.76
Ewes (lactating)			
South Aust. Merino		5.0	0.28
Saxon Merino		5.5	0.16
Corriedale		11.9	0.62
Dorset		11.8	0.44
Angora goats			
Adult wethers		6.1	0.60
Beef cattle (dry, adult)			
Galloway		62	0.75
Shorthorn × Galloway		97	0.87
Hereford × Friesian		104	0.96

Table 16.3. Estimated amount of metabolizable energy (ME) (MJ, above ME for maintenance) needed to increase body condition score (BCS) by one unit in animals fed a reasonable quality pasture (10 MJ ME/kg DM). (From SCARM, 1990; reproduced with permission.)

Type of animal	Live weight change (kg per BCS)	Net energy change (MJ/kg W)	ME required (MJ/BCS)
Adult sheep (scale 0–5)			
Merino	7	21	340
Other breeds	12	21	585
Beef cows (scale 0–5)			
Hereford, Angus	100	21	4900
Dairy cows (scale 1–8)			
Jersey	26	20	1210
Friesian	42	20	1950

Mineral deficiency symptoms are described in each of the National Research Council handbooks (NRC, 2001, 2007a, 2007b, 2016) and in Dryden (2008). Be aware that other nutrients can be involved in a deficiency syndrome, e.g. Mo and S in Cu deficiency, and legume-rich feeds in white muscle disease.

Deficiency symptoms can, with appropriate care, be used to make a tentative diagnosis. However, we

Table 16.4. Symptoms and tests for mineral deficiencies.

Mineral	Deficiency symptom
Ca	Rickets in young animals, osteomalacia in adult animals leading to fragile bones, osteodystrophia fibrosa ('bighead') in horses
Co	Failure to thrive, rough coat, anaemia, difficulty walking, depraved appetite, emaciation which can be extreme *Tests:* blood, or liver (in abattoir specimens) vitamin B12 content; response to vitamin B12 or Co supplement
Cu	Failure to thrive and/or ovulate, pale coat colour (especially around the eyes), rough hair coat, hair loss, fragile bones, difficulty walking and sometimes hind leg paralysis in goat kids, anaemia, diarrhoea Cu excess is poisonous; sheep are the most intolerant of our domestic animals. *Tests:* total plasma Cu content, or caeruloplasmin or superoxide dismutase activities, liver Cu content (in abattoir specimens)
I	Goitre (swelling in the throat as the thyroid gland enlarges), weak or hairless newborns, impaired fertility
Mn	Deformed legs in the newborn, impaired fertility in adults
Na	Abnormal appetite for salt, failure to thrive, reduced feed intake *Tests:* the Na:K ratio in saliva, relative thicknesses of the zona glomerulosa and the cortex in the adrenal gland (in abattoir specimens)
P	Reduced appetite, depraved appetite (pica – eating/chewing bones, carcases, wood, etc.), lameness, fragile bones, pale coat, impaired growth, milk production and reproduction *Tests:* see text
Se	Pale or white lesions in skeletal or cardiac muscles ('white muscle disease'), young animals fail to thrive and show stiffness and/or pain in the legs, growth and reproduction affected Se excess is poisonous *Tests:* blood Se, or the activity of glutathione peroxidase, liver Se content (in abattoir specimens)

often need to confirm this with a more specific test, (such as one of those described in Table 16.4, or below for the P status of grazing cattle, and in Dryden (2008)).

Objective tests for the P status of cattle: There are several possible tests, but none are particularly accurate as the animal's P status is influenced by the P content of its feed, and its ability to draw P from its bones when dietary P is in short supply, a characteristic which is most expressed in lactating cows. Nevertheless, several tests are useful (Dixon and Coates, 2012). These are:

- Blood P content (blood inorganic P, BIP) is not a very sensitive indicator as it reflects the animal's recent dietary history, rather than its underlying P status. Animal age, sampling site, sampling stress, and exercise all influence BIP levels. Nevertheless, BIP has been extensively used to indicate the P status of grazing animals. Blood P can be used, in combination with soil available P contents, to indicate the status of steers and dry cows, but not for lactating cows. Accordingly, one approach is to graze some steers with the lactating cows and to use these as indicator animals.
- Faecal P content reflects the animal's P intake, but the concentration of P in faeces is affected by feed intake level and the amount of endogenous P which is excreted. Faecal P content gives a reasonable indication of feed P content except if the animal is fed a concentrate or a P supplement.
- Bone analysis: this is an invasive test, made by surgically removing pieces of bone from the ribs. It is the best measure of the animal's P status, but the least practical unless done on abattoir specimens.

Planning nutrient supplementation of grazing animals

We should consider financial and welfare outcomes as well as nutritional objectives when deciding on a supplementation programme. To achieve welfare outcomes we must protect the animal from the health consequences of nutrient deficiencies. It is important to differentiate between optimum performance and maximum performance. Optimum animal performance is the more important aim in commercial animal production as it accounts for the economic objectives of the enterprise, whereas maximum performance is solely driven by the objective of achieving an animal's genetic potential. Optimum performance can include keeping an animal alive, or ready to produce (e.g. have a calf) at a later time.

To be successful, a supplement should be:

- nutritionally effective: it provides the first-limiting nutrients;
- reliable: it is accepted by the target animals and intakes are uniform;
- safe: with little risk of poisoning if the delivery system breaks down;
- cost-effective: the cost of the supplement is less than the value of the response; and
- used in appropriate circumstances: supplements should not be used as substitutes for whole feeds.

If animals are supplemented with nutrients which, from pasture analysis, seem to be deficient but which are not the primary cause of reduced animal performance, then we will not improve productivity. The 'leaky bucket' analogy described in Chapter 1 illustrates this. Cattle grazing dormant, dryland range pasture may be deficient in ruminally available N (RAN), energy, S and P, but the first-limiting nutrients are likely to be RAN and energy. Some minerals, e.g. P, Cu, Co and/or Se, may be required year-round if the pasture is growing in mineral-deficient soil.

The safety and cost-effectiveness of supplementation depend on all animals eating the supplement in amounts which are nutritionally effective, and not wastefully excessive or potentially poisonous. But individual animals may not use a supplement, and the intakes of those individuals that do use it are usually very different. Delivery systems are designed to attract as many animals as possible to eat the supplement, but at the cost of excess consumption by some animals. Fortified molasses (M8U, molasses with 8% urea dissolved in it) is an example: most cows will use this supplement and eat 2–3 kg/day or more – this is nearly three times the effective dose of urea and is near the toxic level of urea consumption.

Examples of how urea delivery systems can fail include the internal drum in a rotating drum feeder jamming and allowing animals to drink the molasses/urea/water solution, or urea/molasses blocks becoming soft in hot or wet weather and allowing animals to eat rather than lick the block.

● Supplements cannot replace feeds. Supplements provide specific nutrients, e.g. a mineral or RAN, and they should not be used in situations where a whole feed would be more appropriate. This particularly applies to urea/molasses/protein supplements which are the most likely to be misused in this way. Feeds provide energy, and a range of other nutrients (Chapter 1). Urea/molasses/protein supplements supply RAN and bypass protein and some minerals, but almost no fibre and, except for fortified molasses, are not eaten in large enough amounts to supply enough ME for maintenance let alone to support production.

The decision chart in Fig. 16.1 and the information in Fig. 16.2 will help to identify situations where RAN or mineral supplements will be useful.

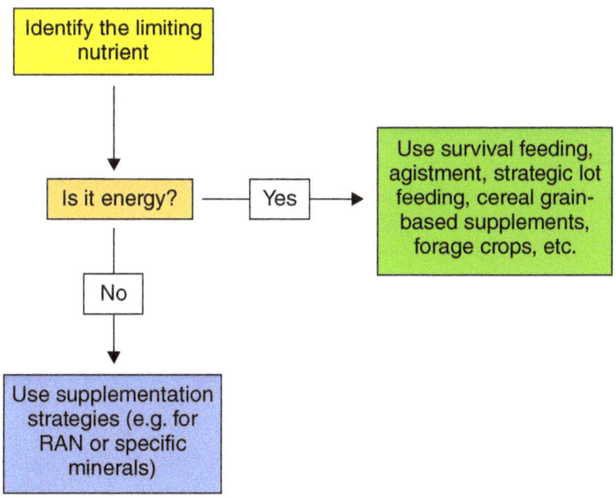

Fig. 16.1. Flow chart for deciding whether to use a specific nutrient supplement or a whole-feed alternative. (Copyright: Gordon McL. Dryden.)

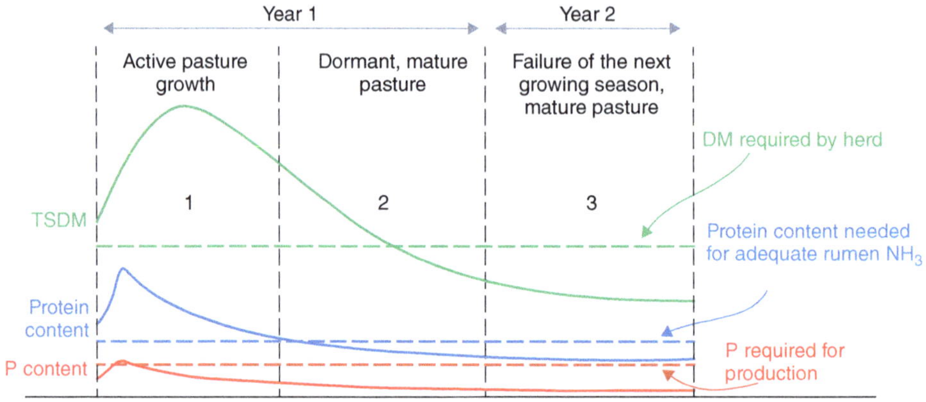

Fig. 16.2. Use of ruminally available N (RAN) and P supplements during the normal growth and maturity cycle of a C4 tropical pasture (Periods 1 and 2), and if the next growing season fails (Period 3). Solid lines indicate pasture total standing dry matter (TSDM), and protein and P contents (not to scale), dotted lines indicate animal requirements. In Period 1 animals may respond to a P supplement because the P content of standing DM falls as the plant ages but protein and energy provided by the growing plant are adequate; in Period 2 a RAN supplement is required because pasture protein content is less than the animals' requirement and RAN becomes the limiting nutrient; in Period 3 additional whole feed (i.e. not just a supplement) is needed because low TSDM means that energy, protein and P intakes are all inadequate. (Copyright: Gordon McL. Dryden.)

Supplement delivery methods

Nutrient blocks are compressed salt or molasses-based blocks which can be used to provide bypass protein, RAN (from urea) and minerals (often Na, P, Ca, Mg, Cu, Co, Se). Some blocks are made with distillers' dried grains and solubles instead of molasses. Nutrient blocks may also provide anti-bloat agents, vitamins, growth promoters, and insecticides designed to kill fly larvae in faeces.

The main advantage of nutrient blocks is their convenience, as no special equipment is needed to use them.

Molasses blocks are made to set (harden) by heating and/or the inclusion of Ca carbonate or Ca oxide. Nevertheless, all blocks which contain urea or potentially poisonous trace minerals (e.g. Cu or Se) must be protected from moisture and high temperatures as they may soften and allow a potentially toxic urea or mineral intake. Both home-made and commercial blocks vary considerably in their consistency and resistance to moisture.

Aqueous solutions are used to deliver urea and minerals to cattle and sheep, and the mixture contains molasses as an attractant. This type of supplement is dispensed from rotating drum feeders – a trough fitted with a rolling drum. The inner, rotating, drum picks up a thin film of the liquid which is licked off by the cow. The supplement dosage is regulated by adjusting the molasses:water ratio. This method has largely fallen out of favour because the solution needs very careful preparation if it contains urea, pumps and vats are needed to prepare it in bulk, the feeding equipment is difficult to use, there can be problems with the supplement fermenting, and steel equipment is liable to corrode when in contact with a molasses/urea supplement mixture.

Fortified molasses is a mixture of molasses containing an amount of dissolved urea, or a mixture of molasses and urea plus added protein meal and minerals. FM is fed from an open trough. Provided that the farm has the necessary pumps and storages the method is not unduly labour demanding and is acceptably safe. Fortified molasses provides amounts of minerals, RAN, undegradable dietary protein (UDP) and ME from the molasses and protein ingredients.

Loose, dry mixes consisting of dry mixtures of salt, dicalcium phosphate and urea, or similar ingredients can be used to provide urea and/or supplementary minerals. Loose mixes are popular in regions where molasses-based supplements are uneconomic because of excessive intake or the high cost of the purchase, delivery and storage of molasses, and they can give results similar to molasses-based mixtures (Bowman *et al.*, 1995).

Water-delivered supplements: minerals or urea are dissolved in water and dispensed through automated dosing equipment into water troughs in the paddock. Delivery in drinking water has these important differences from other methods:

- All animals will consume the supplement, because all drink from the supplied water source.
- Supplement intakes should be more uniform than with other delivery methods (but see below).
- We have to use water-soluble nutrient sources – this is not a problem because there are suitable water-soluble N, P and S sources.
- Special supplement feeding equipment, or expensive carriers (like molasses) are not needed.
- If animals can be supplemented *en bloc*, all the water used by the animals on a property can be treated with the supplement at a single point so we may have to buy and maintain only one dosing apparatus, rather than have supplement feeders for each paddock.

There are important caveats when using water-delivered supplements: supplement intakes will be inadequate or very variable if animals do not drink each day, or if they get some of their water from the feed or from streams or springs. Heat-stressed, thirsty animals drink more than expected amounts of water, and animals have suffered from urea poisoning in these situations. On the other hand, adding urea to drinking water can change voluntary water intake (both increases and decreases have been reported) and this can put animals at risk in hot conditions. Water intake varies between seasons, and at any time there can be substantial variations between animals. For example, coefficients of variation of 55% for weaner heifers and 6–18% for sheep have been reported.

There are some concerns about the stability of supplements dissolved in water which has been obtained from subterranean sources, and possible problems of sedimentation and flocculation, development of concentration layers of supplement in the trough or tank, and algal growth.

Mineral supplementation methods

Minerals which are commonly given as supplements include Ca, P, Mg, Na and S, and the trace minerals Cu, Co, I, Se and Zn. The required minerals vary with soil type, pasture plant species composition and plant age, and animal type and physiological status.

Minerals can be poisonous, even though they are essential nutrients (see Chapter 1) and in some cases we have to take particular care to ensure that dosages are sufficient but not excessive. Excess Cu poisons sheep, while cattle, horses and pigs are tolerant; and Co, I and Se are also potentially toxic. On the other hand, while only a small amount of these minerals is needed, any shortfall can have serious consequences.

Particularly with trace minerals, we should use a delivery method which gives exactly the required dose over several weeks or months. Suitable delivery methods are summarized in Table 16.5. Note that

Table 16.5. Methods of providing macro- and trace minerals to grazing animals.

Delivery method	Suitable for	Comments
Liquid supplements	Na, P, Mg, S	Mineral sources must be soluble; variable intake so not suitable for Co, Cu, I or Se
Nutrient blocks based on salt or molasses	Na, P, Ca, Mg, S	Variable intake so not suitable for Co, Cu, I or Se supplements to sheep
Loose (dry) mixes	Na, P, Ca, Mg, S	Variable intake and difficult to mix trace minerals adequately so not suitable for Co, Cu, I or Se supplements
Fortified molasses	Na, P, Ca, Mg, S	Variable intake so not suitable for Co, Cu, I or Se
Drinking water	Na, P, S	Not suitable for mineral sources which are not water-soluble; potential variable intake may predispose to S toxicity
Oral drench	Co, Cu, I, Se, Zn	Accurate dosage but has to be repeated regularly, not suitable for minerals which are needed in large amounts
Rumen/abomasum bolus	Co, Cu, I, Se, Zn	Accurate dosages for several weeks, months or years but difficult to administer
Subcutaneous or intramuscular injection	Co, Cu, I, Se, Zn	Accurate dosages for several weeks but risk of abscesses with Cu glycinate
Pasture fertilization	Cu, Co, P, Se, Zn	Effective in many cases but expensive and requires adequate rainfall for pasture response; responses may be short-lived depending on the soil type

any method that involves voluntary consumption will give variable mineral intakes (Cockwill *et al.*, 2000; Manzano *et al.*, 2012).

Phosphorus supplements: The most commonly-used P sources are dicalcium phosphate (DCP) and mono-dicalcium phosphate (MDCP, which is a mixture of monocalcium phosphate and DCP). Other sources include phosphoric acid, mono-ammonium phosphate (MAP), superphosphate fertilizer and rock phosphate.

MDCP and DCP are the preferred P sources; they contain 21% P and 20% Ca, and 18% P and 23% Ca, respectively. They are fed in blocks or in dry, loose mineral mixtures. All P sources may contain contaminants such as AS, F, Pb, Cd and Hg so we need to make sure that the product complies with standards for these substances.

Although the other P sources listed above have been used in practice, they all have some potential problems:

- Phosphoric acid has given variable responses when fed to cattle. Holm *et al.* (1981) recorded positive responses when supplementary phosphoric acid was fed to breeding cows, while Playne (1974) found that heifers were adversely affected. Points to watch when using phosphoric acid include the possibilities of inducing a Ca deficiency, poisoning by heavy metals if these contaminate the product, or reduced water consumption if the acid is provided in the drinking water. Phosphoric acid is corrosive and can harm skin and eyes; always use personal protective equipment and always add the acid to water rather than water to acid.
- Commercial grade MAP may contain excess amounts of F and Cd. For these reasons it is best to use technical grade MAP.
- Superphosphate fertilizer can be used to make a P supplement by steeping it in water and discarding the F-rich sediment, but this is not recommended given the availability of other, safer P sources.

P sources can be fed to animals by all of the delivery methods described above. Inclusion rates in feeds rarely exceed 6% due to palatability problems.

Sulphur supplements: The desired N:S ratio in urea supplements is approximately 12.5:1 for sheep and 14:1 for cattle. Molasses provides some S, but not enough to match the RAN provided by most urea supplements. Additional S can be provided from ammonium sulphate or elemental S. Excess S can be toxic.

Non-protein N and protein supplements

These are designed to improve the grazing animal's ability to digest plant fibre in its rumen and thus increase feed digestibility and intake, and protein supplements also increase the amounts of essential amino acids available to the animal.

Rumen micro-organisms require at least 5 mg NH_3/100 ml of rumen liquor for active plant fibre digestion. When ruminants are deficient in RAN (which is the precursor of NH_3) the rate at which fibre is digested in the rumen is reduced and this affects both the obtaining of nutrients from the feed and the animal's feed intake. Deficiencies of RAN occur when pastures have a low protein content and this protein is poorly degradable in the rumen, i.e. when pastures become aged and mature.

The most-used non-protein N supplement is urea, and oilseed meals are often used to provide whole protein supplements.

Urea blocks are available from commercial sources, and there are also recipes for home-made blocks containing urea, protein meals and molasses (Blackwood, 2006; Makkar *et al.*, 2007). Commercial blocks are made in different sizes, from 2 to 100+ kg; home-made blocks are usually 10–25 kg for ease of handling.

The label on a commercial urea block may indicate an 'equivalent protein content'. This is the urea content × 2.87 (urea contains 46.7% N, and this is multiplied by 6.25 to calculate an 'equivalent crude protein content'). This factor assumes that all the N in urea is incorporated into rumen microbial protein and allows for impurities which may be present in the urea.

Urea 'licks' are mixtures of urea, molasses and water fed from a rotating drum feeder. Urea 'licks' have been used in the dry subtropics and tropics for over 50 years.

Molasses was originally included in the lick to attract animals, but it was soon established that a daily molasses intake of about 0.25 kg/head (for cattle) gave optimum results, probably because of the S it contributes. The proportion of molasses used varies between 20% and 60 % (w/w), depending on the experience of cattle with the supplement. The molasses:water ratio should be adjusted to suit individual herds, so as to give an appropriate intake. The urea content is usually about 10% (w/w) and should be adjusted to provide between 30 and 60 g/head daily. Mineral sources, especially for P and S, can be added to the mix.

Fortified molasses: The most usual mixtures are M8U (a mixture of molasses containing 8% urea) and MUP (molasses with 3% urea plus 10% protein meal). FM is fed from an open trough. It is essential that the urea is evenly mixed through the molasses carrier. Fortified molasses is a more reliable delivery method than urea blocks as only 1–2% of a herd refuse the supplement. However, urea intakes are high; some cattle have eaten 6 kg/head daily of an 8% mix. The average intake is 2 kg/head daily, which provides 160 g of urea. This is at least 100 g more urea than is needed and so is a rather expensive method of providing urea. Because of the high urea intakes, M8U must be introduced carefully and slowly.

Urea/molasses supplements, fed from open troughs, are now sold by many commercial suppliers. These supplements can be tailored to each individual herd by adjusting the urea and molasses contents, or by adding an acid to reduce intake. Some manufacturers use a sustained-release urea product (e.g. urea granules covered with a semi-permeable membrane) to enhance safety, and protein meals, vitamins and minerals may be included in the mixture.

Loose mixes: These consist of dry mixtures of salt, dicalcium phosphate, urea and protein meal or similar ingredients, used as a urea/mineral source for cattle. Consumption is variable and there is a risk of poisoning if the mix contains urea unless this is introduced carefully. Feed salt alone for two weeks before adding the urea, and then add all the urea (typically 30–40% of a loose mix) so that its unpleasant taste deters cattle from eating too much of the mix (FutureBeef, 2011). A practical loose mix providing urea, protein and minerals is described by Dixon and Petherick (1996): 380 g salt, 300 g urea, 150 g cottonseed meal, 150 g calcium phosphate and 10 g sulphur.

Water delivery: Because urea is highly soluble in water (1.4 g dissolves in 1 mL water), solutions of urea can be prepared and pumped through the water reticulation system. The usual concentration is 2 g urea/L water (a 0.2% solution). Although this method should give a more uniform urea intake than blocks or licks or dry mixes, there can be problems with this delivery method as discussed above.

Responses to urea and protein supplements

Urea supplements to cattle grazing low-quality, over-mature pasture can reduce the live weight losses experienced by unsupplemented animals (it is optimistic to expect live weight gains) and support better breeding performance.

However, results vary in practice. There are several reasons:

- Variation in supplement consumption between animals.
- Irregular consumption of urea through the day, and rapid metabolism of urea in the rumen.
- Lack of enough forage for animals to be able to express the appetite-stimulating effect of urea.
- Presence of green pasture material if unseasonal rain promotes pasture growth. Cattle will reject urea/molasses supplements in favour of the small amount of green pasture available.

Variation in urea intake: Cattle and sheep must consume an effective dose of urea. This is about:

- 30 g/day for young or small-breed cattle, increasing to about 60 g/day for older, heavier animals; and
- 10 g/day for sheep.

Urea blocks and liquid urea/molasses supplements contain 5–30% urea. An adult cow must eat some 300 g/day in order to obtain an effective urea intake from a urea/molasses supplement containing 10% urea. Intakes of urea supplements vary with supplement type, the delivery system, and animal management (Tables 16.6 and 16.7) and pasture conditions. Consumption of molasses-based blocks by cattle can vary from 150 to 550 g/head daily, but the blocks are not eaten by all the animals in the group (Table 16.7), and acceptance may be as low as 60% of the herd. Nolan *et al.* (1974) found that the intake by cattle of a 3% urea/10% molasses/water mixture given by roller drum varied from 30 mL to 2.4 L /head per day, and that 20% of the animals did not eat the supplement at all.

Lack of synchronicity between RAN availability in the rumen and the intake of forage: If there is not enough volatile fatty acid (VFA) available in the rumen to combine with the amount of NH_3 available to form microbial amino acids, the unused NH_3 will be absorbed from the rumen, detoxified and excreted in the urine. This leads to very inefficient use of the urea-N. Cattle generally visit

Table 16.6. Acceptance and mean intakes of urea supplements fed to sheep. (From Entwistle and Knights, 1974; Taylor and Dryden, 2003; reproduced with permission.)

Supplement	Consumers (% of herd)	Urea intake by consumers (g/head daily)
Merino ewes, grazing dry *Astrebla* sp. pasture		
Low urea mix	84.9	11.7
High urea mix	85.8	14.9
Molasses only	78.5	–
Merino wethers, penned, fed chopped *Chloris gayana* hay		
Drinking water (0.2% urea)	100	5.7
Fortified molasses (M8U)	100	10.8
Dry loose mix	100	4.2

Table 16.7. Supplement intakes by cattle given different methods of urea supplement. (From Dixon and Petherick, 1996; reproduced with permission.)

Category	Intake (g/head daily)		
	M8U[a]	Dry mix	Block
Consumers			
Weeks 1 to 5	1257	176	120
Weeks 6 to 10	1172	145	97
Coefficient of variation (%)			
Weeks 1 to 5	29	85	105
Weeks 6 to 10	26	71	83

[a]M8U is a mixture of molasses and 8% dissolved urea.

a urea supplement only once or twice daily, and as a result they eat doses of urea which are rapidly fermented with the loss of a large proportion of the RAN.

We can resolve some of these problems by careful choice of delivery method and animal management. Modern delivery systems, and especially the use of sustained-release urea, give more uniform intakes, better sustained release in the rumen of NH_3 from urea, and reduce the chance of poisoning.

Deciding when to start a urea supplement: There are three objective tests, all better than simply assuming that animals will respond to a supplement when the available pasture is mature and dry.

- We can measure the animals' rumen NH_3 levels but to do this we need to get rumen liquor samples and carry out a chemical test. This is possible, but not practicable.
- A more feasible option is to analyse the faeces of animals grazing the pasture in question. A response to urea supplementation is likely when the faecal N content falls below 1.3% (DM) (Fig. 16.3).
- A more accurate indicator than simple faecal N content is the ratio of digestible DM (DMD, % DM basis) to crude protein (CP, % DM basis) in the feed. The threshold values which suggest that we might get a response to a N supplement are about 7 for North American range pastures, and 8 or 9 for northern Australian native tropical pastures to 10 for northern Australian Mitchell grass pastures. Preliminary data from Dixon (2007) suggests that the amount of urea needed can also be predicted from the DMD:CP value.

Faecal analysis using near infrared spectroscopy (F.NIRS): We can estimate the feed DMD and CP contents from analyses of faeces using F.NIRS (Dryden, 2003). In addition, F.NIRS analysis has several other uses, provided that we have appropriate prediction equations. For example, we can predict feed nutrient content and diet plant species composition, and also pregnancy and parasite burden. Adoption of F.NIRS technology has been slow, partly because of the work needed to develop appropriate prediction equations, but it has great potential for managing the nutrition of grazing animals. F.NIRS information can help plan grazing management and save money on unnecessary or ineffective supplements.

Sample collection and preparation is very simple. In essence, simply collect at least ten 50 mL samples of fresh, uncontaminated faeces from the paddock the animals are grazing, and either dry (in the sun) or freeze before delivery to the lab. Contact the local provider for detailed instructions.

Warnings about using urea:

- Be familiar with its properties: urea is presented as white crystals, powder or prills (small, spheres), it is highly soluble in water; irritates skin, eyes and respiratory tract; and has a bitter taste.
- Introduce urea carefully. If the target urea content in the supplement is 10% or less (i.e. for FM

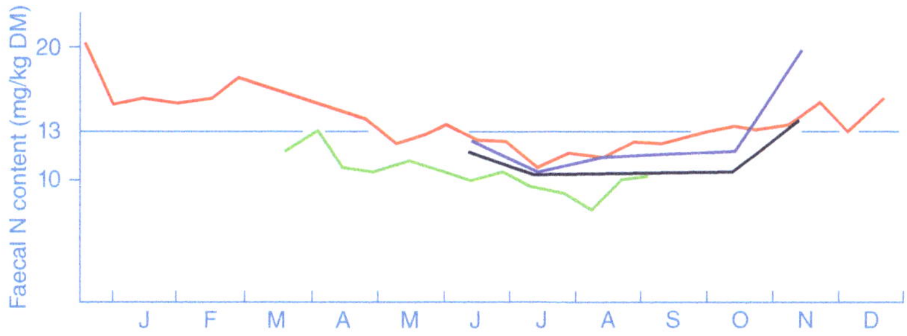

Fig. 16.3. Change in faecal N content as the northern Australian dormant (dry) season continues. (Drawn from data in Addison, 1970; Addison *et al.*, 1984; Foster and Blight, 1984.)

and water delivery), urea should be introduced gradually, over several days or weeks. Loose dry mixes are treated differently because the target urea content is 30–40% and most deaths occur when cattle are given a loose mix containing 10–20% urea.

- Intakes of urea supplements are variable and are affected by the delivery system that is used, different individual animal behaviours, and the environment.
- Urea supplements are not a complete feed, even when they are used with a molasses carrier.
- Urea can be poisonous – a dose of urea equivalent to 30 g/100 kg live weight may be toxic for cattle (Chapter 13). Note that fat animals are less tolerant than lean ones, and that animals which are accustomed to urea are more tolerant than those just starting on a supplementation programme.

Protein supplements: More reliable and greater responses have been recorded with protein supplements such as oilseed meals (Chapter 6) than with urea. These supplements provide bypass protein, some ME, and minerals. They increase animal productivity through more efficient use of dietary ME for live weight gain, increased DM intake without substitution of protein meal for forage (Chapter 7), and possibly increased rumen capacity. Because they are well accepted by animals, they may suit situations when unseasonal rain or temperatures promote a little pasture growth (in contrast to the situation with urea supplements).

Best results are obtained with protein meals which have high UDP contents. Given similar protein degradabilities, the choice of supplement will depend mainly on relative costs, but reliability of supply and the palatability of the supplement should also be considered.

The feeding method is simple. Feed a predetermined amount of the protein meal daily or twice weekly either on the ground, or better still, in troughs. Protein meals are usually palatable, although palm kernel meal should be introduced gradually to accustom animals to it. If there are problems of acceptance, try mixing the meal with molasses. Be aware that some animals will avoid any supplement.

Best results are obtained by feeding beef cattle between 0.5 and 1 kg/head daily. As some animals will find the protein meal very attractive, the supplement should not be fed *ad lib* as the exercise will become very expensive. Protein meals have usually been given as daily feeds but feeding twice weekly will give good results if the protein in the meal has a low degradability. Twice-weekly feeding involves giving half of the total weekly amount in each of the two feeds, e.g. 2 feeds of 2.1 kg/head rather than 7 daily feeds of 0.6 kg/head. Warning: feeding in one amount, 2- or 3-days' supply of a protein-rich, highly ruminally degradable protein meal (e.g. canola or soybean meals) has caused NH_3 poisoning in cattle (DAFQ, 2010–2020).

Do not feed protein meals made from animal products, as these can be a vehicle for prion transmission (see Chapter 12). Feeding animal meals to ruminants is banned in many countries. Suitable protein meals for sheep, goats and cattle are cottonseed meal (43% protein; 0.07% gossypol), soybean meal (47%), canola meal (35%), sunflower meal (35%), copra meal (23%), palm kernel meal (15%; and contains 3% fat) and whole cottonseed (21%; and contains 0.5% of potentially poisonous gossypol; see Chapter 12). Data on the protein and other nutrient contents of these meals are summarized in Chapter 6.

When to stop giving a protein or urea supplement: Stop feeding these supplements when pasture becomes exhausted (see Fig. 16.2). These supplements are designed only to provide the nutrients which are deficient in mature pasture, they are not intended as a replacement for pasture.

Fortified molasses can be used as a survival feed if necessary because under optimum conditions intakes approach 1.5% of live weight/day, which is near to a maintenance feeding level. However, cereal grains are often a cheaper energy source (see Chapter 9 for a method of calculating nutrient costs) than molasses, are accepted by almost all animals, and are easier to store and handle than molasses.

Economics of nutrient supplementation

Although we might get a production response to a supplement, this will not be worthwhile if the supplement costs more than the value of the response.

Growth responses to urea supplements have been reported fairly consistently, but these are almost always reductions in the amount of live weight lost during pasture dormancy (e.g. the dry season in the northern Australian rangelands) rather than actual increases in live weight. Compensatory growth, where unsupplemented animals grow more quickly than previously supplemented ones when given access to good pasture (e.g. in the next pasture growing season), can sometimes remove any financial advantage to urea supplementation.

We can get better results with breeding cattle (e.g. Hennessy *et al.*, 1998). Conception rates have been increased by 5% or more by feeding urea, or more particularly protein, supplements. In one case, pregnancies in maiden 2-year-old cows were increased by up to 40%. Low conception rates in maiden (yearling) heifers, adult cows in poor condition, or cows which had calved in the previous year and were under nutritional stress caused by lactation, have been rectified by supplementation. In some cases, supplementation has allowed up to 75% more cows to hold to service and has reduced the mating period required. Improvements in the growth of suckling calves (about 15 kg heavier at weaning) have been recorded where their dams were supplemented, although this advantage can also be lost through compensatory growth after weaning. But we should note that weaning at the start of the dry/dormant season can be more successful than a RAN supplement (Dixon *et al.*, 2011).

P supplements are economically worthwhile in regions with low soil P contents because pastures growing on these soils are always P deficient. P supplements given to cattle grazing pastures on better soils may give a response when the pasture is growing, but not if the pasture is mature and poorly digestible, and energy is the first-limiting nutrient. In some cases we may need to provide P for more than a year before we see a response. This is because cattle may be able to draw on bone P reserves for a year without supplementation.

In summary, nutrient supplementation is only cost-effective if it:

- keeps an animal alive that might otherwise die, or prevents disorders such as lameness (e.g. P supplements), extreme emaciation (Co), and white muscle disease (Se);
- improves breeding performance;
- improves product quality – e.g. Careful Cu supplementation of sheep prevents 'steely' wool; and
- improves growth during the supplementation period and the animal is to be sold at the end of that period.

Survival feeding

This feeding technique is used in two different situations: in drought when pasture supplies are exhausted and animals have to be given a whole-feed supplement; or if pasture is lost to fire or flood.

Survival feeding is expensive, and in both situations, we should feed the cheapest source of ME, and reduce the feeding level to that which will keep an animal alive, rather than productive. However, there are exceptions: dairy cattle, breeding cows and ewes, and meat-producing animals which are near to finishing, can be fed to maintain production if this is deemed to be financially sound. Determining appropriate levels of feeding is a knife edge and we can easily feed too little with disastrous consequences. Guides to feed types and amounts for survival feeding are provided by DAFQ (2010–2020).

Suitable feeds include forages such as hay or silage, but cereal grains are more often used as these are usually the cheapest source of ME. The gradual loss of pasture in a drought gives time to adapt animals to grain-rich feeds, but rapid-onset emergencies such as floods and fires occur quickly and allow no time to collect adequate feed stocks or adapt animals to a novel feed. Failure of adaptation can cause disorders like rumen acidosis, laminitis and diarrhoea (Chapter 13). To be safe, in these circumstances feed roughage-based rations to ruminants and horses, rather than feeds rich in cereal grains.

Some feeds which are used in droughts are not usually fed under more favourable circumstances. Be aware that failed crops or crop residues can be contaminated with defoliants, pesticides or weedicides (Chapter 6). These chemicals can be absorbed and incorporated into the animal's tissues. Always check novel feeds and observe any withholding periods before selling animals or their products (MLA, 2020).

Fires, floods and droughts inflict social and economic stresses on managers in addition to the stress of dealing with potentially starving animals. Nevertheless, as far as is reasonable, we must give animal welfare a high priority. This may mean destocking and accepting a reduction in future income and the possible loss of prized genetic lines.

Good advice is to 'sell and regret but sell'. Do this early while the animals' condition is still attractive to the market, markets are not inundated with stock for sale, and there is less risk of feeding animals which may subsequently die or may be unproductive when the emergency is over.

References

Addison, K.B. (1970). Management systems on spear grass country. In *Proceedings of the XIth International Grasslands Congress* Brisbane: University of Queensland Press, pp. 789–793.

Addison, K.B., Cameron, D.G. and Blight, G.W. (1984). Biuret, sorghum and cottonseed meal as supplements for weaner cattle grazing native pastures in sub coastal southeast Queensland. *Tropical Grasslands* 18(3): 113–120.

Audigé, L., Wilson, P.R. and Morris, R.S. (1998). A body condition score system and its use for farmed red deer hinds. *New Zealand Journal of Agricultural Research* 41(4): 545–553.

Blackwood, I. (2006). *Making your own protein blocks for cattle*. NSW Dept Primary industries PrimeFact 273.

Bowman, J.G.P., Sowell, B.F. and Paterson, J.A. (1995). Liquid supplementation for ruminants fed low-quality forage diets: a review. *Animal Feed Science and Technology* 55(1–2): 105–138.

Carter, R.A., Geor, R.J., Staniar, W.B., Cubitt, T.A. and Harris, P.A. (2009). Apparent adiposity assessed by standardised scoring systems and morphometric measurements in horses and ponies. *The Veterinary Journal* 179(2): 204–210.

Cockwill, C.L., McAllister, T.A., Olson, M.E., Milligan, D.N., Ralston, B.J., Huisma, C. and Hand, R.K. (2000). Individual intake of mineral and molasses supplements by cows, heifers and calves. *Canadian Journal of Animal Science* 80(4): 681–690.

Commonwealth Scientific and Industrial Research Organisation (CSIRO) (2007). *Nutrient Requirement of Domesticated Ruminants.* Collingwood, Victoria, Australia: CSIRO Publishing.

DairyNZ (2020). *Monitor and mitigate milk fever. TechNote* 13. Available at: www.dairynz.co.nz/media/5789045/technote-13_web.pdf (accessed 30 December 2020).

Department of Agriculture and Fisheries, Queensland (DAFQ) (2010–2020). *Managing Drought*. Available at: www.daf.qld.gov.au/business-priorities/agriculture/disaster-recovery/drought/managing (accessed 30 December 2020).

Dixon, R. (2007). *Utilising Faecal NIRS Measurements to Improve Prediction of Grower and Breeder Cattle Performance and Supplement Management. Project NBP 302.* Sydney: Meat and Livestock Australia.

Dixon, R.M. and Petherick, J.C. (1996). Intake distribution of a range of supplements offered to grazing *Bos indicus* cross cattle. *Proceedings of the Australian Society of Animal Production* 21: 442.

Dixon, R. and Coates, D. (2012). A review of phosphorus nutrition of cattle in northern Australian grazing systems. In Petherick, C. (ed.) *Producer Phosphorus Manual for the Northern Cattle Industry, Appendix 1.* Sydney: Meat and Livestock Australia Limited.

Dixon, R.M., Playford, C. and Coates, D.B. (2011). Nutrition of beef breeder cows in the dry tropics. 1. Effects of nitrogen supplementation and weaning on breeder performance. *Animal Production Science* 51(6): 515–528.

Dryden, G.McL. (2003). *Near Infrared Reflectance Spectroscopy: Applications in Deer Nutrition*. RIRDC Publication No. W03/007. Canberra: Rural Industries Research and Development Corporation.

Dryden, G.McL. (2008). *Animal Nutrition Science*. Wallingford, UK: CAB International.

Earle, D.F. (1976). A guide to scoring dairy cow condition. *Journal of Agriculture, Victoria* 74: 228–231.

Entwistle, K.W. and Knights, G. (1974). The use of urea-molasses supplements for sheep grazing semi-arid tropical pastures. *Australian Journal of Experimental Agriculture and Animal Husbandry* 14: 17–22.

Foster, A.H. and Blight, G.W. (1984). Liveweight response of cattle grazing native pasture in south east Queensland when supplemented with urea molasses in winter and spring. *Tropical Grasslands* 18(3): 131–137.

FutureBeef (2011). *Protein and urea supplementation*. Available at: www.futurebeef.com.au/knowledge-centre/protein-and-urea-supplementation/#typesofurea (accessed 30 December 2020).

Ghosh, C.P., Datta, S., Mandal, D., Das, A.K., Roy, D.C., Roy, A. and Tudu, N.K. (2019). Body condition scoring in goat: Impact and significance. *Journal of Entomology and Zoology Studies* 7(2): 554–560.

Grainger, C., Wilhelms, G.D. and McGowan, A.A. (1982). Effect of body condition at calving and level of feeding in early lactation on milk production of dairy cows. *Australian Journal of Experimental Agriculture and Animal Husbandry* 22: 9–17.

Grain Trade Australia (2018). *Australian Grain Industry – Code of Practice Technical Guideline Document No. 5 Static Grain Sampling – Road Truck*, version 2. Available at: www.graintrade.org.au/grain-industry-code-practice/gta-technical-guidelines (accessed 30 December 2020).

Hennessy, D.W., Williamson, P.J., McLennan, D.J., Farquharson, R.J., Morris, S.G. and Darnell, R.E. (1998). Improved beef production from supplementation of Hereford, Brahman and crossbred cattle grazing low and medium quality pastures in the subtropics of Australia. *Animal Science* 66(1): 93–104.

Holm, A.M., Payne, A.L., Morgan, P.D. and Speijers, E.J. (1981). The response of weaner cattle grazing natural pasture in north western Australia to phosphoric acid, non-protein nitrogen and sulphur in their drinking water. *Australian Rangeland Journal* 3(2): 133–141.

Jefferies, B.C. (1961). Body condition scoring and its use in management. *Tasmanian Journal of Agriculture* 39: 19–21.

Lowman, B.G., Scott, N.A. and Somerville, S.H. (1976). *Condition Scoring of Cattle*. Bulletin No. 6. East of Scotland College of Agriculture, Edinburgh.

Makkar, H.P.S., Sánchez, M. and Speedy, A.W. (eds) (2007). *Feed Supplementation Blocks*. Rome: Food and Agriculture Organization of the United Nations.

Manzano, R.P., Paterson, J., Harbac, M.M. and Lima Filho R.O. (2012). The effect of season on supplemental mineral intake and behavior by grazing steers. *The Professional Animal Scientist* 28(1): 73–81.

Meat and Livestock Australia (MLA) (2020). *Drought Feeding. Residues*. Available at: www.mla.com.au/research-and-development/livestock-production/livestock-nutrition/drought-feeding/residues/ (accessed 30 December 2020).

National Research Council (NRC) (2001). *Nutrient Requirements of Dairy Cattle*, 7th rev. edn. Washington, DC: National Academies Press. Available from: www.nap.edu/catalog/9825/nutrient-requirements-of-dairy-cattle-seventh-revised-edition-2001 (accessed 30 December 2020).

National Research Council (NRC) (2007a). *Nutrient Requirements of Horses*, 6th rev. edn. Washington, DC: National Academies Press. Available at: www.nap.edu/catalog/11653/nutrient-requirements-of-horses-sixth-revised-edition (accessed 30 December 2020).

National Research Council (NRC) (2007b). *Nutrient Requirements of Small Ruminants – Sheep, Goats, Cervids and New World Camelids*. Washington, DC: National Academies Press. Available at: www.nap.edu/catalog/11654/nutrient-requirements-of-small-ruminants-sheep-goats-cervids-and-new (accessed 30 December 2020).

National Research Council (NRC) (2016). *Nutrient Requirements of Beef Cattle*, 8th rev. edn. Washington, DC: National Academies Press. Available at: www.nap.edu/catalog/19014/nutrient-requirements-of-beef-cattle-eighth-revised-edition (accessed 30 December 2020).

Nicholson, M.J. and Butterworth, M.H. (1986). *A Guide to Condition Scoring of Zebu Cattle*. Addis Ababa: International Livestock Centre for Africa.

Nolan, J.V., Ball, F.M., Murray, R.M., Norton, B.W. and Long, R.A. (1974). Evaluation of a urea–molasses supplement for grazing cattle. *Proceedings of the Australian Society of Animal Production* 10: 91–94.

PennState Extension (2016). *Trouble-shooting Milk Fever and Downer Cow Problems*. Available at: www.extension.psu.edu/trouble-shooting-milk-fever-and-downer-cow-problems (accessed 30 December 2020).

Pig Industry Standing Committee (PISC) (2009). *Model Code of Practice for the Welfare of Animals: Pigs*, 3rd edn. Melbourne: CSIRO Publishing.

Playne, M.J. (1974). Detrimental effects of phosphoric acid supplementation of beef cows in northern Australia. *Proceedings of the Australian Society of Animal Production* 10: 111.

Russel A.J.F., Doney, J.M. and Gunn, R.G. (1969). Subjective assessment of fat in live sheep. *Journal of Agricultural Science (Cambridge)* 72: 451–454.

Standing Committee on Agriculture and Resource Management (SCARM) (1990). *Feeding Standards for Australian Livestock. Ruminants*. Melbourne: CSIRO Publications.

Soares, F.S. and Dryden, G.McL. (2011) A body condition scoring system for Bali cattle. *Asian-Australasian Journal of Animal Sciences* 24(11), 1587–1594.

Taylor, S. and Dryden, G.McL. (2003). Responses of sheep to a water-based urea supplement. *Asia-Pacific Journal of Clinical Nutrition* 12: S59.

17 Feed storage and handling

Concentrate feed storage equipment

Silos, bins and bulk bags: Cereal grains, protein meals and macro-minerals such as salt, dicalcium phosphate and limestone are stored in these containers.

Bins have capacities of up to 10 tonnes and are used to store ingredients which are used in relatively small amounts, such as protein meals, milled grain, or the major minerals. In addition, they are used as supply bins immediately upstream of equipment like hammer or roller mills, pellet presses, etc. Bins have a circular or rectangular cross-section, sometimes with internal bracing. They may be open or covered at the top, generally have a sloping floor, and have a discharge chute which is closed with a shutter. Rectangular discharge chutes are better than round ones because protein meals and similar ingredients are less likely to bridge above the outlet. If the bin is integrated into a processing system, the discharge chute may be replaced by an auger – these are called 'live bottom' bins.

Bulk bags (also called 'bulka bags') hold about 1 tonne of minerals, urea and similar feeds. They are convenient for storing this type of ingredient because they can be filled at the manufacturing plant, transported by truck, and then used as storages at the purchaser's premises. They are simple to use, but there are some potential hazards: they are often manually emptied by being suspended by a forklift by the loops at each top corner, with the outlet being untied to let the contents flow out. However, to do this the operator has to work underneath the full bag and they risk being injured if the loops fail or if the product flows in an uncontrolled fashion out of the bag.

Cereal grains are usually stored in silos which hold 20–1000 or more tonnes. Silos are made of plastic or steel, which can be galvanized or painted. Modern silos have a circular cross-section, are roofed and have either a flat or sloping (hopper) floor. Grain is introduced at the top through an inlet chute and removed at the bottom by an auger or other device. Because a silo's inlet is several metres above the ground, they have to be filled by auger, bucket elevator, or pneumatic conveyer (see below).

Angle of repose: If a bin or silo has a sloping floor and we rely on gravity to move the contents when the discharge chute is opened, it is essential that the slope of the floor, i.e. the angle it makes with the horizontal, is greater than the angle of repose of the stored material. If the bin or silo base slopes at less than this angle the material will not move. This also applies to ducts and chutes that are used to transfer feed into bins and silos from bucket elevator discharge points and similar equipment.

The angle of repose is the angle between the side of a stack of bulk (loose) material and the horizontal (Fig. 17.1). Feeds form either a 'piling' or a 'draining' angle; the draining angle is steeper than the piling angle.

The angle of repose is affected by several factors. These are discussed by Xin and Rosentrater (2015) and are summarized below:

- Particle size: large particles flow more readily than small ones and so have a lower angle.
- Moisture content: damp feed forms a pile with a higher than usual angle of repose; e.g. for soybean meal at 10% moisture the angle is about 38° increasing to 45° when moisture content rises to 30%, and for fish meal the angle is about 55° at 10% moisture and 59° at 30%. Feed ingredients absorb moisture from humid air and lose it in dry air.
- Storage period: some materials, such as millrun and soybean meal, compact over time and this can make it more difficult to empty silos or bins as the compacted material has a greater draining angle.
- Particle shape and physical and chemical composition: feeds like meat meals, milled grain and oilseed meals have higher angles than cereal grains.

DOI: 10.1079/9781786394453.0017

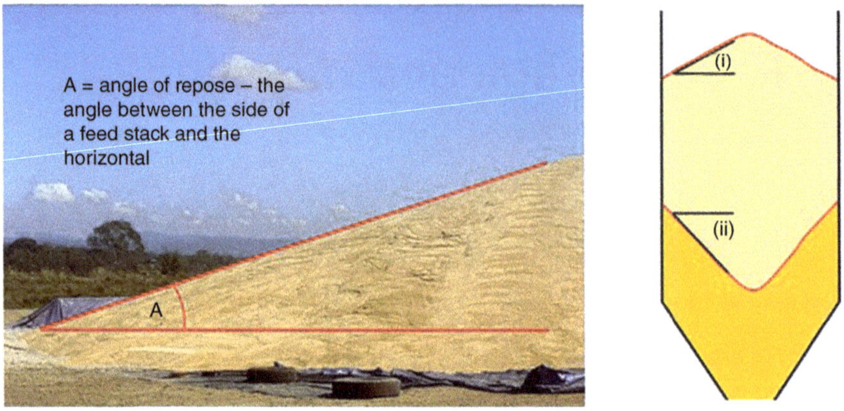

Fig. 17.1. Angles of repose. **(a)** A stack of grain showing a piling angle, and **(b)** a feed bin, showing piling (i) and draining (ii) angles of repose. (Photo courtesy of Julian Gehrke; reproduced with permission. Copyright: Gordon McL. Dryden.)

This is because cereal grains are regularly shaped and have smooth surfaces while the other feeds have irregularly shaped and (in the case of meat meals) sometimes fibrous particles which are more cohesive and do not flow as easily. Ingredients which are rich in fat (as in some protein meals) bind together and form steep-sided heaps.

- Resting surface: the angle of repose is also influenced to a small degree by the surface that the pile is resting on. A rougher surface (e.g. concrete versus steel) gives a slightly higher angle.

Conveying equipment: Concentrate ingredients (e.g. grains, protein meals), prepared loose mix feeds (mashes) and pelleted feeds are transported between storages, processing equipment and feeding equipment in four main ways:

- Augers: these have a continuous metal spiral (the auger 'flight') mounted on a shaft which runs inside a tubular casing. Augers have a boot at the bottom which collects the material which is to be carried into the auger, and a discharge chute at the top. They can be set up to transport material horizontally or vertically, although their efficiency declines as the angle above the horizontal increases. They have flow rates of 10 to 400 tonnes per hour. The auger boot must be protected by a safety screen – because firstly, the auger flight is exposed here because it has to dip into the material in the boot to collect it into the auger body, and secondly, the edges of the flight become very sharp as they become worn.
- Bucket elevators: these are a series of open buckets mounted on a track which rotates around a feed entry point at the bottom (a boot) and a discharge point at the top. They efficiently move material vertically at rates from 20 to 400 or more tonnes per hour.
- Pneumatic conveyers use fans to move feed through flexible tubing at up to 200 tonnes per hour. They are efficient, can transport material horizontally or vertically, and can be easily retro-fitted to existing equipment. However, they tend to demix mash feeds, and the dust-laden air in the system has to be discharged through a form of cyclone (see Chapter 18).
- Chain and disc conveyers have nylon discs attached about 20 cm apart to a stainless-steel chain or wire. They have transport rates up to 1 tonne per hour, are very flexible, and do not damage the feed. They are used in piggeries and poultry sheds to move mash and pelleted feeds from the on-farm storage to the feeding equipment.

Safety when using grain and protein meal storages: There are two important hazards to be aware of – being trapped by falling grain or meal, and poisonous gases produced by microbial fermentation.

A feed stack piled according to its draining angle of repose is unstable and will fall to the piling angle if disturbed. Do not rely on a stack of material showing a high angle of repose to remain stable.

It is dangerous to climb into a bin to dislodge protein meal which has become piled against the walls and will not flow out.

Bulk feeds may 'rathole' as the bin empties, leaving voids beneath surfaces which seem to be firm and stable. Do not walk across grain in a silo as even an apparently stable surface can conceal a void. Falling into a void is fatal as you will be rapidly covered by falling grain.

Poisonous gases, e.g. NH_3, NO_x and CO_2, are produced by microbial action on damp feeds. Never enter a grain silo alone (even an empty one); always have a colleague who stays outside and can rescue you if you are overcome by these gases.

Nutrient losses in stored concentrates and medicated feeds: Cereal grains gradually lose starch in storage if they are stored with higher than optimum moisture contents (McKevith, 2004). This happens quite slowly but is faster in milled grain than in whole grain, especially if it is stored in moist, warm conditions.

Vitamins and medicated premixes lose effectiveness over time – check the expiry date before use. Always store these products in a cool room. Do not store vitamins and trace minerals mixed together, because this can inactivate vitamins.

Storing roughage

Silage: Grass or legume forage is cut when immature, chopped into small pieces (up to 5 or 10 cm long), wilted if necessary to reduce the moisture content from the 80–85% of immature fresh grass to 70–75 %, or 65–70% moisture for maize (corn) silage. This material is then consolidated into silos, stacks or pits (or clamps or bunkers) where it undergoes anaerobic fermentation. Silage pits can be 50 m or more long, 5–10 m wide and 2–2.5 m deep. They can have earth or concrete floors (avoid gravel as this can be scraped up when the silage is removed and can cause rumen impaction) and are covered with an impervious film such as a plastic sheet. This may be protected and secured in place by a covering of earth or old tyres or similar materials.

The cured silage is removed by:

- Opening the face of the clamp and allowing animals to eat it directly from the clamp. This is the least expensive option, but it leads to losses of silage from aerobic spoilage and trampling. Open enough clamp surface to get a depth of about 20 cm eaten into the stack each day (DairyNZ, 2019). A slower consumption rate may allow mould growth and other spoilage.
- Using a silage cutter to remove silage and transport it to the animals.

Silage can also be made by forming the cut forage into round bales and wrapping these with a plastic film, or by compacting the cut forage into a long silage sausage. This material, called 'baleage', has 30–60% moisture. Wrapped bales are fed out simply by taking them to the animals and unwrapping the film. We should take care to repair holes in the plastic film as they occur, and to check baleage for the presence of mould before it is fed. Some authorities recommend vaccinating animals against botulism if wet baleage is used because these products, especially in summer, are suitable substrates for *Clostridia* growth (Clarkson, 2012).

Haystacks and bales: Dried grass or legume is compacted into bales. These are either:

- Small rectangular bales, about 1 m × 60 cm × 60 cm and weighing between 10 kg and 25 kg (the heavier weights are for leafy, green forage; the lighter for cereal straw). The bale is held in place by two strands of baling twine.
- Large rectangular bales weighing 500–600 kg (or up to 700 kg for high density bales) and 2.4 m × 1.2 m × 0.9 m in size, although different balers give a variety of bale sizes. These bales are secured with baling twine.
- Large round bales weighing 350–400 kg (some are only 180 kg) formed into cylinders about 1.2 m long × 1.2 m in diameter. These bales are held together with a plastic mesh wrapping.

Baled hay can be stored in stacks covered by a rainproof plastic film or tarpaulin or stored under cover. This type of storage results in losses of 5% of the hay dry matter (DM) over a year. Round bales can be left in the field, provided that the rounded surface is uppermost to help shed water, but this type of 'storage' will lead to losses of 35% or more of the hay DM over 18 months (Lemus, 2020). For example, if the outer 10 cm of a 400 kg round bale is damaged by rain, this loss represents about 17% of the total bale. Losses of soluble sugars and vitamin A can be 75% or more. Loose hay can be formed into a haystack in the field but again, expect losses at the surface of the stack.

Calculating the amount of storage capacity needed

The amount of feed that we need to store, and thus the storage capacity needed, depends on the number of animals, and their age, weight and physiological state, because these all determine the amount of feed DM that each animal will eat. How these factors influence feed intake is discussed in Chapter 7.

Expected seasonal changes in the availability of cereal grains and other plant feeds, will determine whether we should try to buy, and store, all the feed of that type that we will need until the next harvest. It may be best to consider using an alternative feed of the same type. For example, it might be possible to substitute sorghum for wheat, or replace soybean meal with sunflower meal with possibly added lysine and methionine. The considerations involved in substituting feeds are discussed in Chapter 6.

Seasonal changes in feed ingredient prices reflect the effects of harvest season, growing conditions and crop yields, and whether or not vendors are able to store feeds after the harvest. We can, to some extent, judge how prices are likely to trend before the harvest and thus decide how much feed to buy, and if it would be prudent to stockpile feed or to replace it with an alternative. Stockpiling is expensive – at the least there will be some nutrient loss during storage or from pest damage, and we may have to add the cost of leasing storage to the purchase price. It may well be more economical to replace feeds which are in short supply (and probably expensive because of that) with an in-season substitute.

It is not feasible to store some ingredients for long periods. This applies especially to vitamins and medicated additives which deteriorate over time, especially in hot, damp conditions, and which should not be used after their use-by date. As well, attack by pests and disease organisms will damage feeds (as described below).

Calculating storage requirements: This is a function of the amount of feed needed, and the bulk density of each ingredient.

A cereal grain example: We are finishing 10,000 head of Angus-type steers weighing 400 kg and growing at 1.36 kg per day. The ration is a simple mixture of 75% concentrate (70% cereal grain, 20% oilseed meal, 5% minerals and 5% additives) and 25% cereal straw, all on a DM basis. Thus it contains (75 x 70/100)%, or 52.5% or 0.525 grain, and the grain has a DM content of 90% or 0.9. The NRC (2000) feeding standards suggest that this type of animal will eat 10.2 kg DM per day. We want to know how much grain we have to store to feed these animals for 30 days.

The calculations are:

(a) Amount of grain required:

= {[(number of steers) × (expected DM intake, kg/head per day) × (proportion of grain in the ration, decimal, DM basis)]} / 1000

= (10000 x 10.2 x 0.525)/1000

= 53.6 tonnes DM/day.

To find the amount of grain (as-fed) that we need, convert the grain DM amount to an equivalent as-fed amount by dividing the DM amount by the grain's DM content, and multiply by 30 days:

$= 53.6/0.9 \times 30$

= 1784 tonnes, as-fed (1 tonne = 0.984 UK ton or 1.1 US ton).

(b) The effect of wastage: animals fed this type of feed in troughs will waste about 5% of the feed, by spillage or spoilage.

$$\text{Total amount of grain required} = 1784 \times 1.05$$

$$= 1874\ \text{tonnes.}$$

(c) Bulk storage space for grain needed for 30 days if the bulk density of grain is 750 kg/m^3

$$= \left[(\text{amount of grain, tonnes}) \times 1000\right] / \left(\text{bulk density, kg} / \text{m}^3\right)$$

$$= (1874 \times 1000) / 750$$

$$= 2499\ \text{m}^3.$$

This requires two silos, each 10.3 m in diameter and 15 m tall.

A silage example: We have 200 lactating Holstein/Friesian dairy cattle weighing 680 kg and producing 35 L/day of milk. These cattle eat 22.7 kg DM per day (NRC, 2001) of a total mixed ration which has 40% or 0.4 silage (on a DM basis).

$$\text{Total DM consumption} = (\text{number of cows}) \times (\text{expected DM intake per cow, kg / day}) \times (\text{silage content of the feed, decimal, DM basis})$$

$$= 200 \times 22.7 \times 0.40$$

$$= 1816 \text{ kg DM/day.}$$

The silage DM content is 27% (i.e. 73% water). For enough silage to last 180 days, we need 1816 × 180 / 1000 = 326.9 tonnes of silage DM, or 326.9/0.27 = 1211 tonnes of wet silage. Temperate (C3) grass silage has an average bulk density of 200 kg DM/m^3. Accordingly, we need a storage with a capacity of 6055 m^3. This is equivalent to four silage pits, each 55 m × 11 m × 2.5 m.

Feed storage hygiene

Damage caused by pests: Rodents and birds damage feeds by eating them, but the main damage is by the microbes in their droppings which cause diarrhoea, gastroenteritis and other diseases, and the external parasites such as lice and mites which they carry.

Rats and mice can be detected from their droppings, and footprints and tail marks in dust. Birds leave feathers and droppings, and we might also see dead birds.

It is very difficult to keep rodents and birds out of bulk ingredients. Control of rat and mice infestations is best done with regular baiting, cleaning up feed spillages and dust, and keeping bins and silos in good repair (PoultryHub, 2016). The best way of dealing with birds is to prevent them from entering feed storages; baiting and capturing are not reliable methods (APCA, undated).

Insects infest stored feeds, and their growth is influenced by the feed's moisture content and temperature (HGCA, 2011). These insects breed rapidly at 25–33°C, but most species do not breed at temperatures below 15°C. Most die at temperatures below 5°C or above 40°C.

Signs of insect infestation in animal feed are:

- live insects in or near stored feed;
- exit holes in whole grain (these can be quite large or small);
- pupae cocoons, cast larval skins, silken trails or webs (these may contain faecal pellets, eggs and cast larval skins); and
- an 'off-smell'.

Use insecticides to treat empty storages: we can do this with insecticide sprays and fumigation (if the storages are gas-tight). It is important that we carefully follow the manufacturers' instructions and observe all legal requirements about insecticide contamination of feeds.

Damage caused by micro-organisms: Microbial spoilage occurs when feed becomes damp. This can happen to grain stored in silos when, in humid weather, air-borne moisture condenses on the insides of the silo's walls during the night as the air cools, and this moisture is absorbed by the stored grain and grain dust. This sets up a good medium for mould or bacterial growth.

Bacterial action can cause feeds to heat and catch fire, and *Salmonella* bacteria can cause serious disease in both animals and humans. Mould growth can make the feed that they contaminate unusable. Some moulds produce metabolic products which are very poisonous (Chapter 12) and all mouldy feed should be treated with caution (Whitlow and Hagler, 2008). *Aspergillus* spp. are common moulds, especially on maize (corn) and peanuts, but they will grow on all feeds; these organisms produce aflatoxins, which poison animals and can cause cancer in people exposed to contaminated animal feeds and who eat products from animals fed contaminated feeds.

We can use mould inhibitors where these will not affect the quality of the finished feed. Propionic acid is the most commonly used mould inhibitor, and formic acid is also used. Some antioxidants (e.g. butylated hydroxytoluene or butylated hydroxyanisole) counteract the effects of aflatoxin B1 in poultry (Klein *et al.*, 2002).

Control the moisture content of feeds: This is the most important and practical way to maintain the quality of stored ingredients. 'Air dry' feeds such as grain, protein meals and dry roughages should have less than 13.5% moisture. Minerals generally do not have much moisture unless they are hygroscopic (absorb moisture from the air). Keep hygroscopic materials such as Cu sulphate, Zn chloride and urea in airtight containers.

Aerators are used to control moisture build-up in stored grain – fans suck air in at the base of the silo and blow it up through the stored grain, reducing the moisture load in the grain as it percolates through. But be careful to not introduce humid air into the silo. As well, we should regularly clean storage bins and silos to remove caked, damp residues.

Keep stored feed as cool as is practicable: This can be done by allowing air movement – aerators will help to cool grain, and bagged feed should be stored so that cool, dry air can flow around the bags. Storage design can also contribute – for example, the interior of a white-painted steel silo is about 4°C cooler than in a galvanized one.

Vitamins and medicated additives must be refrigerated.

Feeding equipment

Feeding equipment comes in a wide range of designs, and there is different equipment for roughages (e.g. hay racks) and concentrate feeds and mixed roughage/concentrate feeds (e.g. troughs, also called 'bunks' or 'bins').

Feeding equipment is designed to present feed to animals so that it is easily accessible, wastage is minimized, the consumption rate is controlled, and competition between animals for feed is contained.

To ensure accessibility and reduce waste we must make sure that the sides of troughs and pans are high enough to prevent spillage but not so high as to stop young or small animals or birds from being able to access the feed. Wastage occurs when feed is scattered on the ground, or soiled by trampling, urination and defaecation. Some feeders have roofs or other devices which help to protect the feed from rain and heat, or floors which prevent the feed from falling onto the ground.

Feed can be provided in bulk, but the consumption rate should be controlled. This can be done by using slides in grain self-feeders, or adjusting the rate that feed is delivered to the trough by conveying systems, or by fitting individual animals with transponders which control the access of each animal to a specified amount of feed.

Competition between animals for feed can be reduced either by ensuring that there is adequate feeding space for all animals, or by providing individual feeding stations (e.g. individual teats or subdivided troughs), or by using transponders.

As well as these considerations, well-designed and well-maintained feeding equipment should be:

- Robust: animals will exert substantial pressure on a feeder, especially if they are hungry or are moving to avoid bullying.
- Capable of holding the amount of feed required: calculate the expected feed intake rate of the herd or flock (Chapter 7) and choose equipment which will accommodate that amount without having to be frequently filled. But avoid holding feed for lengthy periods.
- Easy to clean: accumulations of feed meal and dust, especially if damp, are good habitats for bacteria and fungi, and attract pests.
- Allow cattle to feed in a natural 'head down' position; this increases saliva production (Albright, 1993) which helps to maintain rumen health.

Wastage can be a significant part of feed costs. Losses of feed in piggeries varies from 1.5% to 20% of the feed offered (Van Heutgen and Van Kempen, 2010). Wastage of forage and concentrate feed on dairy farms can be as much as 35% when feed is provided in temporary feeders such as under electric fences, in hay rings or on bare ground, or as little as 1% when concentrates are fed in troughs in the milking shed (Dairy Australia, 2009). Feed wastages in storage and feeding are summarized in Table 17.1. Hay losses are similar to those given for silage.

Table 17.1. Estimates of wastage rates (% of amount stored or fed) in storage and feeding out feeds to dairy cattle. (From DairyNZ, 2019; reproduced with permission.)

	Storage			Feeding in paddock[a]			Feeding in bins[b]	
Supplement	Excellent	Average	Poor	Excellent	Average	Poor	Very good	Poor
Grass silage	5–10	15–20	20–40	10	20	40	5–10	25
Maize and cereal silage	6	10–15	20–40	15	25	40	5–10	25
Concentrates	<2	5	15				5	25

[a]Silage losses include wastage at the stack face and during feeding out.
[b]'Bins' are feed pads (for roughages) and milking shed feed troughs (for concentrates).

Feed wastage is caused by poor feeding management:

- Using poorly designed equipment, e.g. feedlot troughs with no head rail (which prevents the nosing of feed out of the trough), or poultry feeder pans with sides that are too shallow.
- Over-filling troughs and hay racks: this, combined with normal animal feeding behaviour, leads to the loss of feed as described below.
- Putting feed on the ground, where it can be trampled and contaminated by soil, faeces or urine, or lost among plant material if it is fed out in a paddock. However, putting it near a fence helps to reduce these losses.
- Using over-fine feed: fine feed particles are often rejected by animals. As well, they accumulate in inaccessible parts of the equipment and are lost as dust when feed is moved from storage to the feed trough.

Animal behaviour is also responsible for feed wastage:

- Animals try to find the most palatable parts of the feed, and they nose among the feed and push or drag it out of the trough. This behaviour is most apparent when they are given a dry mix of concentrate and roughage. The more different the particle sizes are, the more easily animals are able to select between the ingredients, with feed being either pushed out of the trough or not eaten, and subsequently wasted.
- Mash feed fed to pigs can be carried out of the feeding trough as powder stuck to the animal's muzzle.
- When animals are fed long hay in troughs or hay racks, they grasp a piece of hay and pull or jerk it free from the mass. This causes other pieces of hay to be pulled free and fall onto the ground.
- Competition between animals can result not only in different feed intakes but also in wastage. For example, if a cow can climb into a feedlot trough (feed bunk) it may defaecate on the feed and will, in any case, soil it with its hooves.

Equipment for feeding concentrate feeds and concentrate/roughage mixes to ruminants: This equipment is designed to hold and present large amounts of feed to cattle and other ruminants, either grazing or in feedlots.

Grain or mash self-feeders are used to provide concentrate rations to grazing animals. They are large bins (1 or 2 tonnes capacity) which discharge their contents into troughs fitted at the base (Fig. 17.2). The rate at which feed enters the troughs, and thus the daily amount that animals can eat, is controlled by slides. Self-feeders are used in the field and in feedlots. They should be mounted on either skids or wheels so that they can be moved to relieve damage to soil and pasture through the effects of treading, especially in wet conditions. Grain self-feeders are simple to use once the gap between the slides and trough base has been correctly set. However, the feed must be kept dry and fresh – damp feed can bridge in the feeder, and feed will deteriorate if the amount stored in the bin exceeds the rate at which animals can reasonably consume it.

Feedlot troughs (feed bunks) are often made from concrete for robustness, are about 650–800 mm wide, 500 mm high at the back, and 700–750 mm high in the front (Watts *et al.*, 2015). These dimensions

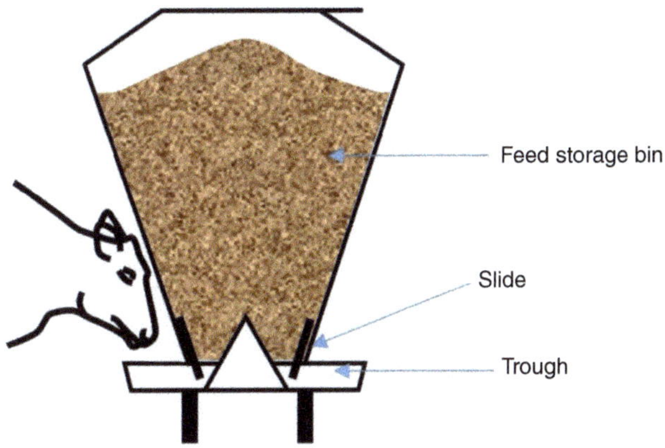

Fig. 17.2. A grain self-feeder showing the grain bin, feed control slides and feeding trough. (Copyright: Gordon McL. Dryden.)

prevent cattle from nosing feed over the front of the trough but allow feed delivery into the trough as they are filled from a feeder/mixer wagon (see Chapter 18) as it travels along a lane outside the pen. Allow 300 mm of linear trough length per animal. The trough must have a head rail which stops animals from climbing into the trough or escaping from the pen. This rail runs either along the fence bordering the trough or along the middle of the trough (Fig. 17.3). It is positioned just above cow head height, i.e. 1000–1100 mm above the bottom of the trough, and it is desirable that it can be raised or lowered to accommodate animals of different sizes. The rail prevents cattle from nosing feed out of the trough as they search for the more palatable constituents. The trough should have drain holes spaced along its length to allow rainwater to drain off.

There is a great deal of stock pressure near the trough and the effects of treading will, in time, remove soil from behind and under the trough. To prevent this, this part of the pen is concreted or gravelled and the feed trough rests on this base.

Feed pads are often used to provide total mixed rations or supplementary concentrate/roughage mixes to dairy cattle. They are simply a concrete floor on which the feed is placed. They can be under cover or in the open, depending on local climatic conditions. Feed wastage by trampling and scattering the material is reduced by confining the cattle behind a fence designed to prevent them from walking onto the feed but allowing them to push their heads between spaces in the fence and thus access the feed. We may have to periodically push the feed back into the eating area as feed is consumed.

Pig feeders: Four forms of feed presentation are used to feed weaner, grower and finisher pigs. Feed is given as a conventional dry diet, either as mash, pellets or crumbles (broken pellets); as a liquid, where the feed is made from liquid ingredients such as whey, sugar syrup, and ethanol distillers' by-products (Shurson, 2009); as a slurry made by mixing a conventional dry mash with water; or by wet/dry feeding where a conventional dry mash is mixed with water which drips from a water point suspended over the feed trough.

Dry and wet/dry feeding are the most commonly used methods. Wet/dry feeding gives more efficient feed use and growing pig performance than dry feeding, and using the water which is spilled as the pig drinks means that we get savings in water use and less effluent.

Whether or not we give pigs free, *ad lib*, access to their feed depends on their genotype (particularly whether or not they may become over-fat), and whether they are weaners and growers (fed *ad lib*) or finishers (sometimes restricted), or pregnant sows (restricted), or lactating sows (fed *ad lib*). Intake is controlled by regulating the rate at which feed fills the trough, or the amount of feed offered to individuals if they are fitted with transponder ear tags or fed manually.

Dry feed and wet/dry feed feeders have a hopper to hold a supply of feed, and a trough to hold the feed as it is presented to the animal. The hopper and trough are made from galvanized or stainless steel, or plastic. The feed hopper can be a tube or a rectangular bin, and is filled either manually or, more commonly in commercial farms, automatically by a conveyer – chain and disc conveyers (see above) are

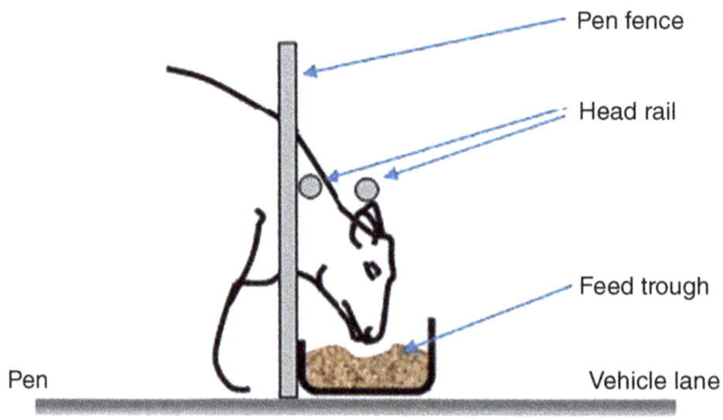

Fig. 17.3. Diagram of a feedlot feed trough (bunk) showing the head rail and design of the trough. (Copyright: Gordon McL. Dryden.)

often used. Troughs can be either rectangular or circular; manufacturers of the latter suggest that they are easier to keep clean because there are fewer places where uneaten feed can accumulate.

Wet/dry feeders have water nipples sited above the feed trough so that spilt drinking water is collected into the dry feed in the trough. Troughs may have drain holes to remove excess water.

When feed is removed from the trough as it is eaten, more feed flows by gravity into the trough from the hopper. The flow rate is usually determined by a shutter positioned between the hopper and the trough. Wheel feeders are a newer design; in these the pig moves a lever sited above the trough or a wheel positioned in the bottom of the (circular) trough. These interact with the feed hopper to dispense an amount of feed determined by the feeder design. Wheel feeders rely on the pig learning to use the device and using it when the trough is empty and they want to eat more.

Recommended dimensions for the feed trough (De Rouchey and Richert, 2010) are shown in Fig. 17.4. The feeder spaces are for feeders designed to accommodate several pigs at a time. The front lip height is set to keep feed in the trough while allowing access to the feed, but also to deter pigs from stepping into the feed.

Poultry feeders: Hatchlings, pullets and broilers are housed in sheds or colony cages and fed *ad lib*, while layers are held in battery or colony cages, or barns. All of these birds are managed and fed in groups, using the four types of feeder described here. The first three are used in commercial poultry farms, in both intensive (housed) systems and in free range systems where the birds are fed indoors and have access to fields outside the shed.

Pan feeders are circular troughs fed from a central hopper or feed tube (Fig. 17.5); they can be used in barns and cages. The feed is delivered by a conveyer (e.g. a chain and disc conveyer) and accumulates in a central well where the height of the accumulated feed is detected by an infrared sensor. When the infrared beam is interrupted the delivery of feed to that feeder stops, and delivery restarts when the feed level falls below the beam. Feed flows from the central well into the pan by gravity and the rate is controlled by adjustable shutters. The pan has a lip 35 to 50 mm high. This allows hatchlings to reach into the feed. As they usually climb into the trough, the troughs may include 'scratch bars' which reduce the loss of feed from the trough. Feeders for older birds have higher lips and bars which cover the pan and prevent birds from climbing into them. Pan feeders can be suspended on cords or chains and raised above the ground as the birds grow. This equipment is made from high-impact plastic, and usually in vibrant colours – red, blue and yellow – to attract birds to the feed.

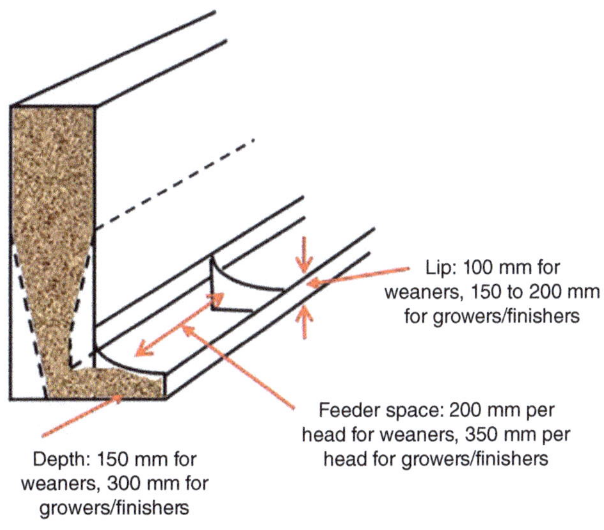

Fig. 17.4. A rectangular feeder for pigs showing the recommended dimensions for weaners and growing/finishing pigs. (Copyright: Gordon McL. Dryden.)

Chain feeders are used in both barn and cage systems. They consist of an endless chain of flat steel links running along the base of a feed trough, and the trough lip is 5 or 10 cm above the barn floor or cage bottom. These feeders can run for many metres along the length of the barn or line of cages. Feed is delivered into the feeder and is taken along the whole length of the chain at a rate of 18 m or more per minute. Chain feeders may have a wire grill superstructure which prevents birds from climbing into the trough and gives individual birds some protection against competition from their neighbours.

Open feed troughs are used with cages. The trough runs externally along the line of cages and feed flows under gravity from a travelling feed hopper which fills the trough as it passes along the line of cages. Birds access the feed trough through the spaces in the side of the cage.

Hopper feeders are suitable for home use. They have a hopper which holds about 5 kg of feed mounted above a trough (similar to the pig feeder design in Fig. 17.4). These feeders may be fitted with a treadle mechanism which, when the bird stands on it, opens a hatch and gives the bird access to the feed. This gives some protection against feed loss to rodents and feral birds.

Feeders for laying hens should provide each bird with at least 100 mm of feed space with linear feeders, or 40 mm of feed space with circular feeders (EU Council, 1999–2017). Broilers are fed *ad lib* for most of their lives and to facilitate this pan feeders should be spaced at about 0.75–1 m intervals along the conveyer track.

Equipment for feeding roughage: A variety of equipment is used to hold roughage and make it easily available to animals.

Hay racks are mesh-sided containers, often with a V shape. The mesh must be fine enough to prevent pieces of hay falling out as the animal eats, but large enough for the animal to get its muzzle through the mesh and take mouthfuls of hay – animals will be prevented from eating if the mesh openings are too small. Some racks have a covering roof, and most have a tray underneath the rack which is designed to catch hay as it is pulled from the rack. All animals, but especially sheep and goats, have difficulty in pulling out pieces of hay from intact bales, especially small rectangular ones which are more tightly packed than large round bales. We must open and break up hay bales before they are put into a rack.

Hay rings (bale feeders) are used to feed round and large rectangular bales. A simple design is to wrap a length of steel reinforcing mesh around the bale, held in position by steel posts. Hay rings are put under considerable pressure from large animals and so must be very robust.

Nets or racks are used to give hay to horses. Nets are made from synthetic cord; they are filled with loose, long hay and hung in the loose box or yard. Chopped hay must be fed in troughs as the smaller particle size of this material cannot be retained in nets or racks.

Feeding roughage in open troughs can lead to wastage, and to the demixing of mixed roughage/concentrate feeds. Hay should be chopped to 10–50 mm pieces if it is to be fed in troughs, and more finely if it is to be mixed with other ingredients. Troughs used for mixed roughage/concentrate feeds should be designed to prevent feed being nosed out of the trough (Fig. 17.3).

Milk and milk replacer feeders: Dairy calves are removed from their dams 36–48 hours after birth and reared on milk or milk replacer. Lambs and

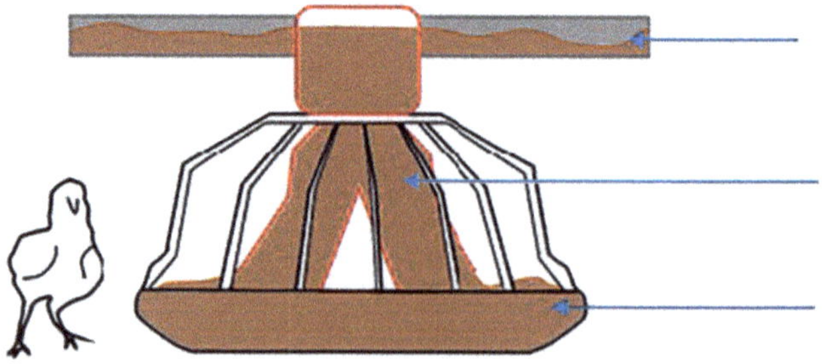

Fig. 17.5. Example of a pan feeder used for broiler chickens. (Copyright: Gordon McL. Dryden.)

kids may have to be artificially reared if they are mismothered, or their dam dies or cannot supply enough milk.

Equipment for feeding these liquid feeds includes:

- A bottle or other container fitted with a teat. These are used when the calf is first being introduced to milk replacer and artificial feeding and can also be used for older calves. Often, these devices are incorporated in a multi-animal feeding station or 'calfeteria'.
- Open troughs can be used if calves are taught to drink rather than suck. However, the reticular groove does not always close when a calf drinks (Ørskov, 1972) and there is a risk of milk getting into the developing rumen where it can cause severe health problems.

Modern calf and lamb feeding equipment can be completely automated. The milk replacer is made by drawing dry powder from a reservoir and mixing it with water, the liquid is heated to the required temperature, individual feed allocations can be set and delivered to each calf or lamb by reading its transponder (contained in an ear tag), and the equipment self-cleans. Almost all automated lamb and calf feeding systems use teats to deliver the feed.

Creep feeding: This is used to provide young, unweaned animals – piglets, lambs, calves, kids and foals – with supplementary feed while preventing the dam from accessing the feed also. The name comes from the way that the trough containing the supplement is protected from adults with a barrier which allows the small, young animal to 'creep' through or under it (Fig. 17.6). These barriers are subjected to great pressure from the dams and must be very robust.

Automated feeding and monitoring equipment: When animals are managed in groups there is always competition between them for feed. This is exemplified by firstborn piglets choosing the best teats, physical aggression by dominant cows over subordinate animals in feedlots, ear and tail chewing in grower pig pens, and feather pecking by birds in barns or cages. Competition is greater when feed is limited, e.g. when the manager wants to control fat deposition by restricting feed intake, or if there is an equipment malfunction.

Ideally, we would either feed all animals individually while still allowing social contact at non-feeding times, or supply an excess of feed so that competition is minimized. Although horses and breeding sows are often housed individually, this option is not viable for other intensively managed animals.

The solution is to set up a system where each animal can access its feed separately from the others in its group. Electronic feeding equipment has gates or other devices which control access to the feed, and the animals wear transponders fitted into a collar or ear tag. As well as removing the effects of aggression at feeding time this equipment allows individual animals to be fed at different rates. The earliest devices were the 'Callan gates' for dairy cattle, and the method has since been adopted in feeding equipment for most types of animals, including pigs, calves and lambs.

Automatic 'walk over' weighing is becoming more commonly used to monitor grazing animals. These depend on using one-way gates ('spear' gates) to force the animal to walk to water or supplementary feed over an electronic weighbridge. This works well provided that the spear gate functions properly. Cattle have been killed when gates

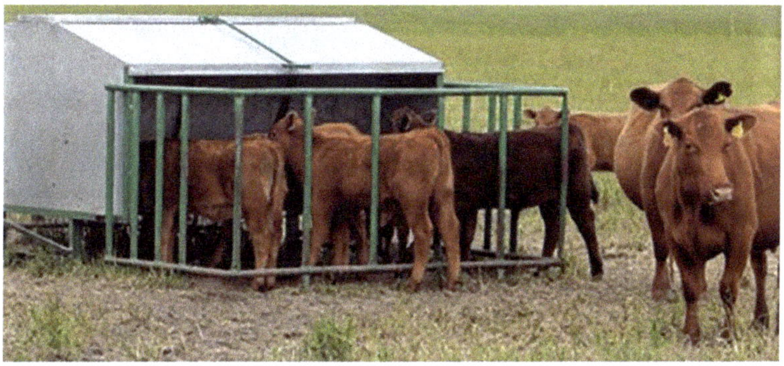

Fig. 17.6. A creep feeding system for beef calves. (From *American Cattlemen*; reproduced with permission.)

have jammed, trapping them in a yard without water. Ideally, spear gates and similar equipment should be continuously monitored.

Equipment to monitor feeding: Animal care regulations, and good animal management, require that we always monitor our animals' welfare. This includes keeping a constant watch on feeding behaviour to make sure that each animal gets its requirement, and that feed and water equipment is working properly. Animals which do not eat their nominated amount of feed can be recorded and the manager alerted.

Remote sensing equipment, including cameras and feed and water level sensors, are useful tools. When combined with individual animal transponders (or even without) we can get a comprehensive, continuous, check on welfare and performance. Currently available equipment includes monitoring by a smart phone app or the internet as a standard. This information can be input into farm system models (see Chapter 10).

Reducing diet selection by animals fed a formulated, mixed ration

If we go to the expense of making a mixed feed which contains all the nutrients that are needed to promote high levels of performance and health, then we do not want animals to eat only part of it. Diet selection among the components of a mixed ration is possible if the different ingredient particles are of substantially different size or density. Minerals and vitamins can segregate from cereal grain and protein meal particles in all rations including pig and poultry feed, while beef cattle feedlot rations, or prepared horse diets which contain both concentrate and roughage ingredients, are very likely to de-mix during handling.

Feeds can be processed to reduce the chance of de-mixing by:

- Making particle sizes as uniform as possible, e.g. we can mill grain to reduce the particle size to something comparable to that of protein meals.
- Chopping hay to allow more intimate mixing with the other ration components.
- Using ingredients such as molasses or tallow to bind feed particles together; note that there are limits to the amounts of these ingredients that we should use. For example, more than about 7% fat will adversely affect rumen function and there are practical limits to the inclusion of molasses in feeds that we want to mix with other ingredients, or convey with augers, etc.
- Processing the mixed feed into pellets: these contain all of the feed ingredients in the proportions that were envisaged in the ration formulation. Pelleting prevents diet selection because the pellets are eaten intact. However, high-roughage rations are difficult, and sometimes impossible, to pellet.
- Transporting feeds in bags rather than in bulk: this is usually not practicable because transporting feed in bags substantially increases the landed cost of the ration.
- Avoiding repeatedly transferring mixed feed between storages: each time a mixture is moved (especially by auger or pneumatic conveyer) the different ingredient particles tend to separate.

It is often difficult to make an intimate and stable mixture of roughages and concentrates even if we chop or mill hay or straw before mixing them with concentrates. Further, finely milling roughages will reduce their effective fibre (peNDF) content for ruminants and can lead to disorders such as rumen acidosis and low milk fat content (Chapter 13). Nevertheless, feeding roughages and concentrates separately is not usually a good option because it allows maximum choice between the two feed types. If this choice varies widely from day to day, we risk digestive disorders such as diarrhoea, acidosis and laminitis.

References

Albright, J.L. (1993). Feeding behavior of dairy cattle. *Journal of Dairy Science* 76: 485–498.

Australian Pest Control Association (APCA) (undated). *Bird Pests.* Available at: www.pestcontrol.org.au/birds.html (accessed 30 December 2020)

Clarkson, N. (2012). Feeding baleage to horses – the ultimate guide. *Horsetalk New Zealand*. Available at: www.horsetalk.co.nz/2012/10/30/feeding-baleage-to-horses-the-ultimate-guide/ (accessed 30 December 2020).

Dairy Australia (2009). *Feed Wastage Study – Summary Report.* Available at: https://cdn-prod.dairyaustralia.com.au/-/media/project/dairy-australia-sites/national-home/resources/2020/07/08/feed-wastage-study-summary-2009/feed-wastage-study-summary-2009.pdf (accessed 22 March 2021).

DairyNZ (2019). *Facts and Figures, A Quick Reference Guide for New Zealand Dairy Farmers*. Available from: www.dairynz.co.nz/media/5791506/facts-and-figures-updated-june-2019-web.pdf (accessed 30 December 2020).

De Rouchey, J. and Richert, B.T. (2010). *Feeding Systems for Swine.* Pork Information Gateway, US Pork Center of Excellence. Available at: https://pork-gateway.org/resource/feeding-systems-for-swine/ (accessed 30 December 2020).

EU Council (1999–2017). *Council Directive 1999/74/EC of 19 July 1999 laying down minimum standards for the protection of laying hens*. Document 31999L0074. Available at: https://eur-lex.europa.eu/legal-content/EN/TXT/?uri=CELEX:31999L0074 (accessed 30 December 2020).

HGCA (2011). *Grain Storage Guide for Cereals and Oilseeds*, 3rd edn. Agriculture and Horticulture Development Board (UK). Available at: www.ahdb.org.uk/grainstorage (accessed 30 December 2020).

Klein, P.J., Van Vleet, T.R., Hall, J.O. and Coulombe, R.A. Jr (2002). Dietary butylated hydroxytoluene protects against aflatoxicosis in turkeys. *Toxicology and Applied Pharmacology* 182: 11–19.

Lemus, R. (2020). *Hay Storage: Dry Matter Losses and Quality Changes.* Available at https://extension.msstate.edu/sites/default/files/publications/publications/P2540_web.pdf (accessed 10 January 2021).

McKevith, B. (2004). Nutritional aspects of cereals. *Nutrition Bulletin* 29(2): 111–142.

National Research Council (NRC) (2000). *Nutrient Requirements of Beef Cattle*, 7th rev. edn. Update. Washington, DC: National Academies Press.

National Research Council (NRC) (2001). *Nutrient Requirements of Dairy Cattle*, 7th rev. edn. Washington, DC: National Academies Press.

Ørskov, E.R. (1972). Reflex closure of the oesophageal groove and its potential application in ruminant nutrition. *South African Journal of Animal Science* 2: 169–176.

PoultryHub (2016). *Rodent control.* Available at: https://www.poultryhub.org/all-about-poultry/husbandry-management/pest-mangement/rodent-control (10 January 2021).

Shurson, J. (2009). *What We Know About Feeding Liquid By-Products to Pigs*. Available at: https://www.thepigsite.com/articles/what-we-know-about-feeding-liquid-byproducts-to-pigs (accessed 10 January 2021).

Van Heutgen, E. and Van Kempen, T. (2010). *Nutritional Effects on Swine Nutrient Excretion and Air Quality*. Pork Information Gateway, US Pork Center of Excellence. Availableat: www.porkgateway.org/resource/nutritional-effects-on-swine-nutrient-excretion-and-air-quality/ (accessed 10 January 2021).

Watts, P., Luttrell, M. and Keane, O. (2015). *Feedlot Design and Construction*. 19. Feeding Systems. Sydney: Meat & Livestock Australia Ltd. Available at: https://www.mla.com.au/globalassets/mla-corporate/research-and-development/program-areas/feeding-finishing-and-nutrition/feedlot-design-manual/019-feeding-systems-2016_04_01.pdf (accessed 10 January, 2021).

Whitlow, L. and Hagler, W. (2008). Mold and mycotoxin issues in dairy cattle: effects, prevention and treatment. *Advances in Dairy Technology*, Vol. 20: Proceedings of the Western Canadian Dairy Seminar, Red Deer, AB, Canada. Available at: https://www.researchgate.net/publication/237455445_Mold_and_Mycotoxin_Issues_in_Dairy_Cattle_Effects_Prevention_and_Treatment (accessed 30 December 2020).

Xin, J. and Rosentrater, K.A. (2015). Factors influencing feed ingredient flowability. In *Agricultural and Biosystems Engineering Conference Proceedings and Presentations*. Dept. Agricultural and Biosystems Engineering, Iowa State University. Available at: https://lib.dr.iastate.edu/cgi/viewcontent.cgi?referer=&httpsredir=1&article=1438&context=abe_eng_conf (accessed 10 January 2021).

18 Feed processing

Feed processing – what it is and why we do it

'Processing' encompasses a range of activities aimed at improving the value of ingredients as components of animal feeds and sources of nutrients, and the way that feed is presented to animals.

Methods of feed processing include procedures which change the physical structure of feeds and/or their chemistry.

Physical changes can be as simple as changing the particle size, as occurs when cereal grains are ground ('milled'). In this process the particle size is reduced from a grain which may be 5 mm or more long and 2–3 mm in diameter, to particles 1–3 mm in size. This change in physical structure has two effects: it gives a particle size which is similar to that of the other major components of animal feeds, especially protein meals and some minerals, and it exposes the grain endosperm to the animal's digestive enzymes. The reduced particle size allows us to make stable mixtures which are less likely to de-mix when they are handled, e.g. when they are moved along an auger or are transported in bulk.

Chemical changes occur when the feed is wetted, treated with an alkali such as ammonia or caustic soda (NaOH), or exposed to heat. These processes gelatinize the starch in cereal grains or degrade the fibrous carbohydrates (cellulose and hemicellulose) of roughages, and in both cases improve the feed's digestibility. In some cases, chemical processing adds nutrients, e.g. treating roughages with ammonia increases the ruminally available N (RAN) content.

Tempering

Tempering is simply adding water to the feed. This discussion deals with tempering of cereal grains. Water can be added most conveniently by spraying the grain as it passes through an auger. By adding small amounts of water to whole grain (i.e. before roller milling) we get (Zinn *et al.*, 1998):

- improved digestibility with about 5% increase in feed conversion efficiency, and up to 10% increase in animal growth;
- reduced power consumption in roller milling by up to 10%; and
- reduced amount of steam needed in steaming and flaking grain.

While there are benefits to grain tempering, note that:

- Tempered grain can only be roller milled as hammer mills cannot process grain with moisture contents greater than about 15%.
- Finished mash products may have to be dried after manufacture (depending on their moisture content) as otherwise there is an unacceptable risk of microbial spoilage.
- Tempered grain tends to produce flakes rather than cuboidal particles when it is roller-milled and these may be difficult to mix into a feed.

Milling/grinding

'Milling', 'grinding', 'sizing', 'rolling' and 'gristing' are synonymous terms for processing which reduces the particle size of feed ingredients. Milling is commonly used to process cereal grains, oilseeds and dried forages.

There are two main types of equipment used for this: hammer mills and roller mills.

All feed processing equipment can be badly damaged by tramp metal (e.g. bolts, nuts, etc. that have broken off harvesting equipment), stones, twine and other contaminants in the feed. To protect our equipment, we must at the very least use a magnet on the feed entry side to trap tramp metal. Sieves which collect stones and other non-ferrous materials are effective, although expensive.

DOI: 10.1079/9781786394453.0018

Hammer mills consist of a set of steel bars, or 'hammers', which rotate rapidly on an axle, and are confined within a casing (Fig. 18.1).

Feed enters the mill through an entry chute which is situated either at the top of the mill, or at an angle at one side. As shown in Fig. 18.1, the feed falls through the path of the hammers and is either broken as the hammers hit it, or when the hammers fling the pieces of feed material against the casing or the screen. Hammer mills which are fitted with 180° screens may have 'breaker plates' situated at the top of the casing, on either side of the entry chute (not shown in the diagram). These are ridged steel plates which provide extra surfaces for the feed pieces to hit and be broken against. Some mills have 'wear plates' – metal skins which cover the inside of the casing and which can be replaced when they become worn by the impact of feed particles against them.

Note that feed is not ground between the hammer ends and the screen; in fact, the hammers must not be in contact with the screen as this would cause excessive wear to both hammers and screen.

The hammer assembly is the core of the hammer mill. This consists of an axle, driven by (usually) an electric motor, which carries rods onto which are threaded the hammers. In most mills the hammers are free to rotate and are separated on the rods by spacers. Typical hammers are shown in Fig. 18.2. One hammer has notched corners and holes drilled at each end so that the hammer can be both reversed (swapped side for side) and rotated (swapped end for end). These modifications allow much longer use of the hammer before it has to be replaced. In addition, some hammers have case hardened tips. In use, the softer steel under the tip wears away and sets up sharp corners.

Hammers rotate at speeds between 1800 and 3600 rpm. In order to maintain these speeds without vibration and possible damage to the mill, it is very important that the set of hammers is balanced, so that the weight of each hammer, and of all the hammers on each hammer rod, vary by no more than 25 g. If we replace hammers it is essential that these are matched for weight and design, including length, thickness and tip profile.

The screen is a perforated metal sheet which is curved to fit the curvature of the casing. It is held in place by a pair of guides at each side. The holes in the screen are usually circular, although sometimes rectangular, and vary in diameter from 0.5–75 mm. In practical use, 3–8 mm holes are used for milling grains, and larger holes are used to roughly mill forages.

The screen retains those particles which are too large to pass through it, so the screen hole size

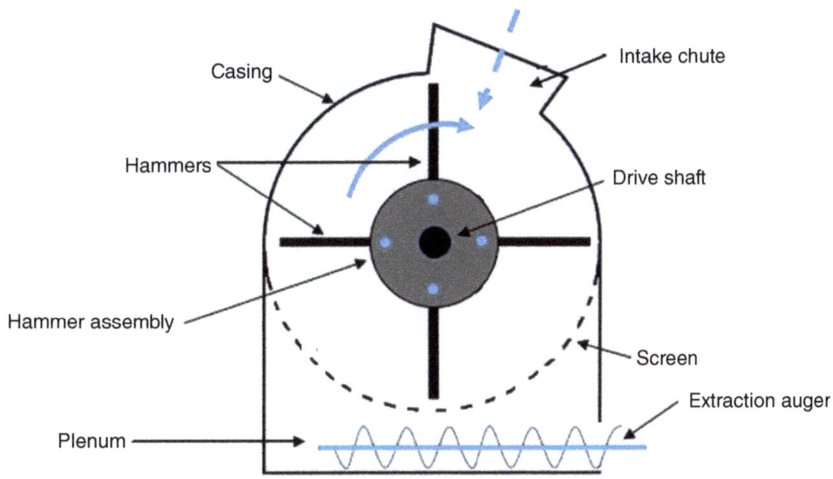

Fig. 18.1. A diagram of a hammer mill showing the design of a mill with a 180° screen and offset entry chute. The direction of rotation of the hammers is indicated by the solid arrow; that of feed entry by the dashed arrow. (Copyright: Gordon McL. Dryden.)

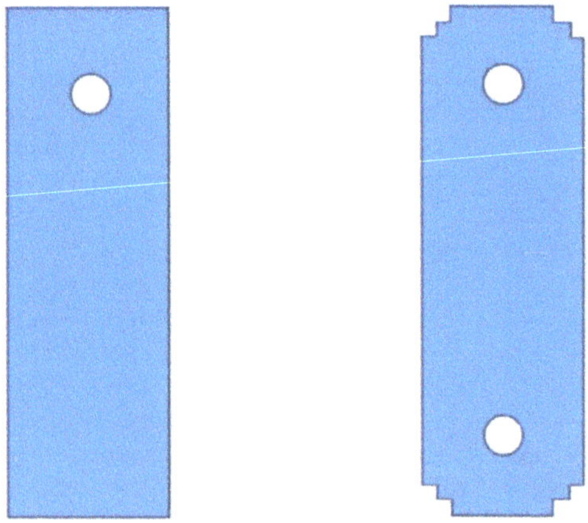

Fig. 18.2. Hammer designs (a) plain and (b) notched. (Copyright: Gordon McL. Dryden.)

determines the maximum size of the milled particles. Feeds such as cereal grains that break into regularly shaped pieces will be milled into particles which have a maximum size similar to the screen hole diameter; those, like forages, that break into needle-shaped pieces will give particles which are able to pass lengthwise through the screen holes, and so their length will often be larger than the hole diameter. Screens with small holes are used to prepare feeds for young animals or which are going to be pelleted (see below).

Figure 18.1 shows a mill with a 180° screen, which is suitable for on-farm use and milling a range of feeds. However, mills are also made with 270° screens where the screen covers almost all of the mill casing circumference. Both configurations have advantages and disadvantages:

- A 180° screen allows the installation of breaker plates and possibly a hay chute. These screens are durable and can be reversed when the working surface becomes worn.
- A 180° screen gives lower processing efficiency than a full-circle screen.
- Full-circle or 270° screens occupy three quarters or more of the mill's circumference. They provide a greater area for the escape of milled material, and typically give higher throughput:power use ratios than 180° screens. These screens can be split so that the descending (entry side) part of the screen and the ascending side can have different hole sizes, with the ascending side holes being larger than the descending ones.
- Full-circle screens have to be flexible to conform to the shape of the mill, so they are thin and light; this means that they are suitable only for materials that are easy to mill, such as grains.

Milled feed is removed from the mill either by a fan which can be set up to draw the milled feed out of the mill, or by mechanical extraction with an auger, or (the best) by a combination of both of these. Because any backflow of air or product into the milling chamber will result in regrinding and slower throughput, a fan must be set up so that it sucks air and milled material out of the mill.

Hammer milling results in the movement of air, as well as milled material, into and through and out of the mill, and this air with its entrained dust has to be removed before the product can be put into storage or taken to the next processing step. Air and dust is removed by passing the product through a cyclone (Fig. 18.3). Here, the air flow direction is abruptly changed, and the air slows down. The entrained fine particles (dust) fall out of the air stream and are collected in a bag; the dust-free air is vented into the environment.

Roller mills have corrugated ('fluted') rolls set in a frame and contained within a housing. Grain enters the top of the mill above the rolls, passes through the rolls where it is broken into smaller particles, and falls out of the mill into a plenum from where it is removed by an auger (Fig. 18.4). Simple roller mills have a single pair of rolls, while mills used in high-capacity mills and flour mills may have as many as three pairs of rolls, set vertically above each other.

The maximum size of the milled particles is set by the distance between the rolls, the type of flutes (corrugations) in the surface of the rolls, and by the relative rotational speeds of the rolls.

The shaft of one of each pair of rolls is fixed, while the other can move so that the distance between the rolls can be altered. When in use, the rolls are set closely together so that the grain kernels passing between them are broken. The rolls must not touch as this would cause expensive damage; most mills have roll stops which prevent this. The small distance between the rolls is called the 'gap', and the area just above the rolls is the 'nip'. The gap is an important factor in determining the maximum size of the milled grain particles.

The two rolls rotate in different directions, i.e. both rotate towards the nip. Obviously, grain would be pushed out of the nip if both rolls rotated

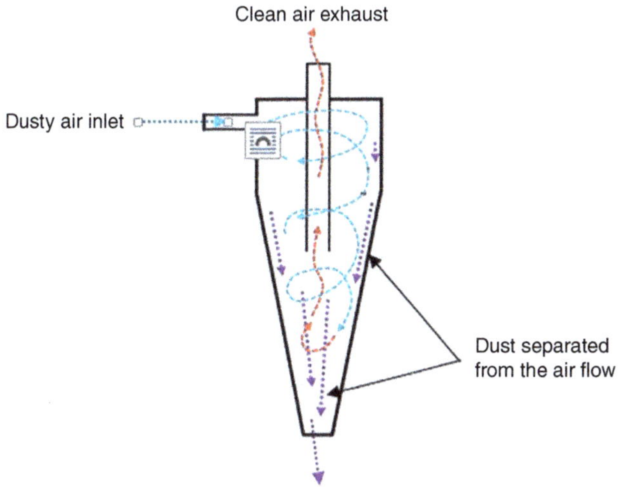

Fig. 18.3. A cyclone dust collector. (Copyright: Gordon McL. Dryden.)

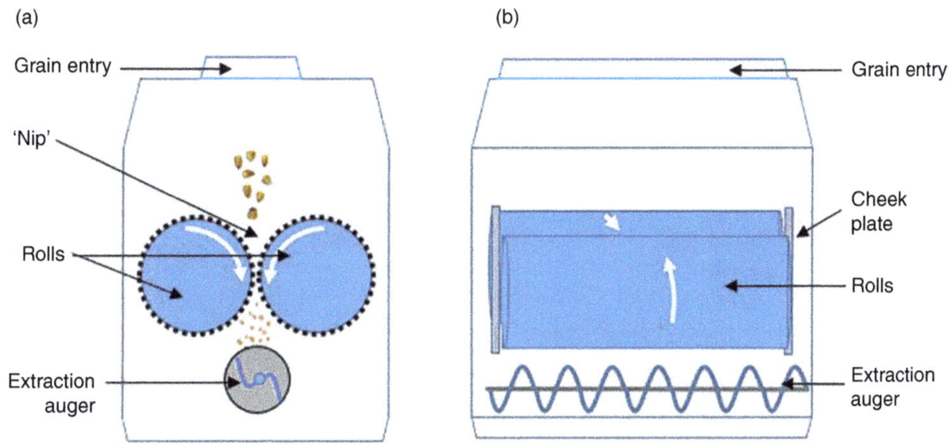

Fig. 18.4. Diagram of a roller mill. (a) End view showing the passage of grain between the rolls, and (b) front view showing a single pair of rolls (rotation shown by the arrows) with the milled grain extracted by an auger. Not shown are the roll drive mechanism, and the mechanisms for adjusting the roll gap (the shortest distance between the rolls) and the roll orientation. (Copyright: Gordon McL. Dryden.)

in the same direction. In addition, they rotate at different speeds. Common speed differentials are between 1:1 and 1:2.5, with many being 1:1.5.

It is very important that the grinding rolls are correctly orientated, i.e. kept parallel and 'in tram'. Parallel is when the roll shafts are in line horizontally, and in tram is when they are in line vertically.

As well as the size of the gap, the final particle size of the milled material is strongly influenced by the type of corrugations, or 'flutes', cut into the rolls. Roll flutes can be cut in many different shapes (Fig. 18.5). The most commonly used profiles in processing grain for animal feeds are the round bottomed V and the Stevens. The LePage ring profile is used to cut pellets into smaller pieces (this is called 'crumbling') without damaging the pellets too much. Flutes are cut either circumferentially or longitudinally. Most roller mills used for animal

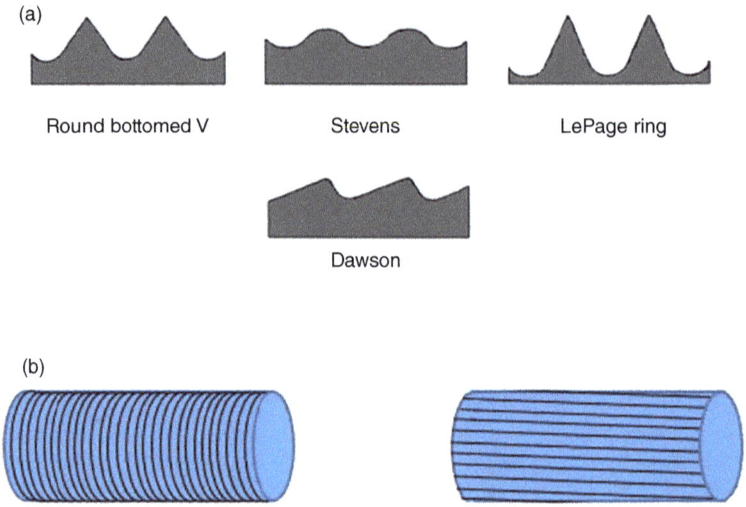

Fig. 18.5. Flute profiles which are commonly used to process grain for animal feeds. (a) Flute profiles. (From Owens and Heimann, 1994; reproduced with permission.) (b) Circumferential (left) and longitudinal (right) fluting, the longitudinal fluting shows how flutes can be cut in a spiral fashion (usually about 2° from the parallel, exaggerated in this diagram). (Copyright: Gordon McL. Dryden.)

feed have longitudinal fluting cut in a shallow spiral so that the flutes in the pair of rolls cross over each other rather than locking into each other as might happen if they were cut exactly parallel to the roll axis. A specialist roll manufacturer will advise when choosing a flute profile.

Milled material is usually removed from the mill with an auger. Roller mills do not need a positive air flow through them to work well, so fans or pneumatic systems are not needed.

Comparison of hammer mills and roller mills: Each type of mill has its own characteristics and uses in animal feed preparation. These are summarized in Table 18.1.

The choice of mill – hammer or roller – depends on the variety of feedstuffs that is to be processed. Hammer mills can be used to process both grains and roughage but they will not easily mill cereal grain or roughage with more than 15% moisture, and compared to roller mills they are less efficient in terms of milling rate and energy use. While roller mills efficiently mill grains and produce a product with less 'fines' (very small particles, or dust) than hammer mills (Fig. 18.6), they will not mill roughage. Hammer mills are probably easier to use than roller mills, and they are more robust. A damaged hammer can be easily replaced, but a damaged roll is expensive to repair.

Milling roughages: Hammer mills and augers are used to reduce the particle size of roughages. The machine of choice depends on the desired particle size.

If all we want is to reduce the particle size to something that we can more easily mix with other ingredients, e.g. in a beef cattle feedlot ration, then we would use a feed mixer wagon or a tub grinder. These machines rapidly and efficiently break up large pieces of roughage.

Feed mixers are a feed box or wagon with two or more counter-rotating augers running the length of the wagon. Long roughage is introduced above the augers, gets trapped between the auger flights, and is cut into short lengths as the augers rotate. The rotation also mixes the chopped roughage with other ingredients as they are added into the wagon. These wagons have electronic scales so that the user can load the wagon with the required amounts of each ingredient and offload the mixed feed in the required amounts.

Tub grinders have a rotating tub which holds the long forage, a hammer mill inset in a stationary base, and a belt conveyer to convey the ground material to a dump or bin (Fig. 18.7). The tub is filled from the top, and its rotation brings new, unground roughage into contact with the hammer mill's rotating hammers which break the material into small pieces. The ground material falls through

Table 18.1. A comparison of roller mills and hammer mills.

Characteristic	Hammer mill	Roller mill
Production rate	Usually between 5 and 12 tonnes/hour	Faster
Particle size control	Limited – relies on particles passing through a screen	Regulated by the size of the gap between the rolls, roll speed, and type of corrugation
Particle size distribution	Wide – varies from particles slightly smaller than the screen hole size to fines of about 100 μm diameter	Narrower – varies from particles which are produced as the grain breaks to fines similar to hammer milling (but less amount of fines than hammer milling)
Specific energy consumption	5–10 kWh/tonne	1.5–5 kWh/tonne
Cost of maintenance	High, as the material being ground abrades the screen and hammers and this wear reduces the effectiveness of the mill; maintenance is continuous	Lower, as the rolls do not experience abrasion from the material being ground, except on the flute edges
Effect of damage	Relatively minor, as hammers and screens can be replaced easily and relatively cheaply	Serious, as corrugations are damaged by tramp iron and stones, and rolls are expensive to repair or replace
Range of materials that can be ground	Any material that can be broken by the impact of fast-moving hammers, and which will pass through the feed chute, e.g. cereal grains, legume or pulse seeds, roughages (hay and straw); will not mill damp materials	Materials which will break under compression and by shearing, e.g. cereal grains, legume or pulse seeds; can process materials which have >16% moisture
Heating during milling	Small increase in the temperature of the ground material	Can slightly increase the temperature of the ground material
Effect on the working environment	Noisy and cause vibration, especially if the hammer assembly is unbalanced; fines may cause a dust problem downstream of the mill	Quieter and cause less vibration

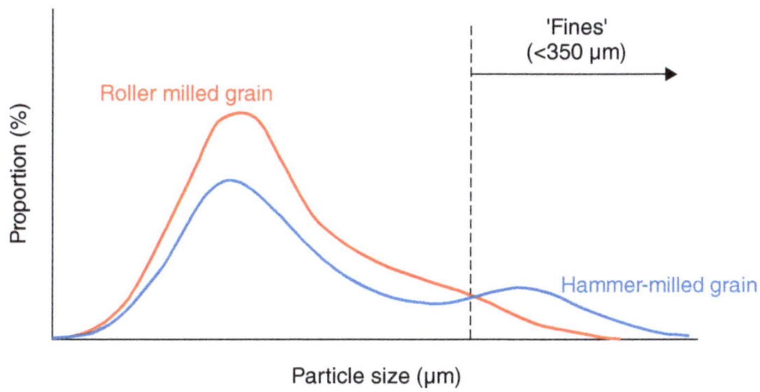

Fig. 18.6. Graph showing the distribution of particle sizes produced by hammer mills and roller mills grinding cereal grain. (Copyright: Gordon McL. Dryden.)

the hammer mill screen onto the belt conveyer which delivers the ground material from the tub.

Tub grinders and feed mixer wagons rapidly cut long pieces of straw or hay into pieces which are about 2–10 cm long. The advantages of these machines are their ability to process roughages of all qualities, their fast processing speed, and the general robustness of the machine. Their main disadvantage is that there is very little (for tub grinders) or no (for feed mixer wagons) control of the size of

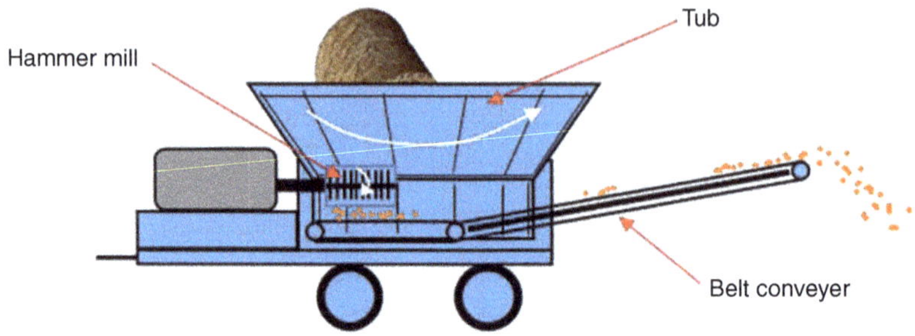

Fig. 18.7. Diagram of a tub grinder showing the tub, hammer mill and product delivery (the directions of tub and hammer mill rotations are shown by the white arrows). (Copyright: Gordon McL. Dryden.)

the resulting roughage particles, although choice of screen size (i.e. the diameter of the holes in the screen) in a tub grinder will set a general upper limit to particle length. Tub grinders produce a quantity of dust because, as we have seen, we have no control over the minimum particle size produced by hammer milling.

Fineness of grind: Cereal grains and dry forages are milled to produce particles which are nearer in size to the other feed ingredients, and which are small enough to readily undergo the pelleting process.

Milling roughages finely is a difficult and expensive process because roughages do not flow easily and they are tough and difficult to break up. Milling roughages so that they can be pelleted or included in a feed mix which is to be pelleted, involves reducing their particle size to about 1 mm in length, from a starting material with particle sizes which are usually not less than 10 cm, i.e. the length of a piece of dried leaf or stem. In addition, they are generally presented for milling in the form of tightly compacted bales. This means that we have to tease out the bale with a 'bale breaker', and possibly mill the material coarsely before a final fine milling.

Although we could reduce feeds, especially grains, to very small particles, we do not do this for these reasons:

- It is very expensive in time and energy to mill feeds to small particle sizes. This is especially the case for forages which have inherently low processing rates.
- The product would contain large proportions of fines (particles <350 μm) which would allow the loss of valuable feed components such as the starch- and protein-rich endosperm and the protein-rich embryo and aleurone layer of cereal grains, and the easily digested non-lignified parts of forages.
- Finely milled feeds are dusty. Dust is a good place for microbes and insects to grow especially if it gets damp, it traps water and sets up rust which can lead to the failure of equipment such as bins and silos, it is a fire hazard, and it makes an unpleasant and unsafe workplace.
- Fine feed particles can cause a number of animal health problems (e.g. oesophageal and gastric ulcers in pigs and horses, and rumenitis in sheep and cattle; Chapter 13), as well as making the feed unappetizing and difficult to eat.

Cattle digest milled grain better than whole grain (Chapter 4) and pigs, horses and sheep also respond to milling although they chew grains more efficiently than cattle (Meyer *et al.*, 1995; Vukmirović *et al.*, 2017). Ruminants given milled roughage eat more, digest it less efficiently, but may produce less CH_4 than when fed chopped hay (Blaxter and Graham, 1956). Horses eat similar amounts of chopped and milled roughage, although they take longer to eat the chopped material (Argo *et al.*, 2002).

Overall, the cost of fine milling, and the nature of animal responses to finely milled roughages, make this processing uneconomic.

Mixing feed ingredients

Most feed ingredients do not have the required range of nutrients present in the required concentrations, so we have to mix a variety of ingredients together to make up a complete ration. To achieve the desired composition, the mixture has to be well mixed, and all the ingredients have to be dispersed evenly throughout the mixture.

Mixers consist of a usually cylindrical body with an auger, or a shaft bearing paddles or blades, running along the long axis of the mixing chamber (Fig. 18.8). Mixers can be vertical or horizontal. Both vertical and horizontal mixers are made for on-farm use, while those used in commercial feed mills are usually horizontal because these are more efficient than vertical mixers. Horizontal mixers have hatches in the top of the mixer which allow the addition of ingredients, and either a hatch or doors in the base of the mixer, where the mixed feed is discharged. Feed is introduced into a vertical mixer either through a hatch at the top or by the action of the mixing auger picking up feed from the bottom.

When using a mixer, consider these things:

- Always have the mixer running before adding any ingredients. This protects the shaft and bearings from damage caused by the inertia of a load of material. If the mixer is used as a batching bin, then make sure that the weighing device can cope with the vibration that is caused by the mixer in motion.
- Avoid over-mixing as this will tend to de-mix the batch. It is best to test a new mixer or new feed by checking for evenness of dispersal throughout the batch by taking samples (from the mixer when stationary) at several different places in the batch, and at different times after starting mixing. Most commercial mixers are run for only about 3 minutes per batch, although this depends on the size and nature of the load and the type of mixer.
- It is difficult to mix liquids (e.g. oils or molasses) into a batch of dry ingredients. We may have to pass the mix through a dresser afterwards to remove any lumps.
- It is difficult to mix small amounts (e.g. 1 or 2 kg) of minor ingredients such as trace minerals or vitamins into a large (e.g. 1 or 2 tonnes) mix because this small amount is virtually impossible to disperse evenly throughout the batch. First mix the amount of minor ingredient with a 'carrier' such as 50 kg of bran or milled cereal grain, and then mix this ingredient/carrier mixture with the rest of the ingredients.

Pelleting

Because pelleting involves the application of heat, both from steam added before the mixed mash enters the press and from friction as the mash passes through the pellet press, there are chemical changes in the feed as well as compaction of the

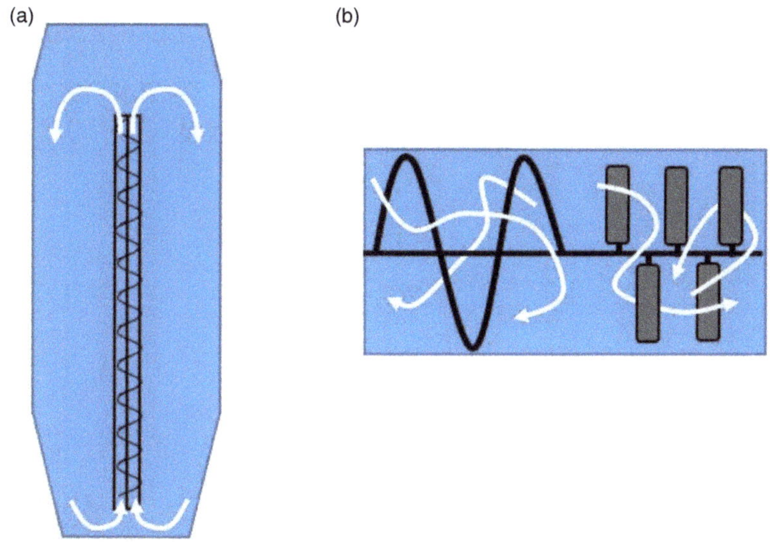

Fig. 18.8. Diagrams of (a) a vertical mixer with a single mixing auger, and (b) a horizontal mixer with a helical mixing blade (left) and paddles (right). The paths of feed particles during mixing are shown by the white arrows. (Copyright: Gordon McL. Dryden.)

ingredients into a pellet. As described below these changes can be beneficial (e.g. gelatinization of starch which makes it easier to digest) or deleterious (e.g. destruction of vitamins).

Five reasons why commercial animal feed manufacturers pellet their feeds:

- Increased digestibility of the starch in cereal grains. This is reflected in an improvement in the feed conversion ratio of pigs (the amount of feed needed to produce a kg of live weight gain) by up to 12%, and growth rate improvements of 13% (Chae and Han, 1998). Although pelleting adds a cost to the feed, this is offset because the animal uses its feed more efficiently.
- Reduced risk of disease pathogens being passed to livestock. The heat applied during pelleting kills a substantial proportion (but not all) of these organisms.
- Loose mixes ('mashes') are prevented from de-mixing, a problem which can happen when vibration separates the large and small particles in a loose mix as it is transported in bulk. Not only does de-mixing waste the time, equipment and money spent on mixing the feed, it also counters the reason for mixing the ingredients in the first place. We mix ingredients to make a complete ration in which the animal will receive all its needed nutrients when the feed is eaten in the recommended quantities. If some of the ingredients are lost from some parts of the bulk, and become concentrated in other parts, we have two consequences: feeding a nutritionally inadequate feed and potentially poisoning the animal from over-consumption of trace minerals (e.g. Cu or Se), urea or medications (e.g. ionophores).
- Allows the use of dry and dusty raw materials such as millrun. When these are used in mash feeds, they will cause dust in farm sheds. This type of ingredient can be included at higher levels in pelleted feeds and this can give significant raw material cost savings.
- Increased weight per volume (bulk density) compared to mash feed. Pellets have a bulk density of 550–650 g/L, which is greater than mash feeds at 500–600 g/L. This facilitates bulk transport and storage and reduces transport costs.

As well as these reasons, there are other advantages and disadvantages of pelleting:

- Increasing the amount of feed eaten or the rate of consumption by increasing the feed's bulk density or by changing its particle size; these both make it easier for the animal to take the feed into its mouth.
- Preventing diet selection: all animals will try to separate out, and eat, those parts of the mixed feed which they find most palatable. When the diet ingredients are packaged in pellets the animal cannot select for palatable (or against unpalatable) ingredients.
- Reducing trypsin inhibitor in soybeans: pelleting has been shown to reduce the effect of trypsin inhibitor on laying birds (although we probably need more evidence on this point).
- Vitamins A, E and K may undergo small (3–10%) losses during pelleting; this is not really a problem because extra vitamins can be included in the premix to allow for this loss, and technology has provided more heat-stable vitamins.

Pellet press construction: The core of a pelleting system (Fig. 18.9) consists of a conditioner and a pellet press. The conditioner is a chamber where the mash which is to be pelleted is mixed with steam. Steam provides heat and added water, which is an essential component of the forces which bind

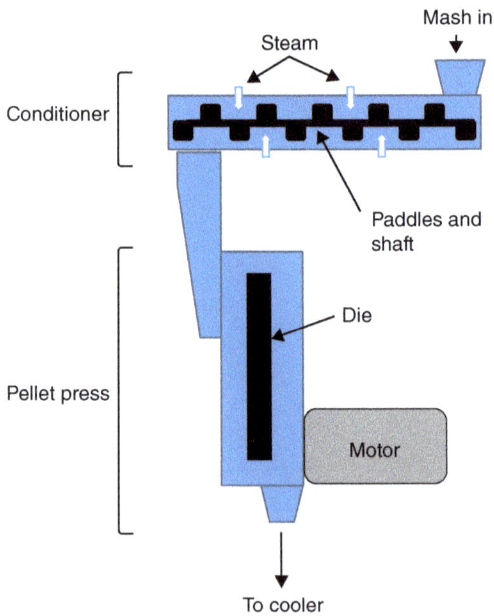

Fig. 18.9. Part of a pelleting system showing a conditioner mounted above a pellet press. (Copyright: Gordon McL. Dryden.)

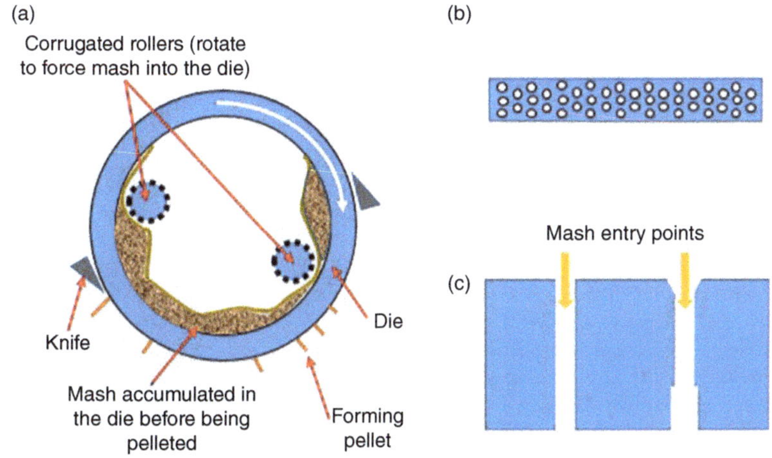

Fig. 18.10. Diagram of a pellet die showing the die, rollers and knives; the mash and forming pellets are also shown. (a) Plan view showing the die, rollers and knives, and direction of rotation (white arrow). (b) Side view showing the die perforations (not to scale). (c) Two pellet die hole shapes: straight (left), and a hole with a counterbore inlet used in processing roughage-rich mash, a straight barrel and a relief bore (right). (Copyright: Gordon McL. Dryden.)

feed particles into a pellet. Steam also reacts with the starches and proteins in the ingredients and makes them easier to digest, and reactions between proteins denatured by heat help to bind the feed particles.

The core of pellet press is a steel ring, the 'die', which is perforated with holes running radially through the ring (Fig. 18.10). Conditioned mash falls into the centre of the die and is forced through the die holes by rollers which rotate inside the die. The shape and size of the die holes determine the diameter and shape of the pellet, and knives set outside the die determine the pellet length.

Pellets and any unpelleted mash or pellet fragments fall from the die and are collected by an auger or moving belt and moved into a cooler. The cooled pellets are then sieved to remove under- and over-sized pieces.

Post-pelleting processing: Fat and molasses are sometimes added to pellets. Both of these ingredients improve the energy content of the pellets, and molasses gives a pleasant odour and taste. However, there are tight limits on the amounts of these ingredients which can be added to the mash before pelleting. The sugars in molasses will char as they pass through the die and this can choke the press. Fat lubricates the passage of mash through the die and we get poorly formed pellets which are liable to break.

However, we can get the benefits of liquid ingredients such as molasses and fat, and solutions of other heat-sensitive ingredients like enzymes and medications, by adding these after the pellets have left the die:

- Fat can be sprayed onto hot pellets as they leave the die, although this is not a very satisfactory method as fat accumulates on the die face.
- Liquid ingredients can be sprayed onto the cooled pellets.
- Vacuum addition: air is pumped out of the tank containing the pellets to form a vacuum. The liquid is sprayed onto the pellets where it remains on the surface, then air is let back into the tank and this forces the liquid into crevices and pores in the pellet surface.

'Crumbling' is a common post-pelleting process. This is where the pellets are passed through a roller mill and cut into small pieces. This retains the advantages of pelleting but reduces the particle size of the product to something that birds and young pigs can easily eat.

Extrusion

Extrusion is a process where conditioned (i.e. reacted with steam) grain or feed mixture (mash) is fed into a barrel and an auger moves and compresses it. The conditioned mash is forced through a die at the end of the barrel (Fig. 18.11). Different dies can form the extruded product into a variety of shapes.

Extrusion has a similar effect on feed chemistry and presentation as pelleting.

Steaming and flaking cereal grain

Steaming and flaking (or steaming and rolling) is a method of processing cereal grains to get the advantages of steam treatment, but at a lower cost than pelleting (Yu *et al.*, 1998; Zinn *et al.*, 2002). Steam-flaked grain is rolled to a thinner flake after more intensive steam treatment (30 to 60 minutes exposure to steam) than is used in steam rolling (10 to 20 minutes exposure). There is less starch gelatinization in steam-rolled grain than in steam-flaked grain.

The steam flaking process is illustrated in Fig. 18.12. It involves passing grain through a conditioning tower where it mixes with steam. After conditioning the softened grain is passed through a roller mill. This mill has plain (uncorrugated) rolls and is designed to flatten, or flake, the grain.

Smaller grains such as wheat, barley and sorghum are processed whole, while maize (corn) may first be coarsely rolled to give smaller particles which will absorb steam more readily than the intact maize kernel. Although this improves steam penetration, the seed embryo can be lost and the extra process introduces an additional cost. Another way of pre-treating maize is to temper it (see above) for about 48 hours.

Steam gelatinizes about 20% of the starch and this, together with the physical effects of rolling on the grain endosperm, increases the grain digestibility. Rolling also prevents the gelatinized starch from retrograding (returning to its original physico-chemical structure) as it cools.

Steamed and flaked grain is used in dairy cattle, lot-fed beef cattle and horse feeds. When used in feedlot rations for beef cattle (Owens *et al.*, 1997) it is not likely to change the growth rates of cattle given any type of grain, but it can lead to reduced feed intakes (12% reduction for maize-based diets, 17% for sorghum and 10% for wheat) and thus improvements in feed conversion efficiencies of up to 10% for wheat-based diets, 11% for maize (corn), or 15% for sorghum.

Steamed and flaked grain has a short storage life as its moisture content allows significant mould growth in 2 or 3 days, so it has to be dried if it is to be used as a component of a feed which will be fed several days or weeks after manufacture. Steamed and flaked grain is very bulky (i.e. it has a low bulk density) and so is expensive to transport.

Alkali treatment of roughages

Cereal straws are produced in very large amounts – almost the same quantity by weight as the grain harvested from a cereal crop. However, this potential feed is not much used because of its low nutritive value. In particular, it is not very digestible (dry matter (DM) digestibilities vary between 40% and 50%) and lacks protein (typically has only 4–7% DM basis). The reason for this is that as the crop matures, the stem and leaves lose cell contents and the residue is rich in the cell wall constituents cellulose, hemicelluloses and lignin (see Chapter 4).

Alkalis like caustic soda (NaOH) and ammonia degrade the cell wall and make the straw much more digestible.

Caustic soda is very effective, but unreacted NaOH can cause ulcers in the animal's mouth, and it loads the feed with excess Na which has to be eliminated from the animal's body and can have adverse effects on soil structure. It is very corrosive – it can injure operators who use it and it will corrode metal objects.

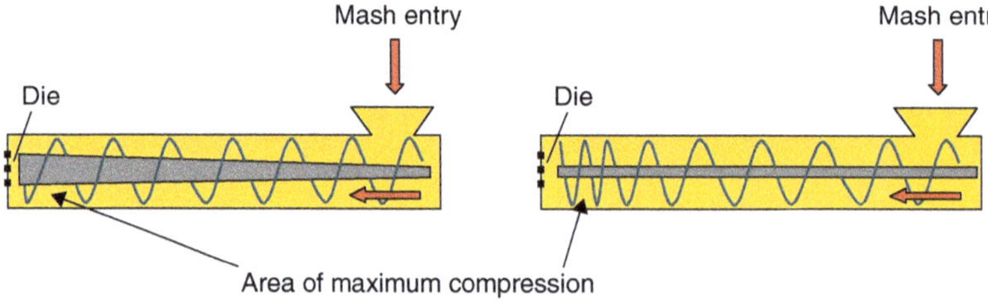

Fig. 18.11. Diagram of alternative designs for a single screw extrusion press. (Copyright: Gordon McL. Dryden.)

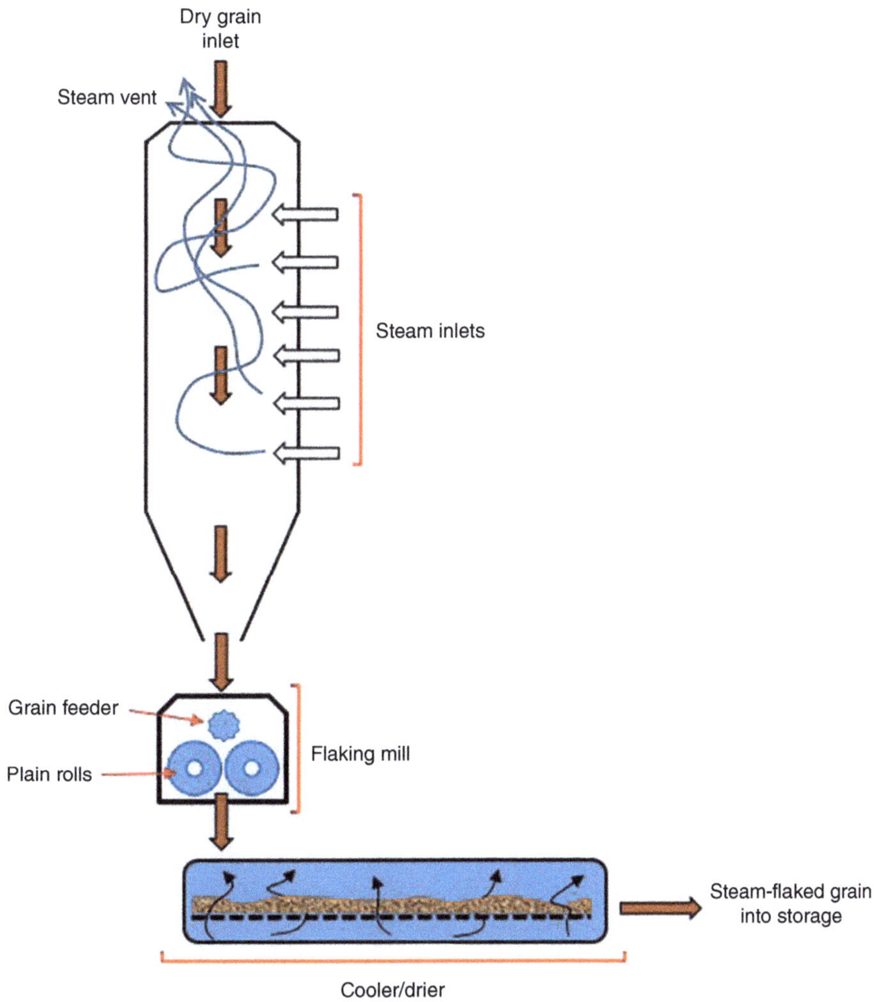

Fig. 18.12. Diagram of a steaming and flaking plant.

Ammonia is effective and less hazardous to use, although the treatment rates are slightly higher than for NaOH and treatment times are longer. The digestibility of cell wall components can be increased from about 48% in untreated barley straw to 65% by treatment with NH_3 at 4.5% of the straw DM. As well as improving the digestibility, ammonia adds water-soluble N, thus increasing its RAN content by up to 300%. The way that NH_3 affects cell wall composition and increases the straw N content are described by Dryden and Kempton (1983), Dryden and Leng (1988) and Sundstøl (1984).

Ammonia can be applied as anhydrous ammonia (NH_3 gas), aqua-ammonia (NH_4OH solution), or urea which breaks down under microbial action to yield NH_3. All of these are readily available and are used as fertilizers. Urea and aqua-ammonia are the easiest to use as we just have to pour the solution over the straw.

To ammoniate straw (treat straw with ammonia):

- Stack the straw to be treated in a compact pile, e.g. a line of round bales or stack of rectangular bales.
- Have a length of impervious film ready to cover the stack – e.g. polythene film, 0.2 mm × 4 m × 50 m,

will easily cover a single row of 38 or 40 round bales. There is no need to have a ground sheet but burying the edges of the plastic sheet in soil will help to seal the stack. Duct tape is handy to repair accidental tears.

- Add NH_3 at a rate equivalent to 3% or 4% of the straw DM. This treatment level assumes that the straw moisture content is the usual 12–15%. There is no need to exceed this NH_3 level as higher moisture contents (e.g. 25%, but see comments about toxicity below) are needed to get an effective uptake of higher levels of NH_3. Unreacted NH_3 simply escapes to the atmosphere when the stack is opened. Ammonia gas can be applied through a perforated pipe laid on top of the row or stack of bales; the gas will permeate through the whole of the stack in a few hours, provided that the stack is correctly sealed. Use a modified anhydrous NH_3 fertilizer applicator rather than trying to dispense the gas from a gas cylinder. Aqua-ammonia and urea solutions are sprayed onto the straw. Again, the NH_3 will permeate through the straw in a day or so.
- Leave the stack sealed for at least two weeks. More time will be needed in cold temperatures.
- When the stack is opened, allow it to air for an hour or so before feeding it out.

However, there are potential risks: NH_3 is a potentially poisonous and corrosive substance and operators must be aware of this. Take care to avoid splashing your skin or inhaling the gas. It is a good idea to invest in appropriate personal protective equipment, including a mask, eye protection and gloves. For an ammonia Safety Data Sheet see Fisher Scientific (2018) or similar.

In addition, forages like grass hays or failed cereal grain crops, which have more cell content material than cereal straws, contain soluble sugars which can react with ammonia to form imidazoles. These are poisonous and can cause a condition called 'bovine bonkers' (Perdok and Leng, 1987). Affected animals become hyper-excited (race around and collide with fences, etc.), uncoordinated, defaecate and urinate frequently, and have muscular tremors. The toxin can be passed on to calves through milk.

Nevertheless, for treating cereal straws, NH_3 is reasonably safe provided that the NH_3 application rate is no more than 3–4%, it is not applied to wet forages, and the temperature within the treated straw does not exceed 70°C, e.g. the temperature which might occur within the stack on a hot summer day. If these adverse effects are avoided, alkali treatment can have a useful place in a farmer's armoury.

References

Argo, C.M., Cox, J.E., Lockyer, C. and Fuller, Z. (2002). Adaptive changes in the appetite, growth and feeding behaviour of pony mares offered *ad libitum* access to a complete diet in either a pelleted or chaff-based form. *Animal Science* 74: 517–528.

Blaxter, K.L. and Graham, N.M. (1956). The effect of the grinding and cubing process on the utilization of the energy of dried grass. *Journal of Agricultural Science (Camb.)* 47: 207–217.

Chae, B.J. and Han, K. (1998). Processing effects of feeds in swine – review. *Asian-Australasian Journal of Animal Science* 11(5): 597–607.

Dryden, G.McL. and Kempton, T.J. (1983). Digestion of organic matter and nitrogen in ammoniated barley straw. *Animal Feed Science and Technology* 10: 65–75.

Dryden, G.McL. and Leng, R.A. (1988). Effects of ammonia and sulphur dioxide gases on the composition and digestion of barley straw. *Animal Feed Science and Technology* 19:121–133.

Fisher Scientific (2018). *Material Safety Data Sheet. Ammonium hydroxide water solution*. Available at: https://fscimage.fishersci.com/msds/00211.htm (accessed 29 December 2020).

Meyer, H., Radicke, S., Kienzle, E., Wilke, S., Kleffken, D. and Illenseer, M. (1995). Investigations on preileal digestion of starch from grain, potato and manioc in horses. *Journal of Veterinary Medicine Series A* 42(1–10): 371–381.

Owens, J.M. and Heimann, M. (1994). Material processing cost center. In McElhinney, R.R. (ed.), *Feed Technology IV*. American Feed Industry Association. Arlington, Virginia, USA, p. 81.

Owens, F.N., Secrist, D.S., Hill, W.J. and Gill, D.R. (1997). The effect of grain source and grain processing on performance of feedlot cattle: a review. *Journal of Animal Science* 75: 868–879.

Perdok, H.B. and Leng, R.A. (1987). Hyperexcitability in cattle fed ammoniated roughages. *Animal Feed Science and Technology* 17: 121–143.

Sundstøl, F. (1984). Ammonia treatment of straw: Methods for treatment and feeding experience in Norway. *Animal Feed Science and Technology* 10(2–3): 173–187.

Vukmirović, D. Čolović, R., Rakita, S., Brlek T., Đuragić, O. and Solà-Oriol, D. (2017). Importance of feed structure (particle size) and feed form (mash vs. pellets) in pig nutrition – A review. *Animal Feed Science and Technology* 233: 133–144.

Yu, P., Huber, J.T., Santos, F.A.P., Simas, J.M. and Theurer, C.B. (1998). Effects of ground, steam-flaked, and steam-rolled corn grains on performance of lactating cows. *Journal of Dairy Science* 81: 777–783.

Zinn, R., Almora, A., Montaño, M.F., Plascencia, A. and Bribiesca, E.R. (1998). Influence of tempering on the feeding value of rolled corn in finishing diets for feedlot cattle. *Journal of Animal Science* 76(9): 2239–2246.

Zinn, R.A., Owens, F.N. and Ware, R.A. (2002). Processing mechanics, quality standards, and impacts on energy availability and performance of feedlot cattle. *Journal of Animal Science* 80(5): 1145–1156.

19 Effects of animal production on the environment

Climate change

Global warming has, and will continue to, put stress on livestock farming, especially pig, poultry and dairy production in the subtropics and tropics. To judge the extent of this we need to know how the global environment has changed over the last decades. According to the IPCC (2019):

> A.2.1
> ... From 1850–1900 to 2006–2015 mean land surface air temperature has increased by 1.53°C (very likely range from 1.38°C to 1.68°C). ...
>
> A.2.2
> Warming has resulted in an increased frequency, intensity and duration of heat-related events, including heatwaves in most land regions (high confidence). Frequency and intensity of droughts has increased in some regions (including the Mediterranean, west Asia, many parts of South America, much of Africa, and north-eastern Asia) (medium confidence) ...
>
> A.2.6
> Global warming has led to shifts of climate zones in many world regions, including expansion of arid climate zones and contraction of polar climate zones (high confidence). As a consequence, many plant and animal species have experienced changes in their ranges, abundances, and shifts in their seasonal activities (high confidence) ...

Global warming effects on both animals and plants are variable, and these observations illustrate the difficulty of predicting the effects of climate change on agriculture and in devising ways of making use of them, or of adapting to them, or of taking precautionary action.

Effect of increased ambient temperature on animals

An animal's or bird's thermoneutral zone (TNZ) is that range of ambient temperatures where it can maintain its core temperature without needing extra energy expenditure. The TNZ is bounded by the upper and lower critical temperatures (UCT and LCT; Fig. 19.1). Considering the effects of global warming, the UCT is most important because it is likely that ambient temperatures, especially in summer and/or in sub-tropical or tropical regions, will exceed the UCT of many types of animal.

Animals respond to rising environmental temperatures by seeking shade, increasing the blood flow and thus heat loss in the blood vessels in their skin, or panting and/or sweating to lose heat by water evaporation. These and other metabolic and physiological mechanisms to control body heat are described by Collier *et al.* (2019). These mechanisms may not be enough to reduce the heat load and once it reaches its UCT the animal becomes increasingly unable to cope and life is threatened.

Similarly, when ambient temperatures fall, animals' first responses are to reduce dermal blood flow, fluff up the coat (piloerection) to improve insulation and reduce heat loss, and huddle together and seek shelter. At temperatures below the LCT, these behaviours cannot cope with the increasing heat loss and so animals begin shivering, and in some cases we get non-shivering thermogenesis (where fat and muscle metabolism generates heat rather than ATP or contraction). These are all energy-demanding processes, so the animal eats more feed and generates more heat as the feed is metabolized. But again, if temperatures continue to fall the animal suffers and may die.

Thermoneutral zones for representative animal types are listed in Table 19.1. These are indicative only, because heat loss is affected by animal breed and strain (e.g. pigs selected for high lean growth have a slightly lower UCT); adaptation to the ambient temperature (differences between acute and chronic heat stress); level of feeding (higher levels lower the LCT); rain, humidity and wind speed (which all affect insulation); insulation

DOI: 10.1079/9781786394453.0019

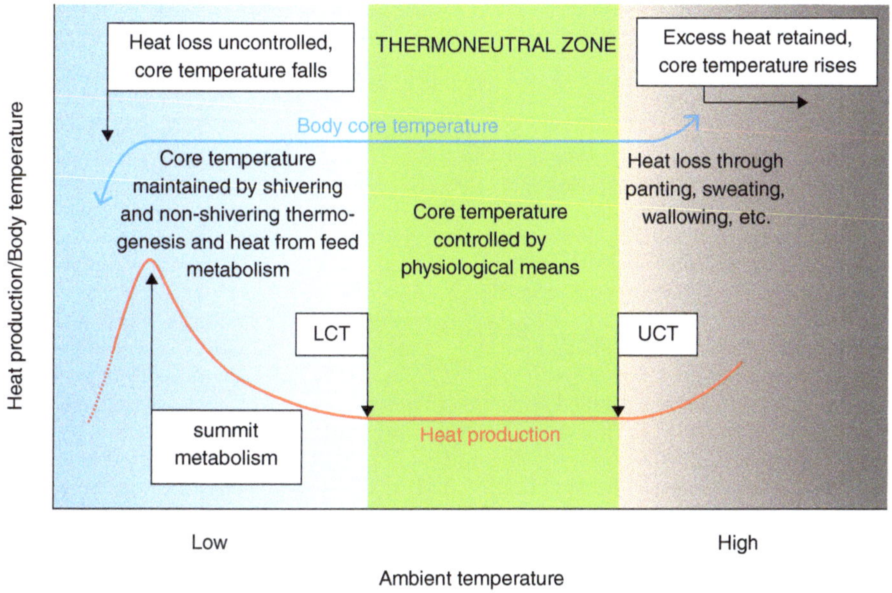

Fig. 19.1. Concepts of heat production and loss from animals. (Copyright: Gordon McL. Dryden.)

provided by carcase fatness, coat length and condition (the range for sheep in Table 19.1 reflects differences between fleeced and shorn lambs); and physiological state (newborn animals have a higher LCT than adults).

High heat loads will reduce feed intake to 75–80% or less of intake under thermoneutral conditions (White and Hanigan, 2016; Chapter 7); impair immunity; affect breeding, e.g. sows have longer farrowing times and more stillbirths; reduce growth in young pigs; impair lactation yield in sows and dairy cows (especially high-yielding cattle), and reduce milk fat and protein contents; reduce egg size and shell quality; and in extreme (but unfortunately not very unusual) cases can result in death.

There are also metabolic effects. Animals suffer oxidative stress, where reactive oxygen species (e.g. peroxides, hydroxides and superoxides) are produced in greater than usual amounts and damage cell lipids, proteins and nucleic acids.

Managing environmental factors and their influence on animal welfare and performance: There are some aspects of the environment which we cannot control – droughts, floods, fires, excessive (high and low) temperatures, rain and wind, etc. But while we cannot control these things, they are not necessarily outside our ability to manage.

Non-nutritional management of heat and cold stress includes providing shade and using fans and water sprays (droplets, not mist) in hot conditions, or providing shelter from wind and rain when it is cold. We may have to erect shelters or plant windbreaks. The insulation provided by the animal's coat is enhanced by preventing feather loss, ensuring that animals are not covered in mud, and not shearing sheep or goats when there is risk of cold weather. Nutritional management simply involves providing adequate, energy-rich feed.

To reduce the effects of high temperatures we can carry out these nutritional strategies:

- Increase the non-energy nutrient concentrations in pig and poultry feeds so that even when these animals eat less feed they still consume the amounts of amino acids, vitamins and minerals that they need.
- Make sure that adequate water is available, and that it is as cool as possible, and non-saline. We might have to install reticulated water, and water troughs.

Table. 19.1. Indicative upper and lower critical temperatures for domestic animals and birds.

Critical temperature	Cattle[a]	Sheep[b]	Pigs[c]	Horses[d]	Poultry[e]
Upper (°C)	25	25 to 30	21 to 25	25 to 30	28 to 32
Lower (°C)	5	–20 to 25	16 to 25	5	10 to 20

[a]McDowell (1972) cited by NRC (1981); [b]Fuquay (1981); [c]NRC (1981); Huynh *et al.* (2005); [d]Morgan (1998); [e]Jini *et al.* (2015).

- Reduce the amounts of roughage in ruminant and horse diets. This will reduce the amount of heat generated by microbial fermentation in the rumen or large intestine. However, we need to be careful about this because all animals, and especially ruminants, need some fibre to maintain digestive tract health (Chapters 1 and 13), and dairy cattle need digestible fibre to ensure that their milk has an adequate fat content.
- Add fat to the diet. This increases the diet's available energy content, and the energy in fat is used more efficiently (with less waste heat production) than that from fibrous feed. Bacterial digestion of fibre in the rumen is impaired when fat is more than 6 or 7% of the diet, but we can get around this problem by using Ca salts of saturated fatty acids (Sukhija and Palmquist, 1990).
- Feed additional Cr, Se and Cu: these help to maintain the tissue's anti-oxidant capacity and added Se and vitamin E increase feed intake and growth rate during heat stress (Chauhan *et al.*, 2016). Inorganic and organic forms of Cr (e.g. Cr-methionine or Cr-propionate) increase feed intake and may improve milk composition in cattle but have inconsistent and minor effects in pigs, and variable and possibly adverse effects in poultry (Bin-Jumaha *et al.*, 2020). Cu (as nano-particles of the oxide) may improve the growth of broilers in hot conditions, but this has to be investigated more extensively. Warning: seek advice on the safe use of these minerals because they all can be toxic in excess.
- Check that the Na, K and chloride (Cl^-) intakes of heat-stressed or intensively exercised horses are adequate. The Na and Cl^- requirements can be met by providing salt *ad lib* (NRC, 2007).

Ambient temperature effects on grazing behaviour: Grazing animals avoid activity in the hottest part of the day. As the surface air temperature rises, animals spend less time grazing and more grazing takes place near dawn and after sunset. This behaviour has been consistently reported for sheep, horses and cattle.

Animals adapt their behaviour to reduce their heat load. When the ground temperature exceeds body temperature cattle will stand rather than lie (this can happen in feedlots in hot conditions where soil temperatures can reach over 50°C in the subtropics), and sheep change their choice of grazing area as ambient temperature changes.

Shade and water are essential in hot conditions. If shade is available, cattle will use this during the hottest part of the day and may prefer to do this rather than graze. Cattle drink during the daytime and may visit water points up to twice a day, with the time between visits decreasing as heat stress increases (Williams *et al.*, 2019). In open pastures (i.e. without shade), cattle will congregate at water points and try to use water to wet themselves, rather than graze, and there may be more aggressiveness between individuals.

There are between-species and between-breed differences in how grazing animals tolerate heat. For example, sheep continue to graze in hot conditions longer than horses (Patkowski *et al.*, 2019); in hot conditions *Bos taurus* cattle (Herefords) have a higher respiration rate, graze for shorter times and seek shade more often than *B. indicus* cattle (Bonsmara × Hereford) (Taborda *et al.*, 2018), and Sahiwal (*B. indicus*) cattle eat for longer in hot conditions than Holstein/Friesians (*B. taurus*) (Kariuki *et al.*, 1999).

When surface water dries up under hot conditions the effective grazing area (Chapter 15) is reduced. This increases grazing pressure on the pasture that can be accessed, with over-grazing of palatable pasture species and possible restrictions on feed intake.

Effects of increased ambient temperature on plants

The expected changes in crop and pasture production and animal performance resulting from global warming are both positive and negative. IPCC (2019) notes that:

A.2.3.
Satellite observations have shown vegetation greening over the last three decades in parts of Asia, Europe, South America, central North America, and southeast Australia. Causes of greening include combinations of an extended growing season, nitrogen deposition, carbon dioxide (CO_2) fertilization, and land management (high confidence). Vegetation browning has been observed in some regions including northern Eurasia, parts of North America, Central Asia and the Congo Basin, largely as a result of water stress (medium confidence). Globally, vegetation greening has occurred over a larger area than vegetation browning (high confidence).

A.2.8.
... yields of some crops (e.g., maize and wheat) in many lower-latitude regions have been affected negatively by observed climate changes, while in many higher-latitude regions, yields of some crops (e.g., maize, wheat, and sugar beets) have been affected positively over recent decades (high confidence).

Changes in pasture composition and nutritive value: Rising CO_2 levels and temperatures influence the distribution of C3 and C4 grasses. C4 plants photosynthesize more efficiently than C3 plants in high temperature/low CO_2 conditions (see Chapter 15), although C3 grasses compete better with C4 grasses at low temperatures or as CO_2 levels rise. The germination rate of C3 plants is less at high temperatures. This means that C3 plants dominate pastures at low temperatures and C4 plants dominate in high temperatures (Lattanzi, 2010) and as global temperatures rise, we will see C3 grasses retreating and being replaced by C4 grasses.

C3 and C4 plants differ in several important characteristics. C4 grasses have more vascular tissue and sclerenchyma than C3 grasses, and they are consequently less digestible (see Chapter 15). They also have lower protein contents than C3 grasses, are less tolerant of hard grazing, and ruminants eating them produce more CH_4 (Crush and Rowarth, 2007). These characteristics reduce feed intake and animal performance. This has already been recorded in African pastoral systems (IPCC, 2019). On the other hand, C4 grasses are more productive than C3 species and give greater pasture dry matter (DM) yields.

Effects of global warming on grain and fodder crop production: We can expect that the yields of C3 crops such as wheat, barley, rice and soybean will be greater as CO_2 levels rise but reduced as temperatures rise. However, C4 crop plants such as maize (corn), sorghum and millet will not respond in this way to increased CO_2, but will be affected, like C3 crops, by rising temperatures. The interplay of these factors is discussed by Wheeler and Reynolds (2013).

How animal production can influence the environment

The expansion of intensive animal husbandry, and production of the pasture and crops needed to support this, is generating increasing amounts of greenhouse gases (GHG) and other pollutants. The main ones are enteric CH_4 and CO_2 gases produced as by-products of carbohydrate fermentation by rumen and large intestine microbes (Chapter 3), and CO_2, CH_4, NH_3, NO_x gases, nitrates (NO_3) and phosphates produced from the microbial breakdown of droppings, manure and urine, and from the breakdown of fertilizers applied to crops and intensively managed pastures.

Enteric CH_4 from ruminants is an important GHG. Global enteric CH_4 production is estimated to have doubled from 1961 to 2012 (Chang *et al.*, 2019) and efforts to reduce the amount of this gas are becoming increasingly urgent, but this conflicts with the increasing demand for ruminant animal products. Alexandratos and Bruinsma (2012) estimate that the global demands for meat and milk are expected to increase by 57% and 48%, respectively, between 2005 and 2050.

Wastes produced by animals and birds enter the environment as gases, or in the runoff from intensively managed pastures and feed lots, and the escape of wastes from piggeries and poultry units. For example, for each 6 kg of pork protein produced it is estimated that about 4 kg of feed N are lost into the environment, and that 68% of this enters water courses as nitrates and other organic N, and 32% is released into the atmosphere as gaseous N compounds (Uwizeye *et al.*, 2019). Grazing animals produce more than 50% of 'man-made' N_2O emissions (IPCC, 2019). Lactating dairy and growing beef cattle retain feed N in milk or beef with efficiencies of only 25–27% and 10–20%, respectively (Hristov *et al.*, 2011). These inefficiencies mean that large amounts of feed N are 'wasted', which increases the cost of feeding, and contaminates the environment when the surplus is released as NH_3, ammonium salts, and NO_3. We find similar situations with P (Chapter 11).

Enteric gases and other pollutants have a range of adverse effects, including:

- Contribution of CH_4, CO_2 and NO_x gases to global warming. The Global Warming Potentials (GWP) of these gases are, respectively, 1 for CO_2, 28–36 for CH_4, and 265–298 for N_2O (USEPA 2020). NO_x gases (NO, N_2O and NO_2) are the next most important GHGs after CH_4. Although they are produced in smaller amounts, their very high GWPs make them serious pollutants.
- Eutrophication, the contamination of watercourses and lakes by NO_3 and other organic N compounds, and minerals especially P. Excess N and P entering watercourses may possibly, be controlled by precision feeding – adjusting feed N and P contents and availabilities to match animal requirements as closely as possible (Chapter 8). This is illustrated in a study carried out on Italian dairy farms by Biagini and Lazzaroni (2018).
- NH_3 combines with nitric and sulphuric acids in the atmosphere to form aerosols, and it pollutes the air in intensive animal housing. Levels of NH_3 in the air are increasing over the USA, Europe and Asia by 2% or more per year (Warner *et al.*, 2017) and this is partly due to intensive animal husbandry and N fertilizer use.
- NH_3 and H_2S cause respiratory distress and injury to the lungs and eyes of housed animals. High concentrations of NH_3 reduce feed intake and thus growth and egg production in pigs and poultry, and can increase mortality rates.
- Producing undesirable odours and attracting insect pests.

Enteric methane is an important greenhouse gas: CH_4 is made by methanogenic archaea (single-celled organisms similar to bacteria), which use the CO_2 and H_2 produced during rumen carbohydrate fermentation (Chapter 3) to synthesize ATP and produce CH_4 as an end-product (Fig. 19.2). Most H and much CO_2 dissolved in the rumen liquor, while the remaining CO_2 not used for CH_4 synthesis, and all of the CH_4, are eructated.

Enteric CH_4 is produced in quite large amounts – about 15% of the total free rumen gas. Sheep produce about 35 g CH_4/day, beef cattle about 290 g/day, and dairy cattle about 395 g/day. Published values vary considerably; those cited here are calculated from Eq 10.21 in IPCC (2006), the estimators of DM intake given in Chapter 7, and assuming a 650 kg live weight dairy cow producing 22 kg milk/day, a 450 kg beef animal and a 55 kg sheep.

Diets which include concentrates produce less CH_4, while roughage diets yield more. This is because

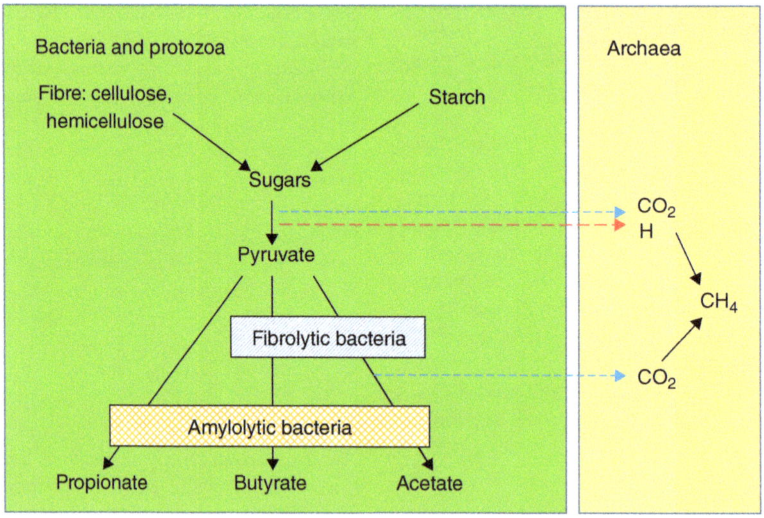

Fig. 19.2. Simplified pathways of H (red dotted line) and CO_2 (blue dotted line) production and methane (CH_4) formation in the rumen. (Fungi also produce H, and a few methanogens use formic acid, acetic acid or ethanol as substrates). (Copyright: Gordon McL. Dryden.)

of the characteristic differences between roughage-rich and concentrate-rich diets in the volatile fatty acids (VFA) produced during rumen fermentation. Acetic acid is a major metabolic end-product of the fibrolytic bacteria, while the amylolytic bacteria produce acetic, propionic and butyric acids (Fig. 19.2; Chapter 3). Propionic and butyric acids are longer-chain VFA than acetic acid, and they have more H atoms. Thus propionic and butyric acids are 'H sinks' and can trap some of the H which is produced by bacteria and protozoa. This trapped H is then unavailable for CH_4 synthesis.

For ruminant animals, CH_4 production has positive as well as negative effects. It removes H dissolved in the rumen liquor which would otherwise accumulate and inhibit the growth and activity of rumen microbes. But on the other hand, CH_4 production accounts for 2–10% of feed energy (IPCC, 2006, use an average value of 6.5% for roughage-fed animals and 3.5% for lot-fed cattle).

Nutritional methods of reducing the production of greenhouse gases and other pollutants

While there are several different ways that we can reduce enteric CH_4 emissions, they may have limited effectiveness, be difficult to implement, or are still in development. However, the concept of CO_2 equivalent (CO_2e) intensity is valuable because reducing this is an approach that we can use immediately and effectively.

Nutritional efficiency reduces the methane intensity of production: If we want to reduce the CH_4 cost of each unit of production (i.e. the CO_2e intensity of production), the first step is to feed a nutritionally adequate diet so as to maximize animal productivity.

The nutritional cost of a unit of product includes the amount of nutrients incorporated in it, plus the energy cost of synthesizing the product, and the share of the animal's maintenance requirement which applies to the product. By improving productivity, we reduce the share of the maintenance cost for each unit, and thus the share of the total CH_4 production.

For example, a 650 kg Holstein/Friesian dairy cow producing 3.5% fat milk requires 43.1 MJ NE_l/day for maintenance and 3.22 MJ NE_l/L of milk (NRC, 2001). If the feed has 6.3 MJ NE_l/kg DM (e.g. a 30/70 mixture of maize grain and timothy hay), then the total DM required is 19.7 kg/day for a cow producing 25 L of milk, and 22.2 kg/day for a cow producing 30 L of milk. The total CH_4 productions are 423 and 478 g/day, respectively (from Eq 10.21, IPCC, 2006). But when we correct for milk yield, the CO_2e intensities are 474 g CO_2e/L for a cow producing 25 L/day and 446 g CO_2e/L for a cow producing 30 L/day.

What we can do to reduce the greenhouse gas cost of animal products: As well as aiming for maximum nutritional efficiency we can reduce CH_4 production by other means. Several of these are discussed by Beachemin *et al.* (2020) and Kumari *et al.* (2020), and a selection is listed here (in order of decreasing current effectiveness):

- Reduce the fibre content of ruminant feeds: as described above, fibrolytic bacteria produce acetic acid as a major end-product, while starch on the other hand, is fermented by amylolytic bacteria which use propionic acid as a H sink.
- Use forages which yield less CH_4 when fermented in the rumen. A practical method for extensive sheep and beef managers is to include tannin-rich pasture plants or feed supplements in the diet. Tannins can improve protein use and control internal parasites (Chapter 12), as well as reducing CH_4. Options include planting *Lotus* spp., sainfoin (*Onobrychis viciifolia*) and sulla (*Hedysarum coronarium*) in pasture mixes, feeding turnip, fodder beet and swede bulbs, or grain legumes, or tree leaves (Chapter 6).
- Use additives which reduce CH_4 production. Some of these are very promising, but this approach requires that grazing animals are fed a supplement, which they must eat in controlled amounts. Additives include unsaturated fats and a range of additives such as ionophores, 3-nitrooxypropanol, tannins, and bromoform (from *Asparagopsis* spp. seaweeds), which will reduce the amount of CH_4 produced by 20–80%. The mechanisms are different for each additive. Unsaturated fats (oils) react with H and thus deny methanogens one of their essential nutrients. Ionophores kill protozoa and reduce H, and thus CH_4 production, whereas tannins inhibit protozoa and fibrolytic bacteria. Tannins

and fats are accepted feed constituents and ionophores are registered for use in feeds. However, the others listed have not yet been approved as feed additives.

- Manage and breed animals for more efficient reproduction: high lambing, calving or farrowing rates reduce the number of breeding animals needed, and potentially improve the ratio of producing animals to breeding stock.
- Breed nutritionally efficient animals: we can reduce the amount of CH_4 produced and the amount of feed used per unit of product by breeding for animals which produce less CH_4 (Pinares-Patiño *et al.*, 2011; NZAGGRC, 2019), or have a negative residual feed index (see Chapter 7), or which are more efficient producers and thus produce more product per unit of CH_4.
- Vaccinate animals against methanogens: this method is still under development. The concept is to establish in the animal antigens to methanogenic organisms; the antigens are secreted in saliva, enter the rumen and inactivate methanogenesis there.

Reducing ammonia and nitrous oxide emissions: Emissions of NH_3 from animal manure can be reduced in two ways. If the protein content of pig, poultry and cattle diets is reduced we get a corresponding reduction in the amount of NH_3 generated from manure and droppings. Reducing the diet protein content by 2–4% units, e.g. reducing the protein content of a weaner pig diet from 18% to 16%, or from 15.5% to 14% for finishing pigs, or reducing the protein in cattle diets by 1.5–5% units, reduces NH_3 emission by 20–65% (review by Sajeev *et al.*, 2018).

Increasing the fibre content of pig diets will reduce emissions of NH_3 (Trabue *et al.*, 2019). A similar effect occurs in poultry. The mechanism may be that protein in fibre is less digested by the animal's or bird's intrinsic digestive enzymes, and so is excreted in manure or droppings as microbial and/or undigested feed protein that are slowly converted to NH_3. When a conventional, concentrate-rich diet is fed to pigs and poultry the protein is more completely digested, the resulting freed amino acids are absorbed, and any excess amino acid-N is excreted as either urea or uric acid which are readily converted to NH_3.

However, these dietary manipulations, especially reducing the feed protein content, are very likely to reduce production rates and feed efficiency. These adverse effects can be ameliorated to some extent by paying attention to essential amino acid intakes (see Chapters 1 and 8) in pig and poultry diets. The idea of ideal amino acid ratios is relevant here (Chapter 5).

Ammonia emissions from dairy and beef cattle are possibly more sensitive to changes in feed protein content than emissions from monogastric animals. To reduce ruminant emissions we must:

- Ensure that ruminally available N intakes are adequate so that fibre is digested as efficiently as possible because this will minimize the amount of feed N voided in the manure.
- Avoid deficiencies of any essential amino acid (lysine, methionine and histidine are often the first-limiting amino acids in dairy cattle diets) and avoid an over-supply of any amino acid. Both of these conditions cause the animal to be loaded with amino acids that it cannot use and which have to be deaminated and the waste N excreted. To achieve these goals, we have to know the rumen degradability of the feed protein (Chapters 1 and 5) and the amino acid composition of the metabolizable protein passing into the small intestine.

Nitrous oxide emissions are mainly from microbial fermentation of manure, but a very small amount is produced in the rumen. Rumen N_2O production can be influenced by the type of diet: protein-rich forages such as lucerne (alfalfa) silage will generate more N_2O than grass hay or maize silage (Gerlach *et al.*, 2018).

Feeding to reduce odour and insects

Odour and insect pests are an unpleasant consequence of intensive pig, poultry and ruminant animal (mainly dairy and beef) production. The odours are caused mainly by NH_3 and H_2S gases, and also by phenols and VFA. These compounds are produced by the action of microbes on uric acid (in bird excreta), urea in urine (voided by animals) and undigested feed protein, endogenous protein, or microbial protein in manure. Flies and other pests are attracted to these volatile organic compounds.

Intensive pig and poultry producers usually use mechanical methods of odour and gas control (e.g. drains and fans). Nevertheless, there are some dietary tweaks that we can use. Adequate cereal grain processing is the best way of reducing the amount of undigested organic matter especially starch, in manure (Miller and Varel, 2002). Cereal grains should be at least milled or ensiled (high moisture grain) to increase their digestibility. Further processing, such as steaming and flaking or extruding (Chapter 18) will also help, although these processes increase the cost of the ration. Another approach is to use a minimum amount of wet ingredients. For example, wet distillers' grains and solubles fed at more than 40% of the feed DM are likely to cause more odours.

References

Alexandratos, N. and Bruinsma, J. (2012). World agriculture towards 2030/2050: the 2012 revision. *ESA Working paper No. 12-03*. Rome, FAO. Available at: ww.fao.org > esa > world_ag_2030_50_2012_rev (accessed 30 December 2020).

Beauchemin, K.A., Ungerfeld, E.M., Eckard, R.J. and Wang, M. (2020). Review: Fifty years of research on rumen methanogenesis: lessons learned and future challenges for mitigation. *Animal* 14(S1): s2–s16.

Biagini, D. and Lazzaroni, C. (2018). Eutrophication risk arising from intensive dairy cattle rearing systems and assessment of the potential effect of mitigation strategies. *Agriculture, Ecosystems and Environment* 266: 76–83.

Bin-Jumaha, M., Abd El-Hack, M.E., Abdelnour, S.A., Hendy, Y.A., Ghanem, H.A., *et al.* (2020). Potential use of chromium to combat thermal stress in animals: A review. *Science of The Total Environment* 707, 135996.

Chang, J., Peng, S., Ciais, P. Saunois, M., Dangal, S.R.S., Herrero, M., Havlík, P., Tian, H. and Bousquet, P. (2019). Revisiting enteric methane emissions from domestic ruminants and their $\delta^{13}C_{CH4}$ source signature. *Nature Communications* 10: 3420. DOI: doi.org/10.1038/s41467-019-11066-3.

Chauhan, S.S., Liu, F., Leury, B.J., Cottrell, J.J., Celi, P. and Dunshea, F.R. (2016). Functionality and genomics of selenium and vitamin E supplementation in ruminants. *Animal Production Science* 56(8) 1285–1298.

Collier, R.J., Baumgard, L.H., Zimbelman, R.B. and Xiao, Y. (2019). Heat stress: physiology of acclimation and adaptation. *Animal Frontiers* 9(1): 12–19.

Crush, J.R. and Rowarth, J.S. (2007). The role of C4 grasses in New Zealand pastoral systems. *New Zealand Journal of Agricultural Research* 50(2): 125–137.

Fuquay, J.W. (1981). Heat stress as it affects animal production. *Journal of Animal Science* 52(1): 164–174.

Gerlach, K., Schmithausen, A.J., Sommer, A.C.H., Trimborn, M., Büscher, W. and Südekum, K.H. (2018). Cattle diets strongly affect nitrous oxide in the rumen. *Sustainability* 10: 3679; DOI: 10.3390/su10103679.

Hristov, A.N., Hanigan, M., Cole, A., Todd, R., McAllister, T.A., Ndegwa, P.M. and Rotz, A. (2011). Review: Ammonia emissions from dairy farms and beef feedlots. *Canadian Journal of Animal Science* 91(1): 1—35.

Huynh, T.T.T., Aarnink, A.J.A., Verstegen, M.W.A., Gerrits, W.J.J., Heetkamp, M.J.W., Kemp, B. and Canh, T.T. (2005). Effects of increasing temperatures on physiological changes in pigs at different relative humidities. *Journal of Animal Science* 83(6): 1385–1396.

IPCC (2006). 2006 IPCC *Guidelines for National Greenhouse Gas Inventories, Prepared by the National Greenhouse Gas Inventories Programme*, Eggleston H.S., Buendia L., Miwa K., Ngara T. and Tanabe K. (eds). Published: IGES, Japan. Available at: www.ipcc-nggip.iges.or.jp/public/2006gl/vol4.html (accessed 30 December 2020).

IPCC (2019). Summary for Policymakers. In: *Climate Change and Land: an IPCC special report on climate change, desertification, land degradation, sustainable land management, food security, and greenhouse gas fluxes in terrestrial ecosystems*. Available at: www.ipcc.ch/srccl/chapter/summary-for-policymakers/ (accessed 29 December 2020).

Jini, D., Bhagawati, K., Bhagawati, R. and Rajkhowa, D.J. (2015). Identification of critical periods environmentally sensitive to normal performance of Vanaraja poultry breed in climatically different locations. *International Letters of Natural Sciences* 46: 76–83.

Kariuki, J.N., Tamminga, S., Gachuiri, C.K., Gitau, C.K. and Muia, J.M.K. (1999). Feeding behaviour of Sahiwal and Friesian cattle under a zero grazing system in a tropical climate. In vanderHeide, D., Huisman, E.A., Kanis, E., Osse, J.W.M. and Verstegen, M.W.A., (eds), *Regulation of Feed Intake.* Proceedings of the 5th Zodiac Symposium, Wageningen, 1998, pp. 215–218.

Kumari, S., Fagodiya, R.K., Hiloidhari, M., Dahiya, R.P. and Kumar, A. (2020). Methane production and estimation from livestock husbandry: A mechanistic understanding and emerging mitigation options. *Science of The Total Environment* 709: 136135.

Lattanzi, F.A. (2010). C3/C4 grasslands and climate change. In Schnyder, H *et al.* (eds), *Grassland in a Changing World*. Duderstadt, Germany: Mecke.

McDowell, R.E. (1972). *Improvement of Livestock Production in Warm Climates*. San Francisco: W.H. Freeman and Co.

Miller, D.N. and Varel, V.H. (2002). An in vitro study of manure composition on the biochemical origins, composition, and accumulation of odorous compounds in cattle feedlots. *Journal of Animal Science* 80(9): 2214–2222.

Morgan, K. (1998). Thermoneutral zone and critical temperatures of horses. *Journal of Thermal Biology* 23(l): 59–61.

National Research Council (NRC) (1981). *Effect of Environment on Nutrient Requirements of Domestic Animals*. Washington, DC: National Academies Press. Available at: www.nap.edu/catalog/4963/effect-of-environment-on-nutrient-requirements-of-domestic-animals (accessed 29 December 2020).

National Research Council (NRC) (2001). *Nutrient Requirements of Dairy Cattle*, 7th rev. edn. Washington, DC: National Academies Press. Available at:www.nap.edu/catalog/9825/nutrient-requirements-of-dairy-cattle-seventh-revised-edition-2001 (accessed 29 December 2020).

National Research Council (NRC) (2007). *Nutrient Requirements of Horses*, 6th rev. edn. Washington, DC: National Academies Press. Available at: www.nap.edu/catalog/11653/nutrient-requirements-of-horses-sixth-revised-edition (accessed 29 December 2020).

New Zealand Agricultural Greenhouse Gas Research Centre (NZAGGRC) (2019). Methane research programme. In *Highlights 2019*. Available at: www.nzagrc.org.nz/page-2019,listing,604,nzagrc-highlights-2019.html (accessed 31 December 2020).

Patkowski, K., Pluta, M., Lipiec, A., Greguła-Kania, M. and Gruszecki, T.M. (2019). Foraging behavior patterns of sheep and horses under a mixed species grazing system. *Journal of Applied Animal Welfare Science* 22(4): 357–363.

Pinares-Patiño, C.S., Ebrahimi, S.H., McEwan, J.C., Dodds, K.G., Clark, H. and Luo, D. (2011). Is rumen retention time implicated in sheep differences in methane emission? *Proceedings of the New Zealand Society of Animal Production* 71: 219–222.

Sajeev, E.P.M., Amon, B. Ammon, C., Zollitsch, W. and Winiwarter, W. (2018). Evaluating the potential of dietary crude protein manipulation in reducing ammonia emissions from cattle and pig manure: A meta-analysis. *Nutrient Cycling in Agroecosystems* 110(1): 161–175.

Sukhija, P.S. and Palmquist, D.L. 1990. Dissociation of calcium soaps of long-chain fatty acids in rumen fluid. *Journal of Dairy Science* 73: 1784–1787.

Taborda, P.A.B., Saravia, C.T. and Espasandin, A.C. (2018) Physiological responses and animal behavior in Bonsmara-Hereford crosses vs. Hereford purebred on environment stress. *Scientia Agricola* 75(6): 479–485.

Trabue, S., Kerr, B. and Andersen, D. (2019). Impact of carbohydrate source on manure and air emissions from swine diets. *Journal of Animal Science* 97(Supp. 3): 388–389.

United States Environmental Protection Agency (USEPA) (2020). *Understanding Global Warming Potentials*. Available at: www.epa.gov/ghgemissions/understanding-global-warming-potentials (accessed: 30 December 2020).

Uwizeye, A., Gerber, P.J., Opioa, C.I., Tempioa, G., Mottet, A., Makkara, H.P.S., Falcucci, A., Steinfeld, H. and de Boer, I.J.M. (2019). Nitrogen flows in global pork supply chains and potential improvement from feeding swill to pigs. *Resources, Conservation and Recycling* 146: 168–179.

Warner, J.X., Dickerson, R.R., Wei, Z., Strow, L.L., Wang, Y. and Liang, Q. (2017). Increased atmospheric ammonia over the world's major agricultural areas detected from space. *Geophysical Research Letters* 44(6): 2875–2884.

Wheeler, T. and Reynolds, C. (2013). Predicting the risks from climate change to forage and crop production for animal feed. *Animal Frontiers* 3(1): 36–41.

White, R.R. and Hanigan, M.D. (2016). Modelling cross-species feed intake responses to thermal stress. *Journal of Agricultural Science* 154: 136–150.

Williams, L.R., Fox, D.R., Bishop-Hurley, G.J. and Swain, D.L. (2019). Use of radio frequency identification (RFID) technology to record grazing beef cattle water point use. *Computers and Electronics in Agriculture* 156: 193–202.

Glossary

These terms and abbreviations are used commonly in animal nutrition and are used throughout this book. They are listed here for convenience. The chapters where these terms are defined are also shown.

Nutritional terms

ADF	Acid detergent fibre; cellulose and lignin of the plant cell wall (Chapters 1 and 4)
AME_n	N-corrected apparent metabolizable energy (Chapter 5)
C3	Temperate, festucoid, grass species (Chapter 15)
C4	Tropical, panicoid, grass species (Chapter 15)
CF	Crude fibre (Chapter 1)
CP	Crude protein (Chapter 1)
DE	Digestible energy (Chapter 5)
dg	(protein) degradability in the rumen (Chapter 5)
DM	Dry matter (Chapter 1)
DDM	Digestible dry matter (Chapter 5)
DMI	Dry matter intake (Chapter 7)
DOM	Digestible organic matter (Chapter 5)
Edg	Effective degradability of feed in the rumen (Chapter 5)
EE	Ether extract (Chapter 1)
FA	Fatty acids (Chapter 1)
FI	Feed intake (Chapter 7)
IU	International unit; for vitamin activity (Chapter 1)
k	Efficiency of use of metabolizable energy (Chapter 5); k_m (maintenance), k_g (growth), k_y (pregnancy), k_{milk} (milk production), k_l (lactating cow).
kp	Efficiency of use of metabolizable protein (Chapter 5); see 'k' for subscripts
LCT	Lower critical temperature (Chapter 19)
Mcal	Megacalories (1000 calories) (Chapter 5)
MCP	Microbial crude protein (Chapter 5)
ME	Metabolizable energy (Chapter 5); see 'k' for subscripts
ME_n	N-corrected metabolizable energy (Chapter5)
MJ	Megajoule (1000 Joules) (Chapter 5)
MP	Metabolizable protein (Chapter 5); see 'k' for subscripts
NDF	Neutral detergent fibre; the total plant cell wall (see Chapters 1 and 4)
eNDF	Effective fibre (Chapter 1)
peNDF	Physically effective fibre (Chapter 1)
NE	Net energy (Chapter 5); see 'k' for subscripts
NFE	N-free extract (Chapter 1)
NPN	Non-protein nitrogen (Chapter 5)
RAM	Restricted animal material (Chapter 6); e.g. meat meals or meat and bone meals
RAN	Ruminally available N (Chapter 5)
RDP	Ruminally degradable protein (Chapter 5)
SFU	Scandinavian feed unit (Chapter 5)

TDN	Total digestible nutrients (Chapter 5)
TDS	Total dissolved solids (Chapter 2)
TME_n	N-corrected true metabolizable energy (Chapter 5)
TSDM	Total standing dry matter of pasture (Chapter 15)
UCT	Upper critical temperature (Chapter 19)
UDP	(ruminally) undegradable protein (Chapter 5)
UFC	Feed unit for horses (Chapter 5)
UFL	Feed unit for lactating ruminants (Chapter 5)
UFV	Feed unit for fast-growing ruminants (Chapter 5)
UR	Pasture utilization rate (Chapter 15)
VFA	Volatile fatty acid(s) (Chapter 3)
W	Live weight (Chapter 8)
$W^{0.75}$	Metabolic size (Chapter 8)

Chemical symbols

Compounds

CH_4	methane
CO_2	carbon dioxide
H_2S	hydrogen sulphide gas
HCl	hydrochloric acid
NaOH	sodium hydroxide (caustic soda)
NH_3	ammonia
N_2O	nitrous oxide gas
NO_X	nitrogen oxide gases

Elements

As	arsenic
B	boron
Br	bromine
Ca	calcium
Co	cobalt
Cu	copper
Cr	chromium
Fe	iron
H	hydrogen
I	iodine
Mg	magnesium
Mn	manganese
Mo	molybdenum
N	nitrogen
Na	sodium
Ni	nickel
P	phosphorus
Rb	rubidium
S	sulphur
Se	selenium
Sn	tin
V	vanadium
Zn	zinc

Index

Note: The page preferences in italics and bold represents figures and tables respectively.

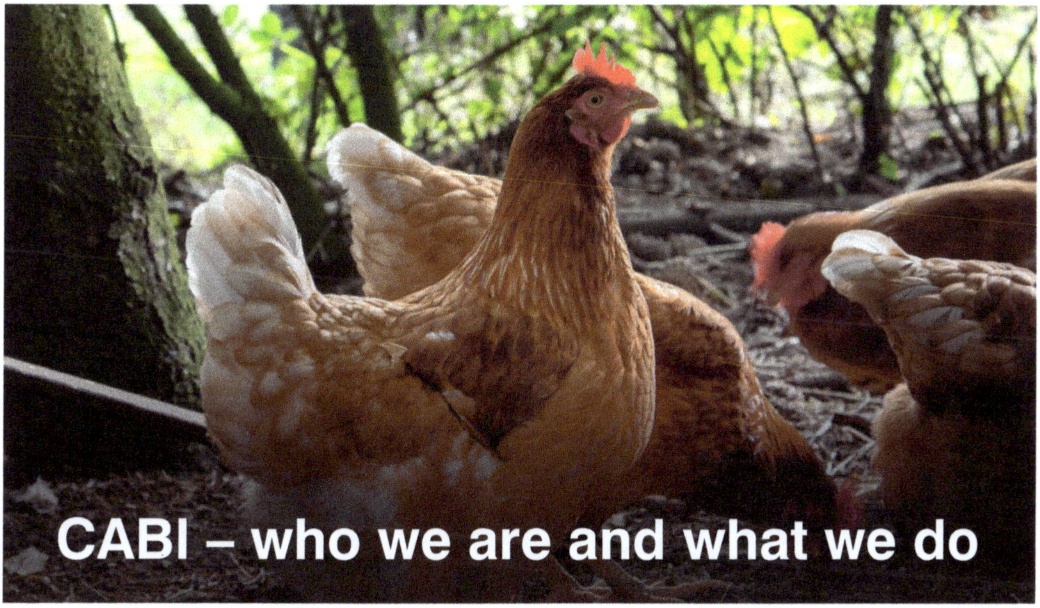
CABI – who we are and what we do

www.ingramcontent.com/pod-product-compliance
Lightning Source LLC
LaVergne TN
LVHW070851210926
848482LV00016B/911